MODELLING OUR FUTURE

POPULATION AGEING HEALTH AND AGED CARE

International Symposia in Economic Theory and Econometrics

Series Editor: ***William A. Barnett***

Volume 14: *Economic Complexity*
Edited by W. A. Barnett, C. Deissenberg & G. Feichtinger

Volume 15: *Modelling Our Future : Population Ageing, Social Security and Taxation*
Edited by Ann Harding & Anil Gupta

International Symposia in Economic Theory and Econometrics Volume 16

MODELLING OUR FUTURE

POPULATION AGEING HEALTH AND AGED CARE

EDITED BY

Anil Gupta

Applied Research and Analysis Directorate, Health Canada, Canada

Ann Harding

National Centre for Social and Economic Modelling, University of Canberra, Australia

ELSEVIER

Amsterdam – Boston – Heidelberg – London – New York – Oxford
Paris – San Diego – San Francisco – Singapore – Sydney – Tokyo

Elsevier
Radarweg 29, PO Box 211, 1000 AE Amsterdam, The Netherlands
The Boulevard, Langford Lane, Kidlington, Oxford OX5 1GB, UK

First edition 2007

Library of Congress Cataloging-in-Publication Data
A catalog record for this book is available from the Library of Congress

British Library Cataloguing in Publication Data
A catalogue record for this book is available from the British Library

ISBN-13: 978-0-444-53005-9
ISBN-10: 0-444-53005-3
ISSN: 1571-0386

For information on all Elsevier publications visit our website at books.elsevier.com

Printed and bound in Great Britain

07 08 09 10 11 10 9 8 7 6 5 4 3 2 1

To my father who taught me the value of education, my mother the spirit of dedication, my wife, the trust in Divine and my daughter, the inner strength. Let the Divine guide all our actions!

Introduction to the Series

The series *International Symposia in Economic Theory and Econometrics* publishes quality proceedings of conferences and symposia. Since all articles published in these volumes are refereed relative to the standards of the best journals, not all papers presented at the symposia are published in these proceedings volumes. Occasionally these volumes include articles that were not presented at a symposium or conference, but are of high quality and are relevant to the focus of the volume. The topics chosen for these volumes are those of particular research importance at the time of the selection of the topic. Each volume has different co-editors, chosen to have particular expertise relevant to the focus of that particular volume.

William A. Barnett
Series Editor

Contents

Part IV: Health Human Resources Modelling

Part V: Data Challenges

Part VI: Overview of Existing Microsimulation and Health Human Resources Models

Dynamic Microsimulation Models

About the Editors

Dr. Anil Gupta
Founding Director, Microsimulation Modelling and Data Analysis Group, Health Canada

For over 20 years, Anil has been on the forefront of popularizing the use of microsimulation in public policy by building and successfully integrating their use in the policy development process in the areas of taxation and health. He played a pivotal role in major tax policy reforms in Canada. He is the founding director of Microsimulation Modelling and Data Analysis group at Health Canada. Among his many notable endeavours, he has worked with Harvard University to develop a summer course on Tax Analysis and Revenue Forecasting where he taught the same during the summers of 1994–2000, and since 2001 at Duke University. He has helped several countries in Asia and Central Europe in building tax analysis and forecasting tools.

He is a recipient of the prestigious Queen Elizabeth 50th centenary gold medal award for distinguished public service in Canada.

Anil is credited with organizing two international microsimulation conferences in USA and Australia. He edited the volume *Microsimulation in Government Policy and Forecasting* in 2000 under the Elsevier series *Contributions to Economics Analysis.*

Anil is a founding member of the Editorial Board of The International Journal of Microsimulation, and an associate editor of Journal of Statistics & Management Systems (JSMS).

Anil holds a PhD in mathematics from the University of Calgary and a masters in systems science from the University of Ottawa.

Professor Ann Harding
Director, National Centre for Social and Economic Modelling, University of Canberra

For the past 14 years, Professor Ann Harding has spearheaded the development of highly sophisticated microsimulation models and databases within Australia, so that policy makers can gain much better information about the likely distributional impact of current and proposed policies. She leads the University of Canberra's National Centre for Social and Economic Modelling, established in January 1993, and is a professor of Applied Economics and

Social Policy at the University. In recent years, with substantial grant funding, Professor Harding has steered microsimulation modelling in Australia beyond its traditional 'tax and social security' focus to such new areas as health, aged care, housing and regional issues, with the goal of extending sophisticated quantitative decision-support tools to policy makers in these areas. Ann has published widely on income inequality, poverty and the distributional impact of government programmes, and is a prolific contributor to public policy debate in Australia, with her work typically being cited every week in the media. In 1996 she was elected a fellow of the Academy of the Social Sciences in Australia and in 2003 was elected president of the International Microsimulation Association.

Notes on Contributors

Jørgen Aasness is a director of research at the Research Department of Statistics Norway. He has a Ph.D. in economics from the University of Oslo and has published articles in *Econometrica*, *The Econometrics Journal*, *European Economic Review*, and in other international journals and books. His key fields of interest are consumer demand, direct and indirect taxation, inequality of standard of living, policy simulation models, and micro/macro links.

Annie Abello is a senior research fellow at the National Centre for Social and Economic Modelling (NATSEM), University of Canberra, Australia. She is interested in issues concerning health and health modelling, the Australian labour market, poverty and inequality. She worked on the development and use of MediSim, a microsimulation model of the Australian pharmaceutical benefits scheme, and is involved in the annual updating of STINMOD.

Cédric Afsa is the head of the division "Redistribution et Politiques Sociales" (Redistribution and Social Policies) which is a subunit of the "Département des Etudes Economiques d'Ensemble" (Department of Global Economic Studies) of the French National Statistical Institute (INSEE).

Kisalaya Basu is a senior economist at Health Canada. Previously, he worked at the State University of New York at Buffalo and at the Centre for Evaluation of Medicines in Hamilton, Canada. He has a Ph.D. in economics from the State University of New York at Albany. His research interests are health human resources, prescription drug coverage and health outcomes. He has published in several health journals. He serves as an associate editor of *Health Policy*.

Marilyn B. Biviano is the director of the Division of Clinical Quality in the Bureau of Primary Health Care in the U.S. Health Resources and Services Administration (HRSA), directing the development of clinical quality health outcome performance measures. Previously, she was the director of the National Center for Health Workforce Analysis (National Center) in

HRSA, where she undertook nursing workforce supply, demand and shortage projections as well as many other health workforce studies.

Laurie Brown is an associate professor and research director, Health Modelling and Research, NATSEM at the University of Canberra, Australia. Prior to joining NATSEM in September 2001, Laurie worked as a senior lecturer in the School of Geosciences, University of Wollongong and at the Christchurch School of Medicine in New Zealand. Laurie has led a number of NATSEM's health and ageing projects funded by the Australian Research Council and the National Health and Medical Research Council and has recently developed a population projection model for estimating the health and economic benefits of preventing type 2 diabetes.

Sophie Buffeteau is a member of the division "Redistribution et Politiques Sociales" (Redistribution and Social Policies) which is a subunit of the "Département des Etudes Economiques d'Ensemble" (Department of Global Economic Studies) of the French National Statistical Institute (INSEE).

Shih-Foong Chin joined NATSEM at the University of Canberra, Australia, in June 2004 from Centrelink, where he managed the Regional Microsimulation Modelling Project in close collaboration with NATSEM. Chin completed his Ph.D. at the University of Queensland in quantitative genetics. Since joining NATSEM, Chin has participated in the development of synthetic social and economic microdata for small areas. To date, his work has focused on re-weighting the 1998–1999 ABS Household Expenditures Survey data to the 2001 census data to produce estimates for statistical local areas.

Adelina Comas-Herrera is a research fellow at the Personal Services Research Unit at the London School of Economics and Political Science (LSE). Most of her work has been on the investigation of the determinants of future long-term care expenditure, in particular dementia and other health conditions, both for the UK and for other European countries. She has worked on developing a methodology for internationally comparable long-term care expenditure projections and investigating the social care workforce implications of the projected increases in demand for long-term care.

John K. Dagsvik is a senior researcher at the Research Department, Statistics Norway. His main research interests include the theory and application of discrete choice modelling, labour supply analysis and stochastic modelling of behavioural relations.

Timothy M. Dall is a health economist and a vice president with The Lewin Group. He works with government agencies, professional associations, hospital systems and health plans on health workforce issues related to clinician supply and demand. He completed his undergraduate work at Utah State University and his graduate work in economics at the University of Wisconsin, Madison.

Robin Darton is a research fellow in the Personal Social Services Research Unit, at the University of Kent, Canterbury, UK. He has a background in psychology and statistics, and research interests in health and social services provision for elderly people and in methodological issues relating to the design and analysis of studies of health and social care. He has been involved in a number of major surveys of care homes, and is currently working on studies of care homes, home care and extra care housing.

Maria Evandrou is professor of gerontology and director of the Centre for Research on Ageing, University of Southampton, UK. Her research interests include inequalities in later life; informal carers, paid employment and resources; and the retirement prospects of future generations of elders, particularly the building and use of different types of policy tools for modelling income, pensions, health, incapacity, demand and supply of formal and informal care among older people in the future.

Jane Falkingham is professor of Demography and International Social Policy at the University of Southampton, UK. Her continuing research interests include demographic change and its consequences for the distribution of social and economic welfare; population ageing and social security; the redistributive effect of the welfare state; and the impact of economic transition on living standards within the countries of the Former Soviet Union.

Dennis F. Fredriksen is research fellow at the Research Department of Statistics Norway. His main research area has been the development, maintenance and use of the dynamic microsimulation model MOSART, including computer programming.

Steve Gribble is currently director of the Social and Economic Analysis and Modeling Division in Statistics Canada. Steve has been active in socio-economic modelling since 1972 and in microsimulation modelling since 1985. His microsimulation projects include SPSD/M, LifePaths and the Modgen microsimulation modelling development environment (www.statcan.ca/english/spsd).

Lin Guohong is the director of the department of economics and management, 359 Military Hospital, Zhenjiang of Jiangsu Province, China. Her research area concentrates on information construction and management of hospitals.

Anil Gupta is the founding director of Microsimulation Modelling and Data Analysis group at Health Canada, where he has worked since 1999. For over 20 years, Anil has been on the forefront of popularizing the use of micro-simulation in public policy by building and successfully integrating their use in the policy development process in the areas of taxation and health. He played a pivotal role in major tax policy reforms in Canada. He has worked with Harvard University to develop a summer course on Tax Analysis and Revenue Forecasting where he taught the same during the summers of 1994–2000, and since 2001 at Duke University. He has helped several countries in Asia and Central Europe in building tax analysis and forecasting modelling tools.

Ruth Hancock is professor of non-clinical gerontology in the Department of Health and Human Sciences at the University of Essex, UK. Her research interests lie in the social, economic and health policy implications of individual and population ageing; and in the analysis of large-scale household surveys, particularly via micro-simulation, to address issues in the areas of financial provision for later life.

Ann Harding is the director of the University of Canberra's NATSEM, established in January 1993, and is professor of applied economics and social policy at the University. For the past 14 years she has spearheaded the development of highly sophisticated microsimulation models and databases within Australia, so that policy makers can gain much better information about the likely distributional impact of current and proposed policies. In 1996 she was elected a fellow of the Academy of the Social Sciences in Australia and in 2003 was elected President of the International Microsimulation Association.

Chantal Hicks has worked on various microsimulation projects at Statistics Canada since 1996. She currently manages the Social Policy Simulation Database and Model (SPSD/M). Other microsimulation projects include various infectious disease models as well as LifePaths.

Einar Holm is professor of social and economic geography at Umeå University in Sweden. His main research field is socio-economic impact studies of population composition and labour market clearing, based on large longitudinal individual databases and spatial microsimulation.

Meng Hong is an associate professor, Faculty of Health Services at the Second Military Medical University, Shanghai, China. Her research area includes synthetical evaluation, data mining and forecast analysis.

Herwig Immervoll is an economist and social policy analyst at the OECD. He is also research fellow at IZA, Bonn; research associate at the Institute for Social and Economic Research (ISER), University of Essex, UK; and research affiliate at the European Centre for Social Welfare Policy and Research, Vienna. His research interests include analysing and monitoring current trends in tax and benefit policies and their effects on poverty, income distribution and labour markets.

Ariadna Juarez-Garcia is a research fellow at the Health Services Management Centre, University of Birmingham. Her interests are in decision analysis and modelling of health technologies, the economics of primary care and micro-simulation of the financial implications of long term care.

Vishnu Kapur is a consultant in the field of microsimulation modelling, actively engaged in the public policy issues concerning social security, taxation and health. Prior to this he was a senior policy analyst at the Department of Finance Canada, where he successfully built a host of microsimulation models in the area of personal income taxation. Later he served as a senior policy advisor with the Microsimulation Modelling and Data Analysis Division at Health Canada. His interests include static and dynamic microsimulation modelling, specifically behavioural aspects of modelling income distribution analysis, poverty analysis and poverty measurement and prescription drug coverage, especially policy issues involved in these analyses.

Simon Kelly is an associate professor at the University of Canberra, Australia, and a principal research fellow at NATSEM. He is currently chief investigator for a five-year research project assessing the social and fiscal policy implications of an ageing population. Simon's research interests are population ageing, labour force trends, household wealth and retirement savings.

Anthony King was the director of Regional Modelling with the NATSEM at the University of Canberra, Australia. He is currently manager of the Participation Modelling Project in the Australian Treasury.

Derek King is a research fellow at the Personal Services Research Unit at the London School of Economics and Political Science (LSE). His areas of expertise are mental health policy and economics, and projecting the demand and financing of long term care.

Marten Lagergren is a research director at the Stockholm Gerontology Research Center. He is also Associate Professor at Stockholm University, department of social work, and has a degree in Mathematics from Stockholm University and in Social Medicine from Karolinska Institute, Stockholm. From 1990 - 2000 he was working as Chief Analyst at the Ministry of Health and Social Affairs, Stockholm. At present he is national coordinator of the large longitudinal study SNAC- the Swedish National Study of Aging and Care. He has published many articles on the development of health and care needs of the elderly.

Urban Lindgren is an associate professor in human geography at Umeå University, Sweden, where he works as a senior lecturer. He has published in the fields of economic geography, population geography and microsimulation modelling.

Xiong Linping gained his Ph.D. in health statistics in 1997, master degree in probability and mathematical statistics in 1991 and bachelor degree in applied mathematics in 1985, China. Now he is a Ph.D. candidate at NATSEM, University of Canberra, Australia. His research areas include medical insurance systems and the application of microsimulation models.

Erling Häggström Lundevaller is a senior lecturer in statistics currently working as a researcher at the department of statistics and the department of social and economic geography at Umeå university. Research interests include socio-economic micro-simulation modeling and simulation of tourism flows.

Juliette Malley is a research officer at the Personal Social Services Research Unit at the London School of Economics and Political Science (LSE). Since joining the LSE she has been working on a study investigating future demand and financial expenditure on long-term care for older people. Her current research interests are in the financing of long-term care and issues surrounding the performance and quality of social services provision.

Mike McCracken is the founder and CEO of Informetrica Limited, an economic research and information company in Canada. He has built a very large econometric model of the Canadian national and provincial economies (currently over 30,000 equations) and operated it continuously since 1974. His microsimulation work uses existing Canadian tools (e.g. SPSD/M) in policy applications.

Richard Morrison has spent his career designing and building policy models that governments actually use. The best known examples include MAPSIT to calculate benefits and taxes as functions of earnings (32 years of use), SIMTAB to perform cross-sectional microsimulation (26 years of use) and DYNACAN to carry out longitudinal simulation of the Canada Pension Plan (12 years of use).

Brian Murphy was an original member of the team that developed Statistics Canada's first microsimulation model in the mid-1980s; the Social Policy Simulation Database and model (SPSD/M). He then managed and developed the SPSD/M project for ten years before taking on his current role as a Senior Advisor on income distribution and taxation at Statistics Canada. Brian has written various journal articles and papers in his areas of interest that include microsimulation, income inequality, low income, and the distribution of government taxes and transfers.

Xisco Oliver is a professor of applied economics at the University of Balearic Island (Spain) where he obtained his PhD in Economics. He has a Master in Applied Economics from the University Pompeu Fabra (Spain). His research has focused on portfolio choice, labour supply and taxation, redistribution of income and social welfare.

Richard Percival is an associate professor and a principal research fellow at NATSEM, University of Canberra, Australia. He has a particular interest in health and dynamic microsimulation models, was a member of the original STINMOD development team and is currently the STINMOD team leader.

Ben Phillips is a senior research fellow at NATSEM, University of Canberra, Australia, where he has worked since 2001, mainly on the creation of regional microsimulation models. Prior to this he worked at the Australian Bureau of Statistics as an economic researcher in the Methodology Division. Ben's experience also includes work for the forecasting unit of the Bureau of Tourism Research.

Linda Pickard is a research fellow at the Personal Social Services Research Unit (PSSRU) at the London School of Economics (LSE), UK. Linda has worked at the LSE since 1996 on a project concerned with future long-term care demand and finance. Linda is particularly interested in informal or unpaid care for older people and has, in collaboration with colleagues at the LSE and elsewhere, conducted research on projections of informal care in future years in the UK and internationally.

Chris Raymond worked as a principal research officer in the Research and Analysis Section of Medicare Australia in Canberra from 2002 to 2006. Currently he is employed in the data and modelling section of the Pharmaceutical Benefits Branch, Commonwealth Department of Health and Ageing in Canberra. He is interested in time series analysis of administrative health data.

Adam Redpath is a programme principal, Information Services, National Services, NHS Scotland. Adam Redpath is a health statistician working to develop statistical information and analysis to support the care of the elderly and patients with cardiovascular disease. He trained as a sociologist at the University of Edinburgh, took a research M.Phil. in social policy (also at Edinburgh) and an MSc in health information at the University of Wales. He has worked for the NHS since 1982.

George Rothman has a Ph.D. in the physical sciences and over 30 years of experience in planning, analysis and modelling work for the Australian Government. He was a foundation member of the Retirement Income Modelling Task Force established in 1992 and has continued to work in the Treasury successor to that Task Force. He has published numerous papers on the dynamics of Australia's superannuation arrangements. He also contributed to various facets of the Australian Government's first Intergenerational Report and to subsequent long-term studies.

Geoff Rowe is a demographer with a Ph.D. from the University of Alberta. He has worked for Statistics Canada for more than 25 years, much of that time devoted to developing statistical models of demographic/socio-economic behaviour using individual level data. Geoff's initial microsimulation experience involved the development of the SPSD/M and he currently heads up the LifePaths project team.

Deborah Schofield is an associate professor and a research leader at the Northern Rivers University Department of Rural Health, University of Sydney. She currently leads a research programme on health, ageing and the workforce. She previously worked for the Australian Treasury where she worked on the Intergenerational Report and at NATSEM where she established the health microsimulation modelling programme.

Amedeo Spadaro is a researcher at Paris-Jourdan Sciences Economiques (PSE), at FEDEA Madrid and professor of public economics at the University of the Balearic Islands, Mallorca. His current research activities are concerned with labour supply and taxation, public finance, income distribution and social welfare, poverty, econometrics and statistical methods and microsimulation, and also include management of several national and international research programmes on evaluation of welfare and tax policies in welfare states.

Nils M. Stølen is a senior research fellow at the Research Department of Statistics Norway. His main research areas have been in macroeconomics, labour market, wage formation, public finance, taxes and pensions. In the last few years his main effort has been in analyses of the effects of reforms of the Norwegian pension system, using the dynamic microsimulation model MOSART and at present he is the head of the MOSART team.

Magnus Strömgren earned a Ph.D. in human geography from Umeå University in 2004. His dissertation analyzes the diffusion of medicine at a distance by means of information technology. Since 2006, Dr Strömgren is a Research Assistant at the Department of Social and Economic Geography, Umeå University. Presently, he is participating in a number of research projects involving large data sets, modeling, and Geographical Information Systems (GIS).

Ruth Studley worked as a health statistician within the Welsh Assembly Government, UK. She was responsible for NHS Statistics including both activity and waiting times. She trained as a statistician at the University of Wales, College of Cardiff and recently completed an MSc in Official Statistics from the University of Southampton, UK. More recently, Ruth heads up the team responsible for Information Standards in health and social care at the Welsh Assembly Government.

Olle Sundberg is a deputy director at the Swedish Ministry of Finance. His main interest is pensions, income distribution and simulation models.

Holly Sutherland is a research professor in the Institute for Social and Economic Research at the University of Essex, UK. Her research is based on building and using microsimulation models and she has a particular interest in developing microsimulation as a tool for international comparative research. As well as coordinating the EU-wide EUROMOD project, her recent activities include research on the gendered effects of re-distribution policies and on child poverty measurement and analysis.

Thor O. Thoresen is a senior researcher at the Research Department, Statistics Norway. Besides his engagement in establishing and applying microsimulation tools, he is involved in various types of tax-policy analyses, such as evaluations of tax progressivity over time, behavioural effects of tax changes and family policy issues.

Linc Thurecht joined NATSEM at the University of Canberra, Australia, in January 2001 having previously worked at the Federal Department of Family and Community Services, where he contributed to the development of the portfolio's budget submissions and led teams with responsibility for forecasting expenditure on income support payments. He holds a bachelor of commerce (honours finance) from the Australian National University and has played a key role in NATSEM's health modelling projects.

Stephen Tise is an economist by training with 23 years of experience as a U.S. Government analyst. During his career, he served in a leadership role for the (U.S) National Center for Health Workforce Analysis where he did most of his health force modeling, forecasting and analysis work. Previously, Mr. Tise was a labor economist at the U.S. Bureau of Labor Statistics and currently he is a senior analyst in health work force emergency preparedness.

Quoc N. Vu is currently a research fellow at NATSEM at the University of Canberra, Australia, after working in the United Nations Development Programme in Vietnam. He also lectured in economics at the National Economics University in Hanoi and worked as visiting research fellow at the Institute of Southeast Asian Studies in Singapore. Vu has a Ph.D. in economics from the Australian National University. His research experience includes social and economic issues and the reform of state-owned enterprise in Vietnam and he is currently working on the STINMOD microsimulation model.

Agnes Walker has extensive experience in applied economic and social research. In her recent work concerning Australia's health sector — health insurance, pharmaceuticals, doctors, hospitals — she extensively used modelling as a policy development tool. Agnes was formerly a principal research fellow at NATSEM at the University of Canberra and is currently at the Australian National University.

Bert Waslander is a consultant and an associate of Informetrica Limited, an economic research and information company. He has developed parts of the DYNACAN model of the Canada Pension Plan and used the SPSD/M in various applications. The main focus of his recent work is on the use of micro data to estimate the impacts of social and economic programs on Canadians.

Paul Williamson is a senior lecturer in the Department of Geography, University of Liverpool, UK. He was awarded a PhD at the University of Leeds for his work on a microsimulation model of health care for the elderly. His principal research focus is on the addition of a spatial dimension to microsimulation, which has found applied expression in the modeling of population change, water demand and housing affordability.

Raphael Wittenberg is a senior research fellow at the PSSRU at LSE, UK. He leads the PSSRU programme of research on the financing of long-term care for older people, which aims to make projections of demand for long-term care for older people and associated expenditure to 2041. Within the programme he has looked at arrangements for financing long-term care in the UK and other countries.

Dr. Michael C. Wolfson is Assistant Chief Statistician, Analysis and Development, at Statistics Canada. This includes responsibility for analytical activities generally at Statistics Canada, for health statistics, and for specific analytical and modeling programs. Prior to joining Statistics Canada, he held a variety of positions in central agencies including the Treasury Board Secretariat, Department of Finance, Privy Council Office, House of Commons, and Deputy Prime Minister's Office with responsibilities in the areas of program review and evaluation, tax policy and pension policy. In addition to his federal public service responsibilities, Dr. Wolfson was a Fellow of the Canadian Institute for Advanced Research Program in Population Health from 1988 to 2003. His research activities have led to published papers in diverse areas, including income distribution, tax/transfer and pension policy analysis, microsimulation approaches to socio-economic accounting and to evolutionary economic theory, design of health information systems, and analysis of the determinants of health. Dr. Wolfson received his B.Sc. in computer science and economics from the University of Toronto, and his Ph.D. in economics from Cambridge University in 1977.

Ma Xiuqiang is currently principal lecturer in the Department of Health Statistics, Second Military Medical University, Shanghai, China. His principal research fields are policy analysis, epidemiology surveys and clinical trial design and data analysis.

Li Yiping is the director of the Balance Center of Health Insurance in Zhenjiang of Jiangsu Province, China, directing the checkout, balance of medical services expenditure of medical insurance participants.

Asghar Zaidi is the director of research at the European Centre for Social Welfare Policy and Research in Austria. Prior to this, he worked at the LSE on the construction of the SAGEMOD dynamic microsimulation model.

Preface

In December 2003, the editors of this volume (and its companion volume) organized a conference entitled "International Microsimulation Conference on Population Ageing and Health: Modelling Our Future" in Canberra, Australia. The conference focused on the recent advances in microsimulation modelling and its direct use in the policy development process around the world. The data challenges associated with the building of these tools received considerable attention at the conference. In addition, two days were dedicated to practical model descriptions and a symposium on modelling efforts in different countries provided further insights into the state of modelling today and its future direction.

The wide spectrum of issues covered and the participation of researchers, policy makers and consultants from around the world at the conference provided a venue for intense discussions. Further, an overwhelming response to the technical workshop on practical models motivated the editors of this volume to take this work one step further through this volume and the companion volume. This volume incorporates the following:

(1) selected papers focussing on health, aged care and other services presented at the 'International Microsimulation Conference on Population Ageing and Health: Modelling Our Future' held in Canberra, Australia in December 2003;
(2) recent thinking in the field of microsimulation as reflected in special contributions by some of the leading experts in the field; and
(3) description of 20 key microsimulation and other models relating to fiscal and health human resource issues concerning sustainability of health and welfare systems around the globe.

We sincerely thank Dr. Kisalaya Basu for his efforts throughout the preparation of the book. We recognize his contribution as an assistant editor of this volume.

The editors wish to thank Michael McCracken and Vishnu Kapur for their very insightful comments on earlier versions of this volume. We would also like to thank Stephanie Pilon and Rachel Lloyd for their outstanding assistance in the organisation of the conference and Rachel for her efforts in the early stages of producing these two volumes. The financial support provided by the following organizations helped the authors to concentrate on the content of the conference and this was largely responsible for making the conference such a success: Applied Research and Analysis Directorate, Health Canada; Australian Bureau of Statistics; Department of Health and Ageing, Australia; Canada Revenue Agency, Canada; National Centre for Social and Economic Modelling, Australia; SAS; and Statistics Canada, Canada.

The editors are grateful to the Hon. Kevin Andrews, Minister for Employment and Workplace Relations, Australia, and Dr. Michael Wolfson of Statistics Canada for their keynote addresses, which contributed greatly in steering the conference towards the key public policy issues and challenges facing world governments today. The editors would also like to thank the session chairs for their valuable contributions, including George Rothman, Michael Wolfson, Jane Falkingham, Maria Evandrou, Lennart Flood, Mark Thomann, Agnes Walker, Marion McEwin, Michael Dunn, Marilyn Biviano, Wendy Stone, Rick Morrison, Michael McCracken, Paolo Roberti, Rachel Lloyd, Michel Lamure, Richard Eason, Michael Dunn and John O'Leary. Particular thanks are also due to the referees, who did an excellent job of reviewing the papers. We have included some of their comments in the introductory chapters and very much appreciated their efforts, which greatly improved the quality of the papers and ensured that this became a refereed volume.

Very special thanks are also due to Monic Gupta, who edited the volumes with enthusiasm and efficiency.

Finally, the authors wish to express to their spouses, Chitralekha Gupta and John Sekoranja, a profound sense of appreciation for their continued support, understanding and patience in the long and arduous task of putting these two volumes together. Their forgiveness and patience brought this work to fruition.

Anil Gupta and Ann Harding

Foreword

There is perhaps no more pressing issue facing advanced economies today than that of the social, economic, and financial ramifications of an ageing population. All of the countries represented in this and the companion volume "Modelling Our Future: Population Ageing, Social Security and Taxation" face the same reality — declining birth rates and an ageing population and improvements in health care that have led to greater life expectancy. The relative size of the working age population will continue to decline in the foreseeable future. All of these conditions lead to an oncoming crisis where the ability of an ageing population to meet its basic needs is put at risk.

But the implications of the impending demographic shift go beyond the social security and the health care needs of an ageing population and they now threaten future economic growth itself. There is particular concern that rising health care costs are straining public sector budgets and will lead to the crowding out of investments in other areas, particularly education and some entitlement programs. Moreover, predicted shortages of health care professionals will further strain the health care system in these countries. Despite differences in the funding of health care systems across OECD countries, the basic demographic challenge is common to these countries thus calling for the cross-country analyses that this volume provides. Similar dire predictions can be leveled at the ability to provide suitable retirement incomes for a growing population, both in terms of universal and individual pension programs.

The microsimulation approach taken by many of the studies in the volume provide an appropriate and much-needed perspective to fully understand the so-called impending social security and health care crises. The lessons learned from the analyses are absolutely indispensable in helping shape the current and future public policy debates in this area. Moreover, the volumes set the stage for cross-country comparisons and provide examples of suitable policies and practices and the ramifications of both.

Carlos E. Santiago
Chancellor and Professor of Economics
University of Wisconsin-Milwaukee
Milwaukee, WI
USA

Chapter 1

Introduction and Overview

Anil Gupta[a] and Ann Harding[b]

[a]*Microsimulation Modelling and Data Analysis Division, Applied Research and Analysis Directorate, Health Canada, Canada*
[b]*National Centre for Social and Economic Modelling, University of Canberra, Australia*

Abstract

Population ageing is posing unparalleled challenges to the foundation of public health systems in the developing world. The cost of health care is spiraling and pharmaceutical costs are increasing at an enormous speed. Furthermore, the challenges are not only economic but also relate to the supply of health human resources (HHRs) in an era of ever increasing demand on the limited health workforce which itself is ageing. This volume tries to put these issues in perspective and to offer a glimmer of hope through insights into the future through careful analysis of needs of the population, factoring in both positive and negative factors affecting the supply and demand of HHRs (e.g. improved health status of the future elderly). After a general introduction, the second section of this chapter examines the modelling techniques used to assess the likely impact of population ageing, including an outline of the different types of microsimulation and other models actively in use today. The third section provides an overview of each of the chapters contained in this volume and ends with a special part on practical models, providing ample information for experts and novices alike to benefit from the progress made in the development and the use of microsimulation models in public policy.

1. Introduction

In December 2003, the Microsimulation Modelling and Data Analysis Division of Health Canada and the National Centre for Social and Economic Modelling organized an international modelling conference on population ageing and health in Canberra, Australia. The focus of the conference was on microsimulation models for forecasting the impact of

International Symposia in Economic Theory and Econometrics, Vol. 16

ISSN: 1571-0386 DOI: 10.1016/S1571-0386(06)16001-9

ageing. The conference attracted participants from some 25 countries. Judging from the wide range of papers presented, the conference more than accomplished its original objectives.

This volume carries the objectives of the conference a step forward. It incorporates selected refereed papers presented at the conference. In addition, it presents papers on recent thinking in the field of health, health delivery, access to health services, and population health using various analytical tools with special emphasis on microsimulation modelling. These papers discuss many of the issues associated with population ageing that are assuming prominence in most OECD countries. These issues include the concerns many governments are having about the likely impact of population ageing upon future government outlays and economic growth.

In Australia, for example, there have already been two major government reports that have attempted to quantify the likely implications of population ageing on government spending. These reports conclude that there will either have to be cuts in current government programs, or increases in taxes, or some combination of these two. The ageing population will also require more health human resources (HHRs) (doctors, nurses, pharmacists, etc.) in an environment where the existing workforce itself is ageing. Economic growth is forecast to slow significantly in future decades due to population ageing, reducing government's ability to rely on an otherwise rapidly growing taxpaying labour force to finance the expected shortfalls.

Not surprisingly, in this environment, governments are attempting to obtain reasonable forecasts of a number of key variables including

- future costs of health, education, aged care, and other services;
- retirement incomes of future pensioners and their ability to help finance their health and aged care needs;
- HHR requirements;
- health status and changing health care needs;
- tax revenues; and
- the labour force, given demographic trends.

We expect that the present volume and the companion volume (Modelling Our Future: Population Ageing, Social Security, and Taxation) will provide timely material to policy makers and researchers across the world. These two volumes incorporate modelling approaches and policy relevant results that are at the international leading edge. They attempt to provide insights into how countries are facing the challenges associated with population ageing. As such, they will provide very useful guidance for the countries that have not yet modelled the impacts of population ageing. They will also provide further insights to those who are actively using microsimulation to simulate impacts of population ageing.

The present volume elaborates upon a number of topics discussed in the introduction of the companion volume (Harding and Gupta, 2006). These include retirement, fertility rates, increasing life expectancies and their impact on the financing of the health systems, the Australian experience, etc. Many topics focus on the critical role microsimulation modelling plays in developing robust forecasts. For the sake of completeness, this overview chapter draws liberally from the material presented in the companion volume (especially the introductory chapter). In addition, it provides some insights from the Canberra conference to demonstrate the important role that microsimulation modelling plays and could play to develop estimates in a changing world. Another useful addition is a special section on practical models that are currently in active use across the globe.

The editors have made every effort to present the material in a cohesive manner to maintain a smooth flow of the book. This volume is intended as a reference text to serve both the established practitioners and new comers to the field of health policy research. The overview section includes comments by referees as we found them most pertinent and revealing. We thank all the referees (see list at the end) for their insightful comments and critiques.

2. The Canberra Conference

In his opening address at the conference, the Honorable Kevin Andrews, the Australian Minister for Employment and Workplace Relations, stressed that the baby boomers will not necessarily create a doomsday scenario; instead, tomorrow's elderly will be in better health and economic state, will live longer, and spend more. He talked of such issues as national pharmaceutical plans, the coverage of services in remote areas, and home care — all of which, in turn, were discussed at length during the conference. He encouraged the researchers to find innovative ways to handle the challenges presented by our changing demography. This and the companion volume provide insights into the current innovative thinking across the globe on this topic.

Michael Wolfson, Assistant Chief Statistician, Statistics Canada, gave the plenary address on 'Population Ageing and Health — Empirical Needs for Effective Foresight'. In his talk, Michael highlighted the relationship between research, the policy process and the statistical agency. He emphasized that policy issues need to be clearly defined in order that statistical agencies can prepare the right data. He stressed the need for statistical agencies to make data readily available to researchers to enable their active engagement in policy analysis. Feenberg and Gupta (2000) stressed the need for timely and easy access to data from statistical agencies to ensure that internal analysis and validation processes do not unduly delay data access to researchers outside.

2.1 Main Conference

Two hundred and twenty participants from over 25 countries attended the conference. There was a balanced participation by policy makers, researchers within and outside governments, academics, and consultants thus providing a wide spectrum of views. The participatory nature of the conference resulted in fruitful discussions on both the traditional and emerging issues facing different governments today — both in the health and the taxation areas and the role taxation could play in the delivery and affordability of health care.

The conference was divided between the main conference (with over 60 presentations from different countries both on Health and Finance issues), followed by a technical workshop and an international symposium.

The presentations at the main conference covered a wide range of issues relating to retirement, taxation, and health among others. For example, using projections from a dynamic microsimulation model, Agnes Walker, an Australian researcher, presented her work (Chapter 5) on the potential labour force impact of emerging trends (e.g. rising obesity rates, improved medical technology) and/or policies, which aim to improve the health of older Australians aged 55 or over. This model could also project the potential impact of improved health on workforce exits through family level decisions — based on the health of each family member as well as the family's income and wealth.

Another example is a contribution from the UK (Chapter 3) that examined demographic change and trends in health and health risk behaviour in Britain to inform future modelling projections, drawing out the implications of these trends for health and social care in later life over the next 20 years. Although the number of older people in the next 30 years can be forecast with some degree of certainty, less attention has been paid to the likely health and socio-economic characteristics of future generations of elders, and how these may differ from previous cohorts of elderly persons. This paper attempts to address these issues by looking back into the past and seeing how the experiences of the generations entering retirement over the next 30 years are likely to shape their future. These and other papers provide further insights into the future while carefully depicting the status quo.

The discussion at the end of the main conference brought together an expert panel on the following eight topics: (1) tax implications, (2) social security and social insurance, (3) health workforce planning, (4) data challenges, (5) forecasting, (6) healthcare and costs, (7) housing and infrastructure, and (8) labour force and economic growth. The key points emerging from these discussions are discussed under the overview section below.

In the formulation and evaluation of policy options, microsimulation analysis is taking on a crucial role. This was corroborated, time and again, by the many key policy advisors from all over the world who participated in the discussions during the conference. An important contribution of the conference was the interaction it generated among modellers and policy makers, which has resulted in an unprecedented dialogue across continents.

2.2 Technical Workshop

The conference devoted one full day to the display and discuss the various policy microsimulation models in use, actively, in participating countries. Thirty-two models from 16 countries were presented at this technical workshop. This was followed by four in-depth two-hour presentations on specific models from Canada, Australia, and European Union. These presentations generated renewed interest in international collaborations in modelling. The last part of this volume presents many of these models.

2.3 Symposium

A one-day international symposium on modelling efforts in different countries, with emphasis on challenges both on the modelling and data front, was held at the end of the conference. Presenters from USA, Canada, UK, EU, Sweden, Norway, Australia, and Denmark gave synopses of the models used in their respective jurisdictions, along with the policy applications of these models in the recent past. These presentations were followed by open discussion on such issues as: (1) data issues and challenges, (2) issues with dynamic models in the context of policy formulation, (3) types of models, (4) model limitation/validation, (5) collaboration or competition, (6) responsiveness to clients, (7) maintenance of models/documentation and ongoing efforts, (8) role of microsimulation in measuring and understanding issues, and (9) international comparison and cooperation. These open and revealing discussions added much to the understanding of the current state of modelling in the developed world. The discussions and work presented at the conference form the basis of the core content of the present two volumes.

The following section is common with Volume I and is included here for completeness sake.

3. Modelling Our Future

There are a wide range of possible methods that can be used to try to simulate our social and economic futures and the impact of policy change. This section first discusses microsimulation techniques, before proceeding to examine cell-based and other techniques.

3.1 Microsimulation

The defining characteristic of microsimulation models is that they analyse the likely behaviour of and the impact of policy change upon *persons* (or households, or firms, or other micro-units). They are often constructed on top of microdata, with sample surveys or administrative data forming typical base datasets for such models. In both cases, the microdata usually contain thousands of individual or micro-unit records, with a host of variables describing the demographic, labour force, income, and other characteristics of each individual or family. Microsimulation models were the brainchild of Guy Orcutt (1957) who, frustrated by the macroeconomic models of the day, proposed a new type of model consisting of interacting, decision-making entities such as individuals, families, and firms.

Static Microsimulation Models

Microsimulation models have traditionally been divided into two broad categories — static and dynamic — although the boundaries between the two have become increasingly blurred. Static models typically use static ageing techniques to update cross-sectional microdata up to the required point in time. These techniques usually involve reweighting the data and uprating monetary values.

When national statistical agencies issue a micro-data file from a national sample survey, they typically attach a *weight* to each individual record in the file, representing the estimated number of comparable individuals in the entire country with similar characteristics to the individual who took part in the sample survey. This weight is the means used to 'gross up' from sample survey results to estimates for the entire population. Reweighting involves replacing these original weights with amended weights, to take account of change in the population structure (by age, gender, labour force status, etc.) between the time the data were collected and the desired time period of the analysis. Uprating involves updating monetary values to reflect changes since the data were collected, such as inflating earnings or private rent paid.

After these two steps, static modellers typically impute the receipt of social security and other benefits and/or income tax or other liabilities, by applying the rules for eligibility or liability to each of the micro-units. Steps may also be taken to make the number of programme participants or taxpayers match to external benchmark data by, for example, simulating less than 100 per cent take-up of a particular payment. At this point, a baseline data file has been generated, which usually shows the current incomes and characteristics of each person or family in the microdata file, plus the imputed current incidence of taxes paid to and cash transfers received from government.

Most static models also allow the analyst to vary the rules of eligibility or liability, and produce output showing the distributional gains or losses for each micro-unit — and the budgetary impact for government — from the policy change. Importantly, the impact can be assessed for the entire population or for relatively large or small population sub-groups (such as sole parent pensioners with two children or the home-owning elderly living in a particular region). Thus these models permit winner/loser analysis of policy changes and thus allow the user to develop policy parameters in line with governments' overall policy objectives. It was these unique features that led an exhaustive review in the United States to conclude 'that no other type of model can match microsimulation in its potential for flexible, fine-grained analysis of proposed policy changes' (Citro and Hanushek, 1991, p. 115).

Static microsimulation models for assessing the distributional and revenue impacts of possible changes in tax and cash transfer policy have been the 'bread and butter' of microsimulation for some decades now. Such models have often played a decisive role in determining the final shape of policy reforms introduced by governments, and they are now widely used across Europe, the US, Australia, and Canada.[1] In recent years, their use has expanded to analyse policy issues in the area of health policy. The recent Nordic microsimulation seminar in Oslo (June, 2006) included a special session on health and microsimulation, where researchers from different countries presented efforts in the areas of pharmaceuticals, health status, and health promotion.[2]

Most static microsimulation models still measure the immediate (or first-round) impacts of policy change, before individuals change their behaviour in response to the policy shock. Yet, in some cases, a policy change may be expected to have a major impact upon behaviour — and may even be designed to do so. Consequently, a growing number of modellers have attempted to simulate the changes *in the behaviour of the individuals directly affected by a policy shock* — for example, by allowing labour supply or consumption patterns to vary in response to a tax change.[3] Yet even these

[1] For example, results from the STINMOD static microsimulation model influenced the final shape of the GST-tax reform package introduced in Australia in 2000 (Harding et al., 2000) while, in the US, the TRIM model has influenced public policy for many years (see http://trim3.urban.org/).

[2] See http://www.ssb.no/english/research_and_analysis/conferences/misi/.

[3] For example, see the MITTS model developed at the Melbourne Institute in Australia (http://melbourneinstitute.com/labour/behavioural/mitts.html) and the wide range of papers presented at the 8th Nordic Seminar on Microsimulation Modelling on labour supply responses (http://www.ssb.no/english/research_and_analysis/conferences/misi). For an example of simulating changes in household consumption as a result of indirect tax changes, see Symons and Warren (1996).

models often remain very much at the micro level, ignoring macroeconomic consequences. For example, they may assume that a cut in marginal tax rates leads to an increase in the labour supply of particular individuals — but what if there are no suitable jobs available for these individuals to fill?

As explained by Citro and Hanushek (1991, p. 178), the behavioural responses in the short or long term by those directly affected by a policy change will subsequently lead to second-round effects — that is, 'to effects that alter the nature of factor or product markets or the level and distribution of consumption, production and employment in the economy or in a sector of it affected by the policy change'. For example, a cut in marginal income tax rates might initially increase labour supply but subsequently lead to cuts in wage rates and changes in output by industry. Consequently, efforts are now also being made to link microsimulation models to macroeconomic models, to capture these other second-round or feedback effects of a policy change (Arntz et al., 2006; Dennis et al., 2006) in the companion volume (Harding and Gupta, 2006).

Dynamic Microsimulation Models

Dynamic models often start from exactly the same cross-section sample surveys as static models. However, rather than using the static ageing procedures described above, dynamic ageing involves 'updating each attribute for each micro-unit for each time interval' (Caldwell, 1990, p. 5). Thus, the individuals within the original microdata or base file are progressively moved forward through time: this is achieved by making major life events — such as death, marriage, divorce, fertility, education, labour force participation, etc. — happen to each individual, in accord with the probabilities of such events happening to real people within that particular country. Thus, within a dynamic microsimulation model, the characteristics of each individual are recalculated for each time period.

There are two major types of dynamic microsimulation models, both of which are illustrated in these two volumes. *Dynamic population* models involve ageing a sample of an entire population, and typically begin with a comprehensive cross-section sample survey for a particular point in time (such as a census). To date, such dynamic models have been used for such purposes as the analysis of retirement incomes, future health status, the long-term impact of social security amendments, and the lifetime redistributive impact of the social security system (e.g. Nelissen, 1996; Wolfson, 1988; Bonnet and Mahieu, 2000; Hancock, 2000; Favreault and Caldwell, 2000; Baldini, 2001; see also O'Donoghue, 2001, for an extremely useful summary of dynamic modelling research).

Dynamic cohort models use exactly the same type of ageing procedures, but usually age only one cohort rather than the many cohorts represented in an entire population. Typically, one cohort is aged from birth to death, so that the entire lifecycle is simulated. For some applications, such models are more cost-efficient than ageing an entire population. Such models have been used to analyse lifetime income distribution and redistribution, lifetime rates of return to education, and repayment patterns for student income-contingent loans (Hain and Helberger, 1986; Harding, 1993a, 1993b, 1995; Falkingham and Hills, 1995; Falkingham and Harding, 1996; Evandrou and Falkingham, 2006).

Like static models, dynamic models face problems when attempting to incorporate either behavioural change by individuals or second-round macroeconomic effects in response to government policy changes. Economists would normally assume that any 'dynamic' model would incorporate behavioural change. However, while dynamic microsimulation models typically do capture some types of behavioural change (e.g. a woman within a model might leave the labour force with the birth of her first child), they do not necessarily allow for changes in the behaviour of individuals or macroeconomic change *initiated by government tax-transfer policy change.*

Recent Developments

Since the early 1990s, microsimulation has flourished. At least three factors have helped to generate this growth. First, the availability of suitable microdata has improved greatly. In Australia, for example, the first public use cross-sectional microdata files were not made available by the national statistical agency until the mid-1980s (with such microdata usually forming the all important base file of microsimulation models). Similarly, the first comprehensive panel study of individuals did not begin in Australia until 2001 (Weston and Wooden, 2002), thus removing a major impediment to attempts to estimate the crucial transition probabilities that underlie dynamic models. In Europe, cross-national data collection efforts such as the European Community Household Panel vastly improved the availability of both cross-sectional and panel data in many member countries. The efforts of Tim Smeeding to develop internationally comparable household level data through the Luxembourg Income Study, along with the initiatives of the Canberra Group, also contributed to improvements in microdata availability and comparability.[4]

A second factor has been the growing demand by policy makers for the types of analyses that only microsimulation models can provide. In many countries, social and tax policies have become ever more complex, with the introduction of new, targeted benefits and the endless fine-tuning of existing programs. As the interactions between the various tax and transfer

[4] See http://www.lisproject.org/links/canbaccess.htm.

programs have increased, it has become more difficult to estimate the impact of policy change from first principles — so that microsimulation models have come to play a vital role in highlighting the (sometimes unexpected) distributional consequences of policy change.

In this environment, static microsimulation has blossomed. Sutherland has played an important role in expanding static microsimulation across Europe, with a series of grants from the European Commission funding the development of EUROMOD for the original 15 EC members and then subsequently its extension to the 10 new EC countries Sutherland (2000). Numerous new country-specific models have also been developed since the early 1990s. Within Australia, NATSEM's STINMOD microsimulation model has flourished and been made publicly available — while Wolfson and others within Statistics Canada have continued efforts to make microsimulation accessible to Canadians, including through the publicly available SPSD/M static microsimulation model (Murphy, 2000). Similarly, Gupta and Kapur (Gupta and Kapur, 1996; Chapter 10 in this volume) have developed such models from within the ministries of Finance (TTSIM) and Health (PHARMASIM) for use in the policy development process in the area of taxation and health. Again with on-going government funding, the Urban Institute in the US developed TRIM-3 and made it accessible through the web (O'Hare, 2000). Among the many other country-specific models, many of which are usefully reviewed in Sutherland (1995), are GLAD-HISPANIA for Spain (Harding and Gupta, 2006, Chapter 14); the LAW model for Denmark (Pedersen, 2000); MODETE and ASTER for Belgium (Decoster, 2000; Capéau et al., 2006) and the FASIT model in Sweden.

Equally important in stimulating the practice of microsimulation has been the growing concern about the social and economic impacts of population ageing. This has encouraged the development of dynamic microsimulation models, which have properties that are uniquely suited to analysing the long-term and future impact of changes in pension and other policies (Harding, 2000). While Orcutt and his fellow researchers had completed construction of the DYNASIM dynamic microsimulation model of the US by the mid-1970s (Orcutt et al., 1976), dynamic microsimulation subsequently languished both in the US and internationally in the 1980s (Caldwell, 1996, p. 506). Some of the models constructed in the 1980s have apparently 'died', including the German SfB3 model (Galler and Wagner, 1986), the Australian HARDING model (1993a), the Canadian dynamic cohort model DEMOGEN (Wolfson, 1988), and the Swedish MICROHUS model (Klevmarken and Olovsson, 1996). (In many cases they have been replaced by newer and more complex models.)

Despite the relatively slow progress made in the 1980s, the picture was very different in the 1990s. Often prompted by concerns about the long-term sustainability of public pension programs, government agencies across the world funded the development of dynamic microsimulation models — including DYNACAN within the Canadian Department of Human Resources, LIFE-PATHS within Statistics Canada (Gribble, 2000), MOSART within Statistics Norway, SESIM within the Swedish Ministry of Finance; PenSim within the UK Department of Work and Pensions; Destinie within the French National Statistical Institute (INSEE); PENSIM within the US Department of Labour; and MINT within the US Social Security Administration (with descriptions of most of these models in this volume). Some of these models borrowed heavily from dynamic microsimulation models constructed in the 1980s and extended in the 1990s — with both DYNACAN and MINT, for example, utilizing much of the US CORSIM model developed by Caldwell (1996).

Outside government — although generally again with public funding — academics also constructed dynamic microsimulation models to answer similar questions, including the SAGE and PSSRU/NCCSU aged care models for the UK, DYNAMOD (and now APPSIM) for Australia (Kelly and King, 2001), SVERIGE for Sweden (see the model description chapters for these four models in this volume) and SMILE in Ireland (Ballas et al., 2005).

Apart from the injection of much-needed funds prompted by concerns about population ageing, another factor assisting the production of microsimulation models was the vast and on-going improvements in computer hardware (and, to a lesser extent, software). These improvements have made the production of microsimulation models and the storage of their results much more feasible.

Technology transfer has also been assisted by regular international gatherings of the world community of microsimulators. Four of those gatherings have since resulted in international edited collections, including from the 1993 conference in Canberra, Australia (Harding, 1996); the 1997 conference at Maine in the US (Gupta and Kapur, 2000b); the 1998 workshop at Cambridge in the UK (Mitton et al., 2000) and the 2003 conference in Australia (this volume and the companion volume). In addition, microsimulation has been strongly supported within the Nordic countries, resulting in five Nordic seminars on microsimulation models being held between 1995 and 2006. Importantly for the future, at the 2003 conference in Australia the International Microsimulation Association was formed and the International Journal of Microsimulation was launched — and a website has since been established through the efforts of Paul Williamson at the University of Liverpool (www.microsimulation.org). The association thus provides an excellent means for the world community to keep in electronic touch.

The Future

Microsimulation appears likely to continue to expand in many directions. Geographically, the discipline is still primarily confined to Europe and the

English-speaking world. However, there is increasing evidence of expansion into both Asian and developing countries — including China, Russia, and Africa and often with encouragement from the UN WIDER institute (Xiong et al., 2006; Davies, 2004; http://models.wider.unu.edu/africa_web/). In a world of limited resources and competing demands, the role of microsimulation is expected to grow more quickly than even in the past two decades. The increased reliance on policies aimed at redistribution of income in a revenue neutral environment point to targeted policies which are most efficiently developed using the tools provided by microsimulation. Lately, there have been concerted efforts to promote the use of microsimulation in developing economies, through the teaching of techniques at such centres as the Duke Centre for International Development, NATSEM and the OECD.

The subject area of microsimulation also continues to expand. There has been an explosion in the cost of public health care across OECD countries and modern governments are concerned about their ability to continue to deliver health services for the ageing population in an environment where the health workforce itself is ageing. Against this backdrop, models of the health system are becoming more common, as this volume makes clear — including models of pharmaceutical subsidies and HHRs (Brown et al., 2006; Gupta and Basu, (Chapter 15); Kapur and Gupta, (Chapter 10)). Similarly, a fast-growing new area is spatial microsimulation, for predicting the local effects of policy change and future small area populations and service needs (Williamson et al., 1998; Voas and Williamson, 2000; Ballas et al., 2005; Brown and Harding, 2005; Chin et al., 2005; Chin and Harding, 2006a; 2006b; Cullinan et al., 2006; King, 2006).

Finally, it is clear that there will be continuing efforts to include both the behavioural responses of individuals and macro-economic effects within the ambit of microsimulation (Klevmarken, 1997). Within Australia, the MITTS model is being used to estimate the labour supply effects of policy changes (Creedy et al., 2002) while, in addition to the chapters contained within this volume, there are ongoing efforts to link macro and micro models (Davies, 2004; Arntz et al., 2006).

3.2 Other Modelling Approaches

This introduction has focused heavily on microsimulation — as dynamic microsimulation, in particular, provides one of the most appropriate methods for examining the lifetime and future impacts of possible policy responses to population ageing. But there are also many other possible modelling techniques that can help to shed light on our socio-economic futures.

Hypothetical or Typical Taxpayer Models

Hypothetical models analyse the situation of an individual (or family), whose particular characteristics are defined by the model user. Thus, a hypothetical model might look at the future superannuation of a single woman earning average earnings and working full-time for 20 years and part-time for 20 years. Such models are very useful for analysing policy outcomes for *particular types of individuals* and can incorporate enormous detail. The RIMHYPO model developed by the Australian Treasury is a good example of this type of model (Gallagher, 1995; http://rim.treasury.gov.au/), as is the Effective Tax Rates Model developed at NATSEM (Toohey and Beer, 2004). Similar models, known as Typical Taxpayer Models (TPU) have been extensively used at the Department of Finance in Canada since the early 1980s. These models are very useful in the early stages of the policy development process, in developing the right parameters to achieve stated policy objectives.

Hypothetical models are especially useful for providing information about how a particular type of family or person is likely to be affected by an existing program or by a possible policy change. What such models cannot tell you, however, is *how many* such families there are in the population. As a result, such models cannot be used to obtain estimates of aggregate budget outcomes or distributional outcomes for the *whole population*.

Group Models

Group (or cell-based) models divide the population into a set of groups defined by characteristics such as year of birth, sex, marital status and labour force status. The extent of diversity is thus effectively constrained by the number and type of groups specified.

The output from such models is again very useful to policy analysts seeking to understand the likely impacts of population ageing. A good example of this approach is the RIMGROUP model developed by the Australian Treasury, for analysing the future impact of superannuation and other policy changes (Bacon, 1999). The chapter by Hossain et al., in this volume also provides another example of this type of approach.

What are some of the limitations of group models? First, there are constraints on the diversity of the groups that can be considered. Suppose, for example, that a modeller wanting to examine future government health expenditure decided to create a group model with 20 cells — 10 age groups multiplied by two genders. Suppose further that research in that particular country had shown that income also played a major role in the usage of health services and that it was important to also include this factor in any model projecting future outlays. If the population was now divided into 10 income deciles, then there would be 200 groups in the model to keep track of in future years (10 age ranges × 2 sexes × 10 income groups). Suppose further that whether or not the individuals were still living with a spouse emerged as another key predictor of future expenditure on nursing homes and health. Then, for each of the 200 groups, there would have to be a further division into married/not married, resulting in 400 groups to keep tabs on. It is thus easy to see how group models can easily become intractable, once more sophisticated modelling is desired. Keeping the number of groups down to manageable levels often means failing to capture the diversity present within the population. And to the extent that such diversity and different characteristics are in fact key predictors of whatever the model is looking at, inaccuracy is introduced into the results.

Another difficulty is that people can generally not move from one group to another. As a result, for example, such models usually cannot cope with changes in circumstances, such as divorce. They also cannot cope easily with fluctuating individual earnings over a lifetime, with people typically being assigned to a lifetime earnings group and then experiencing the average outcomes for their group. Thus, for some population sub-groups of interest — such as sole parents, for example — group models cannot provide comprehensive estimates of likely asset holdings and retirement incomes.

Finally, group models provide details of the *average* experience for each of the groups specified within the model. They do not usually provide details of the degree of dispersion around that mean experience. For example, rather than just showing the average age pension received by a particular group within the model, policy makers might want to know what proportion of that group received no age pension and thus just how skewed the distribution of the pension was.

Despite these undoubted disadvantages, group models have one major advantage relative to dynamic microsimulation models: they are much cheaper and quicker to build. Thus, such models provide a very useful tool for gaining insights into the likely impact of population ageing, without having to wait 5 years for the construction of a full dynamic population microsimulation model.

Stock-Flow Models

The stock-flow approach is used in the forecasting of HHRs. For example, physician services are a flow over the course of a year, delivered by a stock of physicians working at a certain level of intensity. The stock of physicians is best modelled via a stock/flow approach, a common and well-accepted form of modelling. Stocks represent quantities at a point in time, such as the number of active physicians at the end of a calendar year. Flows, on the other hand, represent quantities that change over a period of time (e.g. annually in a model).

Comparing two points in time shows changes in the stock. The change in stock, or net flow, is usually a consequence of a series of contributing flows. For example, for physicians, the key flows are the numbers of physicians entering and exiting the workforce. The flows can be further disaggregated, with outflows being categorized into retirements, emigration, and death and inflows into new entrants and immigrants. Inter-provincial migration, on the other hand, can be either an inflow or outflow. Disaggregating flows allow the supply model to be changed at very detailed levels. Consequently, more control translates into more policy levers. These models are especially useful in capturing both lags and leakages from flows. A critical lag, for example, is how long it takes a new medical school student to graduate and start to practice. Leakages are another form of flow. For instance, the number of students who do not complete their training would be considered a leakage.

Such stock-flow models are very effective policy tools in the planning of HHRs. Biviano and Tise (Chapter 16) describe such a model in the context of nursing resources for the US and Gupta and Basu elaborate on the building of such tools for Canada (Chapter 15). By incorporating both demand and supply in their models, Gupta and Basu are able to project "gaps" in the future supply of physicians and provide policy relevant solutions to fill projected "gaps" using policy levers on the supply side in their model.

Econometric and Statistical Models

A range of other modelling techniques have also been used in these two volumes to examine the impacts of population ageing, including life cycle models of housing tenure choice and savings behaviour and econometric models estimated from both cross-sectional and longitudinal data. Such models provide useful insights into particular aspects of the consequences of population ageing and are much easier and cheaper to construct than full-fledged dynamic population microsimulation models — although, again, they lack the richness of dynamic microsimulation models.

4. Overview of the Volume

This volume presents some of the contemporary research in building microsimulation models for the policy-making process, and the application of these models in measuring the effects of different policies in a number of areas such as health care systems, health and taxation and drug coverage. The main objective of the models is to provide a solid analytical foundation for informed policy making around the world. One of the essential requirements for building such models is demographic, socio-economic, and health-related micro data. However, confidentiality laws often make it difficult to obtain such data at the micro level. Besides, usually there is no unique source of data. Thus, it is important to develop techniques to assemble data from disparate data sources to close the data gaps. Some of these problems are discussed in the closing section of this chapter.

In the opening chapter, Wolfson demonstrates the role of microsimulation modelling in identifying some of the core issues related to population ageing and health. He goes through a variety of examples and delves deeper to bring out the essential for informed policy making, beyond research — the key players who need to be involved, the underlying data, and institutional structures needed to bring it all together. A major example is electronic health care records from hospital and doctor visits, linked to health survey data. The public good potential of these data is enormous; so privacy and related legislation should be responsibly supportive of analytic, research, and statistical linkage and secondary uses of these kinds of very sensitive data.

The main purposes of a good heath care system are twofold. The first is the prevention of disease and, the second, delivery of health care to persons in ill health. Therefore, it is important to have a good understanding of the health status of the population for whom the policies are intended.

Part I of the volume deals with a number of health care issues, including (1) measurement of population health status, (2) relationship between demographics and population health status, (3) health risk behaviour across different cohorts of the population, (4) economics and social experience and their effect on the life course, (5) health inequalities, and (6) the ability of the older population to stay in the work force.

A good health care system must efficiently plan and provide HHRs, necessary prescription drugs, as well as provision for long-term care. The system must be compatible with appropriate public/private health insurance or be publicly funded. Parts II and III present different techniques to build microsimulation models to look at the impact of prescription drug plans, and the application of microsimulation models related to financing healthcare through public/private insurance.

Part IV deals with HHR issues. In particular, it demonstrates the usefulness of models in projecting the future demand and supply of physicians and nurses.

Part V concentrates on data challenges and discusses data quality and confidentiality issues and their impact on analyses using such data.

Finally, Part VI presents various microsimulation models from across the world, to demonstrate the practical operation and use of selected models. This section will enable readers to better understand the operative and the practical sides of various models.

An overview of each of the six parts of this volume follows.

4.1 Part I — Health Status: Overview

The first part of the book focuses on health status. It comprises three chapters. The lead chapter (Chapter 3) explores the implications for policy modelling with respect to demographic change, health, and health risk behaviour across cohorts in Britain. Chapter 4 discusses the development and application of resource forecasting in relationship to the different level of dependency among older people in communities and residential settings in Scotland. The final chapter (Chapter 5) in this part examines health inequalities and the ability of the older Australians to stay in the labour force.

Maria Evandrou and Jane Falkingham (Chapter 3) focus on one of the all-important issues of variable selection prior to the building of a policy-relevant model. It is well known that omitting key variables adversely affects model results. However, difficulties in securing funding for costly model building exercises often results in the selection of bare minimum variables. This chapter reinforces the need to carefully select model variables. It provides a well executed 'template' for other researchers faced with the variable selection problem. The chapter successfully carries out the highly complex task of interpreting data from different sources, each collected for purposes other than the topic of this particular research. It demonstrates that having no single data source available — i.e. no longitudinal data for its time series and cohort analysis — can be overcome through appropriate choice of methodology — i.e. the use of the pseudo-cohort approach in this case. This chapter brings to attention the life course. It highlights the fact that economic and social experiences earlier in the life course have an impact upon prospects in later life. As well, it emphasizes the importance of taking cohort differences into account within projections for social policy planning. The key findings of their work are (1) there will be a rise in solo living among elderly people and it may not necessarily be accompanied by an increase in the availability of care from adult children, particularly among the 1960s baby boomers; (2) it may be premature to assume that tomorrow's elders will be healthier than today's.

Adam Redpath (Chapter 4) presents some measures of dependency among older people in community and residential settings in Scotland. He shows the development and application of the measures in resource forecasting. The objectives of this study are to (1) develop a resource use measure (RUM) which allows care professionals to categorize their elderly service users (over age 65) into a limited number of relative need groups; (2) develop a related set of data, and (3) explore the application of such data in stock and flow models. In his analysis, the final RUM grouping, with nine relative need groups, explained 30 per cent of variation in resource use which was in line with external estimates. The measure has been readily accepted by practitioners as a reliable and easy-to-use tool. Modelling showed the relative impact of rehabilitation and quality of care on residential populations.

Agnes Walker (Chapter 5) uses an enhanced version of the dynamic population microsimulation model DYNAMOD (Model 2) to investigate the likely impact on the labour force of changes in the age of retirement and improvements in health at older ages. The chapter addresses an important and timely issue and will further advance the current debate around policy reforms in the context of an ageing society. The chapter makes a significant original contribution, in that it describes one of the first attempts to include health status within a dynamic microsimulation model and provides an illustration of the application of the model.

Using the model, illustrative scenarios are simulated on the impact that longer working lives may have on individuals and governments. In these scenarios, longer working lives can arise from more favourable labour market conditions facing older Australians aged 65–70 (e.g. greater incentives to stay in the workforce, or general improvements in the health of the population). She found that, if 65–70 year olds had the same employment patterns as 45–64 year olds in 1998, they would have benefited from additional earnings (wages or salaries) totalling around $15 billion ($28 billion in 2018). Also, government expenditure on the age pension would have been around $2 billion lower ($4 billion in 2018 or 3.8 per cent of total outlays). Were it possible to lift the health status of all Australians to that of the richest 20 per cent of the population, then the earnings of 65–70 year olds in 2018 would be 4.0 per cent higher than those with 1998 health patterns.

4.2 Part II — Pharmacare and Health Expenditures Issues: Overview

Part II of the volume brings to light some of the issues and developments in microsimulation modelling with a view to analysing the impact of different factors on drug coverage and drug expenditures. It also dwells on health expenditures in general. Five chapters in this part illustrate the experience of building microsimulation models for prescription drugs plans in Australia and Canada. These papers show how the development of these models adapted to different perspectives and experiences, socio-economic and political structures.

Michael McCracken and Bert Waslander (Chapter 6) review the available models of drug expenditure in Canada. The topic is timely as Canada does not yet have broad-based public insurance for pharmaceuticals. Models which provide robust costing and distributional analysis would be valuable policy tools. The chapter also reviews policy challenges and proposed solutions using various tools of analysis — including microsimulation models to evaluate several proposals for prescription drug plans. They report some results and key strengths and limitations of the various approaches, and suggest extensions and improvements. The chapter concludes with some observations on the use and utility of micromodels.

Deborah Schofield and George Rothman (Chapter 7) project Commonwealth Health Expenditure in Australia's First Intergenerational Report (IGR) 2002–2003, which provides a basis for considering the Commonwealth's fiscal outlook over the long term and identifies emerging pressures. Health expenditure was identified to be a source of very significant future spending pressure, with spending on health projected to increase from about 4 per cent of GDP in 2001–2002 to about 8 per cent in 2041–2042. The pharmaceutical benefits scheme (PBS) was projected to be the fastest growing component, increasing about fivefold as a percentage of GDP. Technological change and increased use and cost of services were found to be the main drivers of Commonwealth health spending, with population growth and ageing being much less significant drivers of growth. Projections are presented for the main components of health spending and the sensitivity of the projections to demographic and other assumptions is assessed. To capture the significant uncertainties associated with projecting expenditures, revenues and overall economic performance over such an extended period, the authors perform a sensitivity analysis of various parameters.

Brown et al. (Chapter 8) use a microsimulation model (PharmaSim) to examine the effects on older people of a recent change in the eligibility threshold, and level of co-payment, for the Australian PBS. The chapter provides an important illustration of the usefulness of such microsimulation tools for policy analysis. This chapter examines government outlays on Australian PBS, which have increased rapidly over the past 10 years. The study examines the impact on the costs to government and patients of PBS listed medicines and estimates the distributional effects of the policy change, particularly for older Australians.

Chris Raymond and Brett Parsons (Chapter 9) discuss modelling of two important pillars of the health care system in Australia, the medicare system and the PBS. This is an important topical issue today, not only for Australia but also for most of the developed world. The tools presented in the paper are policy oriented; thus, they are useful to those concerned with the increasing cost of health care. This work has its value in both its policy applications and the knowledge about the tool.

The model uses standard forecasting procedures from SAS and thus makes them accessible to others facing similar challenges. A logical extension of this work would be to incorporate changing health status and its impact on the overall utilization of health resources. This is partially addressed in a paper by Lagergren (Chapter 13). However, this issue needs special attention as the health status of the future elderly is improving, which potentially means some relief to the otherwise pressured health care systems. Using microsimulation techniques, we need to do sensitivity analysis of the requirements under different assumptions of health status of individuals on the one hand and the policy options of the governments on the other.

Vishnu Kapur and Anil Gupta (Chapter 10) present the development of a Microsimulation Model for Pharmacare and illustrate its usefulness in analysis and policy applications. Drugs are emerging as an increasingly important part of health care system in Canada, where the proportion of health care expenditures devoted to drugs has been rising faster than other components. Two recent reports on Health Care in Canada — the Kirby report and the Romanow report — focus on relief to families for rising cost of drugs. This work could make a useful contribution to the international literature on pharmaceutical modelling. There are only few examples internationally where microsimulation has been used to model health policy effects (Brown et al., 2004; Harding et al., 2004).

The chapter describes the process of building a microsimulation model for drug-related programs including a pharmacare program. The chapter describes the methodology used to create a database at micro level from disparate data sources and the process of building the microsimulation model. Database construction is a major task that could have an impact on the capacity/validity of the model. The authors have extended their work, described in Gupta and Kapur (2000a), to include more health-related variables for policy simulation. Exactly the same task of statistically matching a health and an income survey was undertaken by NATSEM (Brown et al., 2004), and the reader may find it useful to apply the best practices from these very successful approaches. Finally, the chapter presents results of a simulation of a hypothetical drug benefits program and the cost and distributional impact of the simulation, analysing those impacts on a number of socio-economic and demographic variables.

4.3 Part III — Financing, Caring and Health Delivery: Overview

Part III of the volume brings forth the issues related to financing of health care. The lead chapter (Chapter 11) presents a microsimulation model to look at the impact of medical insurance reform of government employees and workers in China. Chapter 12 presents an analysis, using the Canadian LifePaths model, of the changing characteristics of people who are in a 'sandwich generation' — people who have children living at home and a parent aged 65 years or over. Chapter 13 examines the future needs of long-term care of elderly persons in Sweden using a simulation model. The last chapter (Chapter 14) from Australia provides a new perspective on the use of microsimulation models. A regional microsimulation is used to look at the impact of changing preferences on the use of Income Support services by clients.

Xiong Linping et al. (Chapter 11) present a microsimulation model of medical insurance reform of government employees and workers in China. This is a very interesting paper for a number of reasons. First, it documents one of the first microsimulation projects to come out of China. For that reason, it is of particular importance in a volume on microsimulation. Second, it reports on a health microsimulation model, which is one of the interesting new directions in which microsimulation modelling is expanding — i.e. beyond the more traditional domains of taxes and cash transfers. Third, the results suggest that the current medical insurance system in China is not affordable in the long run. It may require some specific reform measures which are not likely to be politically popular. The paper thus provides a good illustration of the ability of microsimulation models to help policy makers, in providing estimates of how programs are likely to evolve some years before major problems actually emerge.

Hicks et al. (Chapter 12) present an analysis, using the Canadian LifePaths model, of the changing characteristics of people who are in a 'sandwich generation' — people who have children living at home and a parent aged 65 years or over. The analysis compares the characteristics of four cohorts of these people: those born in the 1930s, 1950s, 1970s and 1990s.

Marten Lagergren (Chapter 13) examines the future needs of long-term care of elderly persons in Sweden. The paper deals directly with the use of resources in the future by the elderly. Through the use of appropriate data from different sources, the author provides evidence that the resources required in the future would be relatively lower when we take into account the improved health of the future elderly. This is a common concern of many OECD countries. The paper demonstrates the sensitivity of projections of long-term care needs to assumptions about the future health status of older people. In an effort to estimate the future needs of publicly financed long-term care of frail elderly persons, a new model has been presented in this chapter.

Anthony King (Chapter 14) outlines an approach to the forecasting of the use of local welfare offices by pensioners, who claim a means-tested state-funded pension in Australia. The chapter outlines the elements required to construct such a model, explaining the various assumptions and data inputs required. The chapter concludes with a few illustrative examples of forecast results. The principal novelty the model introduces is spatial disaggregation of overall service demand. Forecasting of service demand at a sub-regional level is a problem faced by many analysts across the world. In this sense, the chapter is clearly of interest to a wide international audience.

4.4 Part IV — Health Human Resources Modelling: Overview

This part of the volume focuses on HHRs. It comprises two very elaborate chapters on the development, issues, and application of HHR models in a policy environment. Given the looming shortages of HHR in the wake of population ageing, the planning tools presented in this part are very timely and can assist planners in not only identifying the projected gaps in the supply of HHR but also in finding practical solutions to fill these gaps. The lead chapter by Gupta and Basu discusses the importance of HHR forecasting models and their usefulness for HHR planning in the Canadian context. Biviano and Tise (Chapter 16) elaborate, with examples, the thinking behind the projected demand and supply of registered nurses (RNs) and subsequent shortages as projected by the Health Resources and Services Administration for USA.

This part introduces models other than microsimulation models to complete the picture — both the economic sustainability and the HHR needs in an ageing society. Today, we are faced with unprecedented shortages of HHR and, to accentuate the problem, maldistribution of HHR both inside countries and around the world makes the problem even more severe. If present trends continue, these shortfalls will only increase. To make the right choices, both in terms of forming HHR and ensuring their right mix and deployments, policy makers require planning tools. The next two chapters provide practical tools to deal with this problem for the two most important of these resource types, physicians and nurses. These tools also provide a framework for planning other HHR such as pharmacists.

Both chapters use utilization as a proxy for demand of HHR. This allows the models to create realistic projections of these resources in the near to medium term. The nurse demand, in particular, is derived from the demand for other health care services as the functions of nurses are not easily distinguishable in a setting where physicians are the first point of contact. The authors make a point that future nurse workforce will be influenced by the combination of supply and demand.

Gupta and Basu (Chapter 15) emphasize the building of policy-relevant HHR models. The development of workforce supply and demand models for physicians and nurses in Nova Scotia is well documented in this paper. These models will be an important tool for medical workforce planners for many years to come, providing an informed basis on projected needs and shortages for provincial as well as federal policy makers in Canada. The paper does an excellent job in laying out the models and explaining how they work.

The methodologies for the models are quite appropriate and easy to apply in other situations — for example, for another province in Canada. The demand model methodology, as mentioned above, is based on utilization (by specialty), where utilization is defined as a function of current population utilization patterns projected out for future population projections. The demand projections are in terms of full-time equivalents (FTEs) by specialty. Supply models are stock and flow models with resultant projections in FTEs again by specialty. The authors claim that, given the world-wide concern about HHR and the common problems in building policy-relevant models, the lessons distilled from their work will prove useful to those facing similar challenges elsewhere in the world.

Marilyn Biviano and Steve Tise (Chapter 16) provide an excellent example of the application of modelling in the health field. They provide an elaborate framework for building such tools for nursing resources from their experience in the US context. They tackle the distribution issue head on to demonstrate that the smaller states in US will bear the brunt of the shortfall in the coming years.

This chapter describes the construction and application of two models — one generating annual, state-level projections of the RN supply and the other the demand for RNs. The chapter outlines the structure of the models, the data, methods and assumptions, and briefly discusses some of the limitations.

While these models are developed for the US, they have general applicability and will be of widespread interest. Nursing workforce shortage is an international phenomenon and there is urgent need for good workforce planning models that can assist policy makers in ensuring adequate future supply of nurses, especially at a regional level. The chapter uses the US case to illustrate some very common nursing workforce issues — such as difficulties in recruitment and retention, an ageing workforce, regional disparities, etc. The authors assume a fairly standard approach to workforce modelling — including in their projections of supply, recruitment, attrition, and workforce participation rates, and a variety of key health care organizational, economic, population, and geographical variables in modelling demand. They found that in 2000, the national supply of FTE RN was estimated at 1.89 million, while the demand was estimated at 2 million (a shortage of 6 per cent). Using internally developed demand and supply models and exploiting the estimated trends in demand and supply the shortage by 2020 is estimated to increase fivefold.

4.5 Part V — Data Challenges: Overview

Part V focuses on demographics, data, and modelling. It comprises two chapters. The lead chapter discusses data quality and non-response effects by using Logistic Regression in the Welsh Health Survey. The second chapter focuses on confidentiality and the importance of synthetic data.

Ruth Studley (Chapter 17) concentrates on data quality and non-response effects by using Logistic Regression in the Welsh Health Survey. The aim of the second Welsh survey (Government Statistical Service, 1998) was to collect information from groups within the population representing those with a range of illnesses or disabilities and also representing healthy people — without using any medical records. The results provide a picture of health of the people of Wales, the way the National Health Service is used and areas where service could be improved. This chapter aims to discuss issues surrounding the data quality and the adjustments used for non-response bias.

Paul Williamson (Chapter 18) deals with statistical disclosure control practices (DCPs) and microdata quality issues. Against scenarios foretelling 'worst case' conditions and an environment characterized by increasing concern for confidentiality, he considers that a real danger exists that the informational content of released microdata will be degraded by the use by national statistical agencies of increasingly aggressive disclosure control measures. He recognizes that disclosure control is not a free lunch. It has a cost in terms of quality, associated with standard statistical practices (e.g. multivariate analysis and very small sub-groups, sampling errors, population weights, and rounding error), data protection laws, confidentiality, and associated risks of disclosure (aggregation and suppression practices). As always, however, there is choice and different costs can be associated with different methodologies. In a nutshell, it is important for researchers to be able to grasp the limits of microdata that are made available to judge whether they meet 'modellers' needs' or whether they can be met by making different choices or following different courses. Since different DCPs can have different costs for researchers it is important to investigate ways to control and optimize choices among alternatives DCPs. Williamson's article leads to a positive answer, which it can only be hoped that national statistical agencies will ponder when they weigh confidentiality-disclosure-microdata quality.

As data access is being 'liberalized', the quality costs imposed by confidentiality are apparently on the rise. Williamson's paper, therefore, suggests that it is not justifiable that more microdata should be hidden and a hidden cost paid in terms of quality — nor that anonymization may be a sufficient reason at the cost of quality. The academic community should express its concern on confidentiality and allied statistical practices which 'artificially' lower the quality of the micro data made available to them.

4.6 Part VI — Overview of Existing Microsimulation and Health Human Resources Models

The objective of this section is to demonstrate the practical operation of selected models currently in use around the world. The motivation for the inclusion of this section in the book came from discussions and appreciations received at the technical session at the microsimulation conference in Australia in December 2003. One whole day was dedicated to the presentation of 32 models from different countries. Many modellers have shown interest in knowledge about the operative or the practical side of models.

This part follows upon a similar approach included in an earlier volume by Gupta and Kapur (2000a). This time around, we gain by the inclusion of health-related models, pension models, spatial microsimulation models and a long-term forecast models. We hope the modelling community around the world will find the material helpful in their modelling work.

Part VI starts with a lead article by McCracken and Gupta, which provides a perspective on the stage of modelling in the world today and attempts to synthesize lessons from each of the models. This is followed by a short chapter on each of the 22 models included in this part. The selection of these models is based on a number of considerations. First, we intend to cover as a wide spectrum of use as possible (tax, transfer, and health). Second, we attempt to cover a wide geographic range. Third, we try to cover many types of models (e.g. static and dynamic). Each chapter provides background information and working details of the model and also demonstrates its usefulness in the policy process. The model description generally follows the following format:

- *Introduction*: Describes the purpose and scope of the model;
- *Overview*: The type of model — Static, Dynamic, Hybrid, Stochastic, Longitudinal, etc. Who owns the model and some details about the difficulties and challenges faced during its construction?
- *Data issues*: The underlying data (administrative, survey, synthetic, or hypothetical taxpayer data); agency responsible for the data; data construction and data ageing details (imputation, under-reporting adjustment, and re-weighting; merging; updating; projection component; micro-macro links);
- *Technical particulars*: Language, system requirements, typical run time, whether interactive;
- *Usage and usability*: When last used and for what type of simulation?
- Availability of model; Does the model have an educational value?

The model descriptions are divided into four groups: dynamic microsimulation models; static microsimulation and macro–micro approaches, HHR models, and spatial microsimulation models.

The remaining part of this section provides an overview of each of the models in the chapter sequence.

Dynamic Microsimulation Models

MOSART (Norway)

- MOSART is a Dynamic Microsimulation model from Statistics Norway, primarily devoted to pension issues. It starts with 1 per cent of the

Norwegian population in 1993 and has extensive income and other information on these individuals. The data are drawn from administrative records and thus the model and the data are only accessible to Statistics Norway. The primary users of the model are the Ministry of Finance and the Ministry of Labour and Social Inclusion.

- The model has a good user interface but has no real outside users. All the analysis is performed by analysts at Statistics Norway and any work for outsiders (including the media) is highly scrutinized before being passed on to external clients. We feel that with good planning there is scope for sharing the model with outsiders while respecting the confidentiality of data at the same time.
- The model is written in Simula, an object-oriented language, developed in Norway in the 1960s, but the output from the model can be manipulated in SAS. There are a range of languages for models in the book. Both C and C++ are common choices but some models are written in Turbo Pascal and some are developed by organizations in a local language. One common feature seems to be the availability of SAS, Excel or some other better known platform for manipulation of results and model output for further analysis.

DYNAMOD (Australia)

- This is a dynamic microsimulation model for taxes and transfers. The authors claim that the probability calculations and alignments are achieved in a unique manner. The model uses transitional probabilities, exploits macro–micro linkages and survival functions. In its earlier version, the developers tried to incorporate in the design an integrated macroeconomic model. This became too ambitious for the team and virtually resulted in a major break for the project. This provides some useful lessons for modellers, for example, contain the project, be practical, develop step by step, and do not be overambitious.
- The model is based on a 1 per cent sample from the 1986 census, a common feature of many dynamic models.

SAGE (UK)

- This is a dynamic microsimulation model aimed at policy analysis in the areas of social policy, pensions, and health and long-term care needs. The model incorporates health and disability status and thus will help the policy makers in this important area of public policy.
- The model uses a sample of the British population (0.1 per cent) from the 1991 Census as its base. The authors rightly argue in favour of a representative sample even at the cost of missing some key variables. In their

view, this avoids initial biases in the data building processes. As has been the experience of most of the authors in the volume, it is almost impossible to find one source of comprehensive data for modelling. The modellers have, therefore, taken recourse to working with disparate data sources. This involves statistical matching, imputation, massaging data in many ways, etc. before moving on to the modelling part.

- The authors use a variety of data sources to determine the transitional probabilities. The population in the model is updated using these transitional probabilities at fixed 1-year intervals.

LifePaths (Canada)

- The LifePaths simulation model is a longitudinal microsimulation model from Statistics Canada. It is in turn the basis for a number of more specialized longitudinal microsimulation models used in the areas of health policy, time use analysis, and intergenerational equity.
- The model is a dynamic overlapping cohort model. The unit of simulation consists of a 'core' individual whose complete lifetime is simulated from birth to death.
- LifePaths is implemented using the Modgen language developed at Statistics Canada. Modgen is an object-oriented extension of C++, and provides the model developer with an integrated environment for creating microsimulation models. Generated models run on Windows 32-bit platforms.
- A public release version of LifePaths is available on the Statistics Canada web site together with other supporting software.

SESIM (Sweden)

- The Scandinavian countries have been relatively more successful in both building and using microsimulation models, especially dynamic microsimulation models. SESIM is focused on estimating the impacts of population ageing on the public finances. In addition, the model has been extended to analyse the health status of the elderly. This makes the model very useful as the elderly tend to consume a disproportionate amount of health care services.
- The model allows simulation both at the individual and the household level. This is quite important when dealing with the care of the elderly. The model has information on geographic distances between the elderly and their relatives (care givers) and other information such as the number of days the care is needed. In addition, the model has extensive information on income and taxes. This allows the use of tax instruments for developing health policy options and potential health programmes.

- The model code is readily available through their website. This should provide an incentive for both the novice and the experts to develop and enhance their own models. The model could potentially be used at universities (in Sweden) for learning and limited policy analysis work.

DYNACAN (Canada)

- This model is based on the structure developed by Steven Caldwell's CORSIM model at Cornell University in the 1970s. The author puts great emphasis on alignment and provides a good example of how to do it right. The model is built for the government to forecast Canada Pension Plan (CPP) outlays and number of recipients. The micro data behind the model is a 1 per cent representative sample of the Canadian Census of 1971. Like other models, the model lacks some key data that are available only through other surveys and aggregate administrative data (e.g. CPP program data).
- The model is written in the C language. It uses SAS for extraction of results and analysis. Because of the highly technical nature of the code, the model is handled primarily by the Dynacan team. The model is for use of clients within the government only.
- The model has a potential for education as it provides a powerful test bed framework for examining demographic evolution in Canada. But for this to become a reality, the model would have to be made available to outsiders.
- The next phase of Dynacan is expected to expand to include after tax implications of government policies to estimate the net impact of policy changes in the area of CPP. This will be an extremely important enhancement of the model capability as it is the after-tax impact of policy changes that matters to individuals.

DESTINIE (France)

- DESTINIE is a stochastic, dynamic microsimulation model built by the French National Statistical Institute (INSEE). The main purpose of DESTINIE is to analyse the effect of alternative pension rules on the participation rate and the amount of pension of successive cohorts. The age of retirement in the model is endogenously determined according to a labour-leisure trade-off. The main data source is the individual level data from the 1998 Financial Asset Survey by INSEE. As usual, these data are supplemented by imputation of certain variables from other sources. The data in the model is aged to 2050 using a mix of approaches — deterministic rules, behavioural responses, and random transitions.
- The model language is Turbo Pascal but, like other models, the output from the model can be further manipulated using SAS and Excel.

- Recently, the model was extensively used in the French Pension reform. The future development of the model is aimed at analysis of the French health care system.

Static Microsimulation and Macro/Micro Approaches

GLADHISPANIA (Spain)

- This is a university-based static microsimulation model for tax policy analysis. It derives its data from the Economic Community Household Panel (ECHP), the part belonging to Spain. The model is fully interactive and does extensive tax policy analysis of the Spanish tax system. The web version of the model is coded in Java. The model has behavioural responses to labour supply especially in response to policy changes. Recently, it was used to simulate the impact of an option replacing the existing Spanish tax system with a new flat tax with a vital minimum (an amount of income considered as subsistence and thus not taxed). The model is actively used as a teaching/learning tool in a university environment.

STINMOD (Australia)

- This is Australia's tax and transfer static microsimulation model. This model is publicly available with a user-friendly interface. The model is built on data from several sources. Thus, it requires merging of information from disparate sources as well imputation of some missing variables. An important aspect of STINMOD is the inclusion of the institutionalized population in the model database. This is important for policy impact analysis because of the high incidence of cash transfers to this group. NATSEM routinely uses this model as a training tool for the 'Microsimulation techniques for social and economic analysis' course under the University of Canberra's Management Program.

EUROMOD (E.U.)

- EUROMOD is a multi-country static model representing the tax-benefit system of 15 European countries. It will soon be extended to include new members since 2004 raising the number of countries to 25. The model is a tax policy analysis tool for measuring comparative impact of changes to the tax benefit system of one member country vis-à-vis all other countries. The model is also used by members to do their respective country specific tax modelling. This should be a motivation for a similar model for Canada–USA–Mexico, given that these countries are closely connected through trade.

- The model is written in C++ and is readily available both as an academic tool and a policy analysis tool to students of policy analysis and researchers alike.
- Another project, 'Accurate Income Measurement for the Assessment of Public Policies' (AIM-AP), under EUROMOD, has attracted a large network of researchers across Europe. This program is designed to improve the comparability, scope and applicability of tools, methods and data for the measurement of income and the analysis of the effects of policies on inequality, poverty and social inclusion. These initiatives will definitely help improve the use of the evidence base in policy-making across nations.

PSSRU and CARESIM (UK)

- The PSSRU long-term care finance model for the UK makes projections of future long-term care demand and expenditures. CARESIM analyses the current and projected future distributional effects of alternative ways of financing long-term care. They are linked for two purposes. The first is to improve the apportionment of total expenditure between the private and public sectors in the PSSRU model. The second is to weight CARESIM results to take account of the fact that older people who need care are not a random sub-sample of the older population.
- The PSSRU Long-Term Care Finance model was constructed as part of a project on long-term care finance. It answers two related policy issues on the funding of long-term care for older people. The first is whether expenditure, and specifically public expenditure, on long-term care will remain sustainable over the coming decades. The second is what should be the balance between public and private expenditure on long-term care. The model has been actively used for various important initiatives including projections for the Department of Health, the Royal Commission on Long-Term Care, the Institute for Public Policy Research, the European Commission, the National Assembly for Wales, the Nuffield Foundation, and the Joseph Rowntree Foundation.
- CARESIM aims to provide information relevant to assessing the distributional effects of alternative care charging regimes. It is a dynamic microsimulation model which uses data on a sample of older people's income and assets to simulate what each older sample member would be required to pay towards his or her care costs should he or she need care.

SPSD/M (Canada)

- The SPSD/M is a static microsimulation model. It is comprised of a database, a series of tax/transfer algorithms and models, analytical software and user documentation. It was developed by Statistics Canada, with participation of other federal government departments through a steering committee, to provide state-of-the-art microsimulation capability to the wider policy-making community.

- The SPSD is a non-confidential, statistically representative database of individuals in their family contexts, with enough information on each individual to compute taxes paid to and cash transfers received from both federal and provincial levels of governments.
- It has been used to study every major change in the Canadian tax/transfer system since 1984 including several tax reforms, unemployment insurance reforms, and special issue areas such as intergenerational equity
- The SPSD/M is written in C++. The full program requires PC with 220-Mb available disk space running under Windows 2000 or Windows XP.
- Since 1987, the SPSD/M has been available to the public. The database and model are provided on a licensed basis as either a single use version or a site licence.

OECD — Tax and Benefit Model

- This is another multi-country modelling of tax-benefit analysis across OECD countries. However, in this case the unit of analysis is a household and a comparative analysis on five typical households (single person, one or two-earner couples with or without children) under tax-benefit systems of 29 member countries. The model can simulate practically all policies relating to the tax-benefit situation of these typical households and thus provide a comparative analysis of the tax burden on same household under the tax systems of different countries.
- The 'model household' approach used in this model is similar to the so-called 'Typical Taxpayer Analysis' approach undertaken by the Department of Finance in Canada. Such an approach is critical in the early stages of the policy development process. Coupled with the microsimulation approach, the policy makers can fully appreciate both the revenue and the distributional impacts of policy changes and their impact on typical households.
- The model uses STATA and is accessible to all countries through an online system.

PHARMASIM (Canada)

- The Pharmasim microsimulation model deals with policy impact analysis of the provincial drug plans in Canada. The model fully simulates the Canadian tax system and has separate modules for each of the provincial drug plans. Like many other models, the real challenge lies in building a comprehensive database from disparate data sources. The model uses various survey data sources and also aggregate data from administrative sources. The model does analysis of health-tax issues and could be used to design and evaluate a potential national drug plan.

- The output from the model can be further analysed to fully understand the distributional impact of policy changes. The model has an innovative way of modifying otherwise very complex provincial plans through a special file structure, the flex files. Through these files the model is linked to Typical Pharmacare User Model (TPU); similar in idea to the OECD model described above. The Pharmasim and TPU then provide a complete analysis in the development of new policy options in the above areas.

LOTTE (Norway)

- LOTTE is the Norwegian static tax-benefit model based on tax records. This model has been in operation since the 1970s. The later versions include commodity taxes and a behavioural component. The database used by the new version includes expenditure data drawn from the household expenditures survey. Other household information is also added to the database. The combined data are then projected to future years based on macro estimates from Finance and Statistics Norway. The model is actively used in budget making and budgetary reforms.

Health Human Resource Models

IPDSM (Canada)

- IPDSM is a physician supply and demand forecasting model at the Department of Health in Canada. Health care in Canada is a provincial subject. However, the federal government is responsible for the Canada Health Act that lays down a number of principles for health care. Besides, the federal government plays a lead coordinating role in many areas including supply and demand of health personnel. The supply component of IPDSM is national but the demand side of the model is presently limited to the province of Nova Scotia because of lack of data. The supply model follows the stock-flow approach and the demand is based on current utilization of health care services at the individual level. One of the challenge facing policy makers is to eradicate the overall shortages of physicians. Another problem is to overcome the uneven distribution of physicians across regions of the country. IPDSM has an inter-provincial migration component that accounts for such moves based on historical data and future trends. The model accommodates such movements while projecting supply numbers into the future.

- In the population ageing context, given that the physician work force is also ageing, the model provides a practical tool for HHR planning. This model could be adapted to work for other provinces in Canada. It could also be adapted to work for other countries.

NSM and NDM (USA)

- NSM and NDM models work under the mandate of the United States Health Resources and Services Administration (HRSA). These models forecast the supply of and demand for nurse resources in the United States. Both models use data on nurse workforce collected through the quadrennial Sample Survey of Registered Nurses (SSRN). NDM is a national model and data limitations do not allow estimates at the state level. On the other hand, NSM is built on state level data directly and the national estimates are obtained through the summation of state level estimates.
- The NDM forecasts future demand for healthcare services in six types of settings: inpatient, outpatient, and emergency departments in general and short-term hospitals; non-general and long-term hospitals; nursing facilities; and home health care. It is a utilization-based model and the demand is projected in full-time-equivalent (FTE) nurse resources.
- The NSM follows a stock-flow approach similar to the IPDSM model described above. Apart from regular in and out flows, inter-state migration is also modelled. This is also true of IPDSM where the model explicitly simulates the impact of inter-provincial migration on the future supply of physicians by province.

MediSim (Australia)

- MediSim simulates changes to the Australian Pharmaceutical Benefit Scheme (PBS) at individual and household level while estimating the revenue and distributional impacts of options for possible policy reforms. This model was developed by NATSEM and is used both by the government and non-government agencies interested in policy analysis in this area. The underlying database for the model is constructed using the 2001 National Health Survey (NHS) as the starting point. A number of variables are added to this base data from other sources through statistical merging and imputation processes. The sample for the NHS excludes about 3 per cent of the Australian population living in institutions. However, the resultant micro data is re-weighted to represent the entire population of Australia.
- The model and its underlying database permits modelling at the drug level, i.e. type of drug, level of use, and its price. This makes the model

extremely useful for policy formulation. MediSim's chief utility has been in quantifying the use and cost of PBS medicines under different policy settings, and the distributional effect of such policy options. The model can measure the impact of changes in other model parameters such as medicine prices or supply, or demographic changes (such as population ageing). PHARAMASIM (Model 12) lacks this capacity in its present form.

- The only hands-on users of the model are the members of the MediSim team. To date, results from the model have been used primarily by Medicines Australia.

Spatial Microsimulation Models

SVERIGE (Sweden)

- SVERIGE (*System for Visualizing Economic and Regional Influences Governing the Environment)* represents a family of a spatial, dynamic micro simulation model representing all individuals and families in Sweden with a high level of spatial resolution. This is a national model but allows analysis and results for any spatial division, county, municipality, or (for some versions) $100\,m^2$ of space area in Sweden. The model updates itself on an annual cycle. However, certain modules are event-based and are updated once an event is triggered. The model is based on 100 per cent population. Thus, there is no need for the imputations necessary for most of the other models in the volume. The only time some information is imputed is when a user requires some specific information on individuals such as attitude. The model was developed in a university environment and thus has potential as a teaching tool. At present, the restriction on data sharing precludes any such arrangements. The developers have ideas on how to make it happen but that will take time.

NSW Hospital Model (Australia)

- This is an innovative spatial microsimulation health model. The model performs distributional analyses of patients treated in NSW hospitals and is used to project future hospital use and the related costs. The model has also been used to determine the split of use between public and private hospitals. The model uses administrative hospital data from all hospitals in Australia for the period 1996–1997 to 1999–2000. The novelty of this model is that it has imputed SES at an individual level. (with most earlier work having made such imputation at a spatial area thus making an assumption that SES is uniform for all individuals/families in that spatial area). The linking of patient records from different hospitals along with some probabilistic matching resulted in a unique identifier for each patient for all hospital separations at different hospitals.

CuSP (Australia)

- Centrelink is the Australian agency responsible for the delivery of a range of government services including income support payments and associated services. Thus, it has a large customer base that uses different channels to contact the agency, ranging from walk-in offices to email. The CuSP model is a static spatial microsimulation model designed to generate small area projections of Centrelink customer numbers and characteristics and their associated channel use. This is another innovative application of spatial microsimulation from NATSEM.
- The CuSP model is primarily used by Centrelink as a decision support tool. The model enables them to predict into the future the usage of Centrelink's many services down to the small area level. Centrelink is also able to simulate the impact on these services of changes to government social security policy and the impact changes in different demographic and economic conditions.

SpatialMSM (Australia)

- SpatialMSM is a spatial microsimulation model used to generate estimates of household characteristics within small areas and to model the spatial impact of policy changes in income tax and cash transfer programs. It was developed by the National Centre for Social and Economic Modelling (NATSEM) at the University of Canberra, starting in 2003, and represents part of NATSEM's continuing attempts to develop small area microsimulation models. The spatialMSM system has been used to generate small area estimates of such variables as wages and salaries, disposable income, income tax paid, social security and family benefits received, personal wealth, poverty rates, and housing stress.
- The methodology employed by the spatialMSM system involves two major steps. Step one creates household weights for small areas using a core technique called 'reweighting'. Step two applies the SLA household weights thus created to the selected output variables generated by NATSEM's static model STINMOD, to create the small area (SLA) estimates of the desired outputs (such as housing affordability and household income poverty).

5. Conclusions

Orcutt's dream is gradually being realized. There have been considerable advances in the development and use of microsimulation modelling, as

Orcutt envisioned in his seminal paper. The use of microsimulation has now expanded to health care and to spatial applications. The near future is expected to see its advancement to almost all public policy areas that directly influence the welfare of citizens, for example, education, agriculture, city planning, and so on. However, before the use is fully integrated into the policy-making processes, modellers will have to come up with approaches that increase the confidence of policy makers in the estimates produced by these models. Such approaches may involve development of models that integrate the simplicity of static models and the power of dynamic models. One of the objectives would be to estimate second level impacts of policy changes resulting from behavioural responses. This objective is not hard to realize in the short to medium run horizon.

There has been a sizeable increase in the need to blend health and tax simulation capabilities in OECD countries, which have a host of health-related tax deductions. We need to continue to develop innovative ways to blend health policies with tax policies in a world with competing demands and limited financial resources. Through microsimulation modelling, we can develop tools that simulate realistic policy options, balancing program objectives with fiscal constraints to help maintain solidarity of public programs. This is our hope!

References

Arntz, M., Boeters, S., Gürtzgen, N. and Schubert, S. (2006). *Analysing Welfare Reform in a Microsimulation-AGE Model: The Value of Disaggregation*. Paper presented at the 8th Nordic Seminar on Microsimulation Models, Oslo, 7–9 June (available from www.ssb.no/misi).

Bacon, B. (1999). Ageing in Australia: Some Modelling Results and Research Issues, *Policy Implications of the Ageing of Australia's Population*, Productivity Commission, Melbourne.

Baldini, M. (2001). Inequality and Redistribution over the Life-Cycle in Italy: An Analysis with a Dynamic Cohort Microsimulation Model. *Brazilian Electronic Journal of Economics*, 4(2).

Ballas, D., Clarke, G. and Wiemers, E. (2005). Building a Dynamic Spatial Microsimulation Model for Ireland. *Population, Space and Place*, 11(3), 157–172.

Bonnet, C. and Mahieu, R. (2000). Public Pensions in a Dynamic Microanalytic Framework: The Case of France, in Mitton, L., Sutherland, H. and Weeks, M. (eds), *Microsimulation Modelling for Policy Analysis*, Cambridge University Press, Cambridge.

Brown, L., Abello, A., Phillips, B. and Harding, A. (2004). Moving Towards an Improved Micro-Simulation Model of the Australian Pharmaceutical Benefits Scheme. *Australian Economic Review*, 37(1), 41–61.

Brown, L., Abello, A., Phillips, B. and Harding, A. (2006). The Australian Pharmaceuticals Benefit Scheme and Older Australians: Changes in Government Outlays and Consumer Costs from the 2002–2003 Federal Budget Measures, in

Gupta, A. and Harding, A. (eds), *Modelling Our Future: Population Ageing, Health and Aged Care*, International Symposia in Economic Theory and Econometrics, North-Holland, Amsterdam.

Brown, L. and Harding, A. (2005). The New Frontier of Health And Aged Care: Using Microsimulation to Assess Policy Options. *Quantitative Tools for Microeconomic Policy Analysis*, Productivity Commission, Canberra (available from http://www.pc.gov.au/research/confproc/qtmpa/index).

Caldwell, S. (1990). *Static, Dynamic and Mixed Microsimulation, Mimeo*. Department of Sociology, Cornell University, Ithaca, New York, July.

Caldwell, S. (1996). Health, Welfare, Pensions and Life Paths: The CORSIM Dynamic Microsimulation Model, in Harding, A. (ed), *Microsimulation and Public Policy*, North-Holland, Amsterdam.

Capéau, B., Decoster, A., De Swerdt, K. and Orsini, K. (2006). Distributional Impact of Shifting the Base of Financing Social Security from Personal Contributions to Indirect Taxes. Paper presented at the 8th Nordic Seminar on Microsimulation Models, Oslo, 7–9 June (available from www.ssb.no/misi).

Chin, S.F. and Harding, A. (2006a). *Regional Dimensions: Creating Synthetic Small-Area Microdata and Spatial Microsimulation Models*. Technical Paper no. 33, National Centre for Social and Economic Modelling, University of Canberra, May.

Chin, S.F. and Harding, A. (2006b). SpatialMSM, in Gupta, A. and Harding, A. (eds), *Modelling Our Future: Population Ageing, Health and Aged Care*, International Symposia in Economic Theory and Econometrics, North-Holland, Amsterdam.

Chin, S.F., Harding, A., Lloyd, R., McNamara, J., Phillips, B. and Vu, Q. (2005). Spatial Microsimulation Using Synthetic Small Area Estimates of Income, Tax and Social Security Benefits. *Australasian Journal of Regional Studies*, 11(3), 303–336.

Citro, C.F. and Hanushek, E.A. (1991). *The Uses of Microsimulation Modelling, Vol. 1: Review and Recommendations*. National Academy Press, Washington.

Creedy, J., Duncan, A.S., Harris, M. and Scutella, R. (2002). *Microsimulation Modelling of Taxation and The Labour Market: The Melbourne Institute Tax and Transfer Simulator*. Edward Elgar, Cheltenham.

Cullinan, J., Hynes, S. and O'Donoghue,C. (2006). The Use of Spatial Microsimulation and Geographic Information Systems (GIS) in Benefit Function Transfer — An Application to Modelling the Demand for Recreational Activities in Ireland. Paper presented at the 8th Nordic Seminar on Microsimulation Models, Oslo, 7–9 June (available from www.ssb.no/misi).

Davies, J. (2004). *Microsimulation, CGE and Macro Modelling for Transition and Developing Economies*. Discussion Paper no. 2004/08, World Institute for Development Economics Research (UNU/WIDER), Helsinki (available from www.wider.unu.edu/publications/discussion-papers-2004).

Decoster, A. (2000). ASTER, in Gupta, A. and Kapur, V. (eds), *Microsimulation in Government Policy and Forecasting*, North-Holland, Amsterdam.

Dennis, F., Heide, K.M., Holmøy, E. and Solli, I.F. (2006). Macroeconomic Effects of Proposed Pension Reforms in Norway, in Harding, A. and Gupta, A. (eds), *Modelling Our Future: Population Ageing, Social Security and Taxation*, International Symposia in Economic Theory and Econometrics, North-Holland, Amsterdam.

Evandrou, M. and Falkingham, J. (2006). Demographic Change, Health and Health Risk Behaviour Across Cohorts in Britain: Implications for Policy Modelling, in Gupta, A. and Harding, A. (eds), *Modelling Our Future: Population Ageing, Health and Aged Care*, International Symposia in Economic Theory and Econometrics, North-Holland, Amsterdam.

Falkingham, J. and Harding, A. (1996). Poverty Alleviation vs. Social Insurance: A Comparison of Lifetime Redistribution. In: Harding, A (Ed.), *Microsimulation and Public Policy.* North-Holland, Amsterdam.

Falkingham, J. and Hills, J. (1995). *The Dynamic of Welfare: The Welfare State and the Life Cycle*. Prentice-Hall, New York.

Favreault, M. and Caldwell, S. (2000). Assessing Distributional Impacts of Social Security Using Microsimulation, in Gupta, A. and Kapur, V. (eds), *Microsimulation in Government Policy and Forecasting*, North-Holland, Amsterdam.

Feenberg, D. and Gupta, A. (2000). Some Perspectives on Data Issues in Microsimulation Modelling, in Gupta, A. and Kapur, V. (ed), *Microsimulation in Government Policy and Forecasting*, North-Holland, Amsterdam.

Gallagher, P. (1995). *The Policy Use of the Products of the Retirement Income Modelling Task Force*. Conference Paper 95/3, Retirement Income Modelling Task Force, Canberra (available from www.rim.treasury.gov.au).

Galler, H.P. and Wagner, G. (1986). The Microsimulation Model of the Sfb3 for the Analysis of Economic and Social Policies, in Orcutt, G.H., Merz, J. and Quinke, H. (eds), *Microanalytic Simulation Models to Support Social and Financial Policy*, North-Holland, Amsterdam.

Government Statistical Service. (1998). Welsh Health Survey, Her Majesty's Stationery Office. National Assembly for Wales, Wales.

Gribble, S. (2000). LifePaths: A Longitudinal Microsimulation Model Using a Synthetic Approach, in Gupta, A. and Kapur, V. (eds), *Microsimulation in Government Policy and Forecasting*, North-Holland, Amsterdam.

Gupta, A. and Kapur, V. (1996). Microsimulation Modelling Experience at the Canadian Department of Finance, in Harding, A. (ed), *Microsimulation and Public Policy*, Elsevier (North-Holland), Amsterdam.

Gupta, A. and Kapur, V. (eds). (2000a). *Microsimulation in Government Policy and Forecasting*, North-Holland, Amsterdam.

Gupta, A. and Kapur, V. (2000b). Introduction and Overview, in Gupta, A. and Kapur, V. (eds), *Microsimulation in Government Policy and Forecasting*, North-Holland, Amsterdam.

Hain, W. and Helberger, C. (1986). Longitudinal Simulation of Lifetime Income, in Orcutt, G.H., Merz, J. and Quinke, H. (eds), *Microanalytic Simulation Models to Support Social and Financial Policy*, North-Holland, Amsterdam.

Hancock, R. (2000). Charging for Care in Later Life: An Exercise in Dynamic Microsimulation, in Mitton, L., Sutherland, H. and Weeks, M. (eds), *Microsimulation Modelling for Policy Analysis*, Cambridge University Press, Cambridge.

Harding, A. (1993a). Lifetime Income Distribution and Redistribution. Applications of a Microsimulation Model, North-Holland, Amsterdam.

Harding, A. (1993b). Lifetime vs. Annual Tax-Transfer Incidence: How Much Less Progressive? *Economic Record*, 69(205), 179–191.

Harding, A. (1995). Financing Higher Education: An Assessment of Income-Contingent Loan Options and Repayment Patterns over the Lifecycle. *Education Economics*, 3(2), 173–203.

Harding, A. (ed). (1996), *Microsimulation and Public Policy*, North-Holland, Amsterdam.

Harding, A. (2000). Dynamic Microsimulation: Recent Trends and Future Prospects, in Gupta, A. and Kapur, V. (eds), *Microsimulation in Government Policy and Forecasting*, North-Holland, Amsterdam.

Harding, A. and Gupta, A. (eds). (2006). *Modelling Our Future: Population Ageing, Social Security and Taxation*. International Symposia in Economic Theory and Econometrics, North-Holland, Amsterdam.

Harding, A., Warren, N., Robinson, M. and Lambert, S. (2000). The Distributional Impact of the Year 2000 Tax Reforms in Australia. *Agenda*, 7(1), 17–31.

Kelly, S. and King, A. (2001). Australians over the Coming 50 Years: Providing Useful Projections. *Brazilian Electronic Journal of Economics*, 4(2), 1–23.

King, A. (2006). Providing Income Support Services to a Changing Aged Population in Australia: Centrelink's Regional Microsimulation Model, in Gupta, A. and Harding, A. (eds), *Modelling Our Future: Population Ageing, Health and Aged Care*, International Symposia in Economic Theory and Econometrics, North-Holland, Amsterdam.

Klevmarken, N. (1997). *Behavioral Modelling in Micro Simulation Models: A Survey*. Working Paper no. 31, Uppsala University (available from www.nek.uu.se/Pdf/1997wp31).

Klevmarken, A. and Olovsson, P. (1996). Direct and Behavioural Effects of Income Tax Changes: Simulations with the Swedish Model MICROHUS, in Harding, A. (ed), *Microsimulation and Public Policy*, North-Holland, Amsterdam.

Mitton, L., Sutherland, H. and Weeks, M. (eds). (2000). *Microsimulation Modelling for Policy Analysis*. Cambridge University Press, Cambridge.

Murphy, B. (2000). SPSD/M, in Gupta, A and Kapur, V. (eds), *Microsimulation in Government Policy and Forecasting*, North-Holland, Amsterdam.

Nelissen, J.H.M. (1996). Social Security and Lifetime Income Redistribution, in Harding, A. (ed), *Microsimulation and Public Policy*, North-Holland, Amsterdam.

O'Donoghue, C. (2001). Dynamic Microsimulation: A Methodological Survey. *Brazilian Electronic Journal of Economics*, 4(2).

O'Hare, J. (2000). TRIM3, in Gupta, A. and Kapur, V. (eds), *Microsimulation in Government Policy and Forecasting*, North-Holland, Amsterdam.

Orcutt, G. (1957). A New Type of Socio-Economic System. *Review of Economics and Statistics*, 58(2), 773–797.

Orcutt, G., Caldwell, S., Wertheimer, R., Franklin, S., Hendricks, G., Peabody, G., Smith, J. and Zedlewski, S. (1976). *Policy Exploration Through Microanalytic Simulation*. The Urban Institute, Washington, DC.

Pedersen, T. (2000). Distributional Outcomes of the Danish Welfare System, in Gupta, A. and Kapur, V. (eds), *Microsimulation in Government Policy and Forecasting*, North-Holland, Amsterdam.

Sutherland, H. (1995). *Static Microsimulation Models in Europe: A Survey*, Microsimulation Unit Discussion Paper, MU9503, University of Cambridge.

Sutherland, H. (2000). EUROMOD, in Gupta, A. and Kapur, V. (eds), *Microsimulation in Government Policy and Forecasting*, North-Holland, Amsterdam.

Symons, E. and Warren, N. (1996). Modelling Consumer Behavioral Response to Commodity Tax Reforms, in Harding, A. (ed), *Microsimulation and Public Policy*, Elsevier, Amsterdam.

Toohey, M. and Beer, G. (2004). Financial Incentives for Working Mothers Under A New Tax System. *Australian Journal of Labour Economics*, 7(1), 53–69.

Voas, D. and Williamson, P. (2000). An Evaluation of the Combinatorial Optimisation Approach to the Creation of Synthetic Microdata. *International Journal of Population Geography*, 6, 349–366.

Weston, R. and Wooden, M. (2002). HILDA Has Arrived! *Family Matters. Australian Institute of Family Studies*, 63(Spring/Summer), 66–70.

Williamson, P., Birkin, M. and Rees, P.H. (1998). The Estimation of Population Microdata by Using Data from Small Area Statistics and Samples of Anonymised Records. *Environment and Planning A*, 30(5), 785–816.

Wolfson, M. (1988). Homemaker Pensions and Lifetime Redistribution. *Review of Income and Wealth*, 34(3), 221–250.

Xiong, L., Ma, X., Li, Y., Meng, H. and Lin, G. (2006). Microsimulation Model of Medical Insurance Reform of Government Employees and Workers in China, in Gupta, A. and Harding, A. (eds), *Modelling Our Future: Population Ageing, Health and Aged Care*, International Symposia in Economic Theory and Econometrics, North-Holland, Amsterdam.

Chapter 2

Population Ageing and Health — Empirical Needs for Effective Foresight

Michael C. Wolfson

Statistics Canada, Canada

Abstract

This chapter is adapted from an introductory keynote speech for the conference. It provides brief sketches and examples from a series of analyses and projections related to population ageing and health. The first purpose is to illustrate some of the core issues in these two topical areas of public policy. The second purpose is to go behind the examples, and indicate what it takes to produce these kinds of quantitative results — the key players who need to be involved, the underlying data, and institutional structures needed to bring it altogether. The general premise is that public policy is much improved if its development and evaluation is accompanied by systematic empirically grounded analysis, and "what if" modeling — which together are in essence the foundation for effective foresight.

1. Introduction

Population ageing and health are two broad empirical and policy domains where microsimulation modeling offers tremendous analytical opportunities. In this chapter we begin by illustrating some of the core issues related to population ageing and health. While we shall be using Canadian examples, many of the issues are very similar in other developed countries. Indeed, some of the chapters presented in the present volume go much further into these issues.

Secondly, our discussion goes beyond the examples, and talks about what it takes to produce these kinds of results — the key players who need to be involved, the underlying data, and institutional structures needed to bring it altogether.

International Symposia in Economic Theory and Econometrics, Vol. 16

ISSN: 1571-0386 DOI: 10.1016/S1571-0386(06)16002-0

2. Will an Ageing Population Leave Enough Workers?

There is a long history of demographic projections showing that we can expect growing numbers of elderly in our population. One dramatic way to show the impact of this trend had been by subdividing life expectancy into a traditional triad — a sequence of three phases of the life cycle, namely school (and pre-school), work, and retirement. These earlier analyses used a simple extension of the demographer's trusty tool, the period life table.

The results shown in Table 1 are from Gnanasekaran and Montigny (1975) for the years 1921–1971, and from Bélanger and Larrivée (1992) for 1986. In all cases, these results (other than age at death) are based on comparisons of a sequence of tabulations of cross-sectional labor force survey data, no actual transition probabilities from longitudinal data have been used. And all but the last row uses the simplifying assumption that labor force entry and exit flows are equal to the net changes in stocks from one year to the next. The last row uses an increment–decrement life table approach combined with gross flows from the Labour Force Survey.

The table shows the substantial increase in life expectancy of men in Canada over most of the 20th century (the middle column showing average age at death). At the same time, there is a near tripling of the length of time spent "retired".

This is rather scary for those concerned with the financial base for funding public pensions and health care — in fact the results shown in this table were central to launching a large, horizontal policy research exercise in Canada about a decade ago in 1996 (Policy Research Initiative, 1996).

However, the life table methodology underlying these results is rather crude, not least because it focuses only on males, thereby ignoring the major increase in female labor force participation, but because it treats each calendar year of life as dichotomous — either a year of work or not.

Table 1: Standard Working Life Table Results

Year	Average age at			Number of years	
	LF Entry	Retirement	Death	Working	Retired
1921	17.5	62.7	67.6	45.2	4.9
1931	18.0	63.0	68.4	45.0	5.4
1941	18.2	63.1	69.1	44.9	6.0
1951	18.5	62.9	70.4	44.4	7.5
1961	19.2	93.0	71.2	43.8	8.2
1971	19.8	62.3	71.3	42.5	9.0
1986a	20.0	65.5	73.8	44.6	8.3
1986b	20.0	60.3	73.8	39.4	13.5

In contrast, we have developed much more sophisticated estimates of working lives for Canada, using Statistics Canada's LifePaths microsimulation model (Model 12). The two graphs below, with results for men on the left and women on the right, show overall life expectancy at age 50, year by year, over the whole of the 20th century (Figure 1). Importantly, these are cohort rather than period expectancies. We clearly see rising life expectancies for both men and women — the black lines at the top.

In addition, we have subdivided this last quarter century or so of life, starting at age 50, between times spent in working for pay and time not in paid work. (To be precise, we have assessed the expected sojourn time in the states 'employed' or 'self-employed' rather than the expected time at work.)

This perspective raises different questions than the original working life tables above. Paid working years have declined significantly for men attaining age 50 between 1950 and the mid-1980s. Since that time, this trend has halted, and may have modestly reversed. Women, on the other hand, show growth in working time after their 50th birthday, closing in on, but not quite converging with men.

However, combined with the increases in life expectancy, these graphs show continuing increases in *non*-working years, to as much as 20–30 years after attaining age 50.

These are remarkably long periods of time, certainly in the context of the working life table results shown in Table 1. Part of the discrepancy is due to

Figure 1: Work, and Non-Work Life Expectancies (LE) at Age 50, Cohorts Born 1900–2000

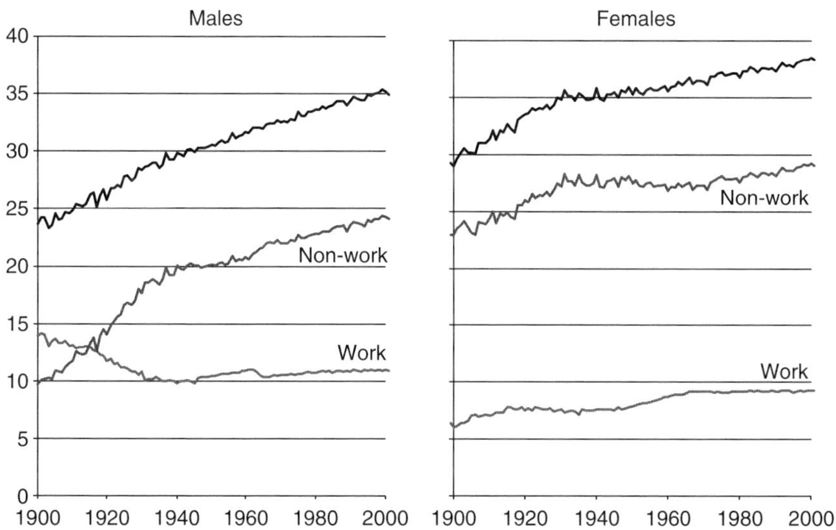

the fact that these are cohort rather than period life expectancies. Another turns on the way a "year of work" is being counted. The earlier analyses counted a person as working during an entire year if they had worked at least some minimal time during the year. This LifePaths analysis, in contrast, using much richer data, distinguishes sub-annual periods in or out of paid work.

The lines indicating non-work clearly show a growing duration of life outside the paid labor force after age 50, but one that was already far larger than the earlier cruder analyses would suggest.

These "data" are actually a blend of historical "fitting" to a wide range of data sources — plus a set of projections of a coherently related set of socio-demographic factors, including mortality, fertility, nuptiality, educational attainment, and of course, participation in paid work. This is offered as one example of the kinds of results policy makers need in order to think through the implications of an ageing population. It is important to note that a proper presentation of these results, as well as other projections shown below, would also include sensitivity analysis to the key assumptions underlying the projections.

The conventional question raised by results like the ones discussed here, is to ask how large the remaining population is to support this "burden" of senior individuals who are not working in the paid labor force. The usual response is to compute demographic "dependency ratios" — either counting only the elderly, or both the elderly and the school and pre-school age population in the numerator.

These two dependency ratios are shown on the left-hand graph (Figure 2). The unsurprising result is that the old age dependency ratio is increasing,

Figure 2: Two Views of the "Ageing Burden"

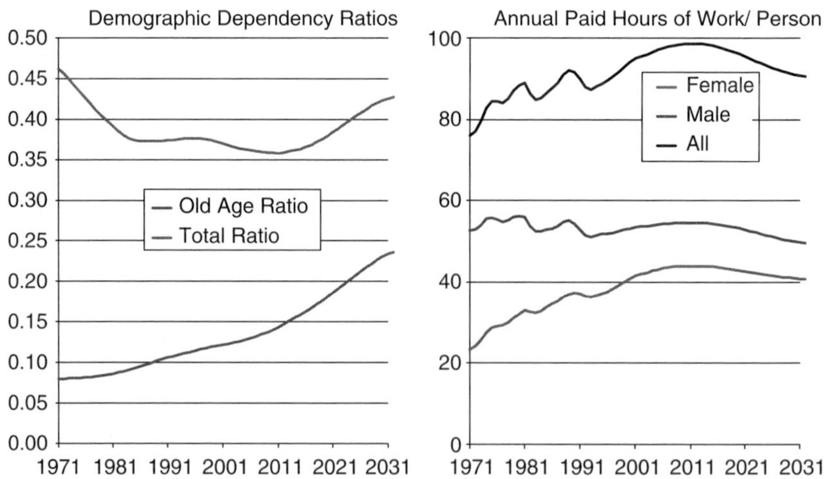

and will do so at an increasing pace as the baby boom cohort begins reaching age 65 around 2011.

However, the total dependency ratio will continue to decline in Canada, albeit very gradually, until the end of the decade. Still, from a government fiscal policy point of view, this is not very comforting, because typically, much more of the cost of bringing up children is born privately than the costs of caring for the elderly.

But more interestingly, the graph on the right-hand side shows a form of "economic dependency ratio": Instead of counting people using only a simple classification by age, it shows the total number of paid hours of work in the economy per capita — an idea we first encountered in a paper by Jane Falkingham perhaps 20 years ago. Rather than dividing the "dependent" population mechanically by age, when thinking about the economic "burden" individuals place on society, it is better to take account of whether or not the individual is in paid work, and hence contributing to national output.

Our estimates and projections suggest that this figure will also peak in about 2011 at just under 1,000 hours. The trend in per capita paid hours is similar to the total dependency ratio. But the rise is not as steep and is more stable, reflecting mainly increased female labor force participation. And the decline in paid hours per capita after 2011 is also not as sharp.

For example, by 2031, the total dependency ratio is projected to reach the same level as in the mid-1970s; while the paid hours per capita ratio projected for 2031 is similar to that in the late 1990s. This latter comparison should be considerably less frightening, from the perspective of the demo-doomsayers, than the simplistic demographic dependency ratio.

At the same time, the paid hours per capita indicator reflects behaviours that are more amenable to public policy. There is no (acceptable) way government can change the pace at which its citizens attain age 65 — a key input to the demographic dependency ratio. On the other hand, there are a number of policy levers that can influence the economy's paid hours per capita — including the age of entitlement to public pensions, and tax and regulatory provisions with regard to retirement age and early retirement in employer-sponsored pension plans.

Indeed, in a speech by the Australian Assistant Treasurer (Assistant Treasurer, 2003), anticipating the attainment of a population of 20 million in Australia in 2003 and building on an earlier "intergenerational report", the Treasurer referred to similar projections by the Australian Bureau of Statistics (ABS), and canvassed the main policy options facing government, including higher taxes, lower spending, increased immigration, deficit financing, improved productivity, and greater labor force participation among mature age workers.

These sorts of indicators are important for effective foresight with regard to the policy implications of population ageing. And to produce these graphs requires a sophisticated statistical and modeling infrastructure, as well as partnerships among the policy process, the research community, and the national statistical office or agencies. In particular, the LifePaths model, which underlies these projections, is the result of major efforts in data analysis and synthesis, primarily by Statistics Canada analysts, building on a wide variety of studies in the published academic literature, and the needs and priorities of Canadian government policy ministries (Wolfson and Rowe, 2001; Rowe, 2003; Rowe and Nguyen, 2004).

3. Ageing and Health

One of the reasons population ageing is of such a great public policy interest is health care. Figure 3, drawing on data from the Canadian Institute for Health Information (CIHI, 2003), shows recent per capita health care costs broken down by age group and by main kind of expenditure. Overall, there is a dramatic increase especially after age 65. This increase is driven mainly by hospital and nursing home costs ("other institutions").

Naïve projections of the impacts of an ageing population use these kinds of age-specific per capita costs, holding them fixed into the future. Such projections quickly reach very frightening conclusions that health care costs can be expected to escalate dramatically as the baby boom cohort moves into its senior years.

Figure 3: Per Capital Health are Costs by Age Group, 2000

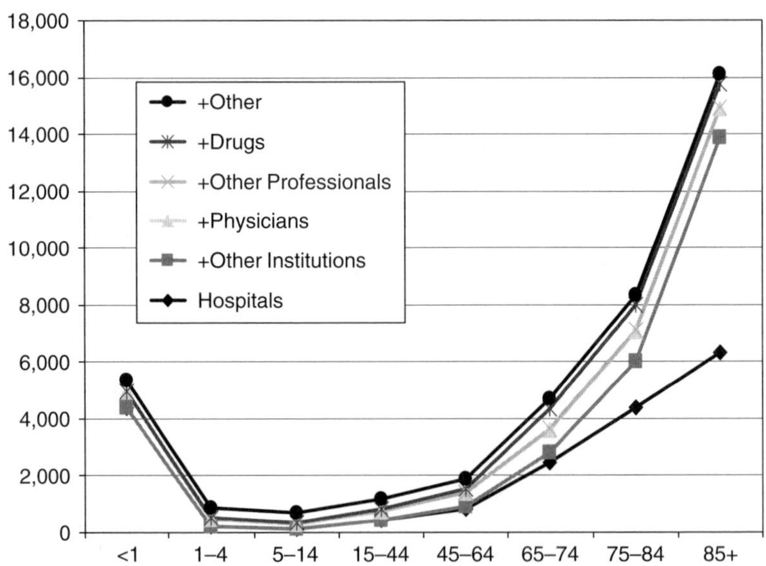

Figure 4, again drawing on data from CIHI (2003), shows the time series of nominal health care expenditures, again broken out by the main kind of expenditure. Overall, costs have risen substantially with the notable exception of hospital costs in the early 1990s — related to major efforts at deficit reduction.

The asterisk notes a bit of numerology — drug costs that historically were in 3rd place after physician and hospital costs, moved into 2nd place in Canada after the mid-1990s.

These trends are a major source of concern not only for health ministers, but also for finance ministers. The worry is that, unchecked, the exponential growth in health care budgets will eat up all the fiscal resources of government.

However, it is important to emphasize that these changes in expenditures are occurring at a pace that is too rapid to be blamed on the demographic force of population ageing.

One possible explanation for these expenditure trends can be gleaned from this graph (Figure 5). It shows a scatter plot of sub-provincial health regions, and focuses on individuals who suffered a heart attack. The horizontal axis shows the mortality rate after one year in each health region for heart attack victims, while the vertical axis shows the rate of revascularization, either or both angioplasty or heart bypass surgery, for these same individuals.

The black line, reassuringly, shows that there is some positive association between being revascularized quickly, within 14 days of a heart attack, and one year survival. But there is a very substantial variation across this set of health regions, both in mortality rates (between 10% and 27%) and in revascularization rates (from almost nil to 25%).

Figure 4: Per Capita Health Care Costs over Time by Use (Current $)

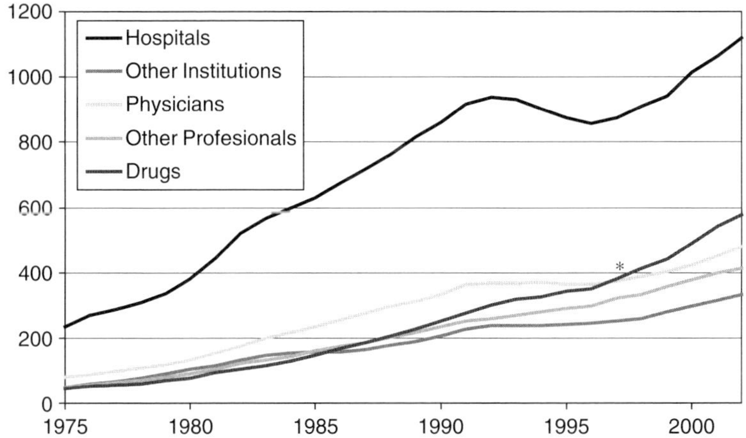

Figure 5: One Year Mortality Rate vs. % Revascularized Within 14 Days, AMI Patients in Health Regions with Populations Over 100,000, 4 Provinces, 1995–1996

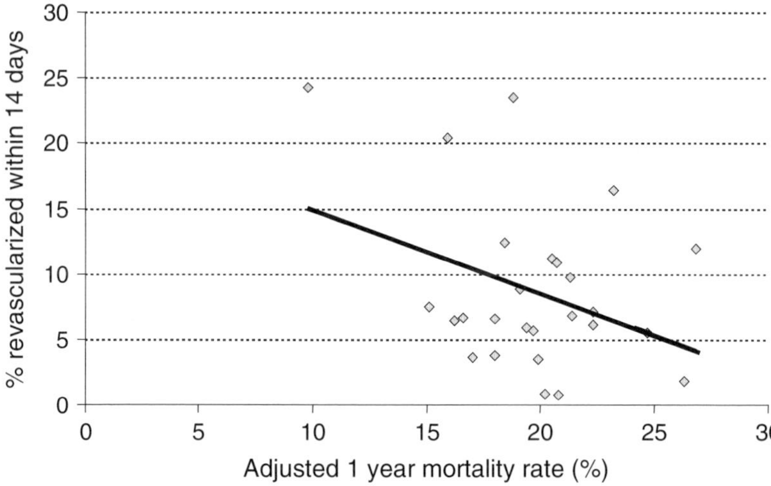

Source: Johansen et al. (2002), Stats Can, (2001)

This is an instance of the well-known finding of "small area variations" in the health services research literature. But it represents a fundamentally important extension, because the rate of surgery has been linked to a health outcome, in this case one-year mortality.

These are disturbing results — so much variation, both in procedure rates and in survival rates after a heart attack — and not a terribly strong link between the two.

Key implications of these results are that the health care system is not spending money on treating heart attacks as wisely or effectively as it could, and that it lacks the basic information to understand why and what to do about it.

In turn, these results suggest that controlling the future costs of the health care system will likely have to depend far more on in-depth data systematically linking health care interventions to health outcomes, on understanding the sociological and economic incentives driving practice patterns among health care practitioners, and on managing the diffusion of new treatments and health care technologies. Growing numbers of elderly in our populations is not likely to be the main issue.

And again, underlying these results was an excellent degree of cooperation and partnership among Statistics Canada, colleagues in the health research community, and provincial health ministries — since this analysis used computerized patient microdata from provincial health care systems, linked to death certificates on a national basis by Statistics Canada.

The fact that most important determinants of health lie outside the health *care* system is widely accepted, but not nearly as widely acted upon.

Figure 6 shows estimates of the effects on life expectancy of two major risk factors — smoking and physical activity. In addition, life expectancy is broken down by whether or not the individual can expect to spend those years of life moderately or severely disabled.

Not surprisingly, smoking and physical *in*activity are each bad for overall life expectancy as well as for disability-free life expectancy.

In turn, these estimates suggest major prospective benefits from interventions, as part of the "health system", defined more broadly than the "health *care* system", not only to reduce tobacco smoking, but also to increase physical activity, among others of the broad determinants of health. Thus, interventions based outside the formal health *care* system might have beneficial effects in mitigating rising health care costs.

But this raises the question of how one constructs the analytical tools to assess the trade-offs and opportunity costs of alternative strategies for improving population health. The WHO's Global Burden of Disease estimates (Murray and Lopez, 1996) as well as those made by the Australian Institute for Health and Welfare (Mathers et al., 1999) are leading examples. There is work underway in Canada in this area. This is a very challenging task, but one that is essential to empirically based foresight.

As shown earlier in Figure 4, drugs have moved into 2nd place in Canada in terms of health care expenditures, now ahead of doctors, but still well behind hospitals. There is no way that demographic factors in Canada can account for these increased expenditures. Rather, the continual innovation

Figure 6: Female Life Expectancy at Age 45 by "Lifestyle" and Disability

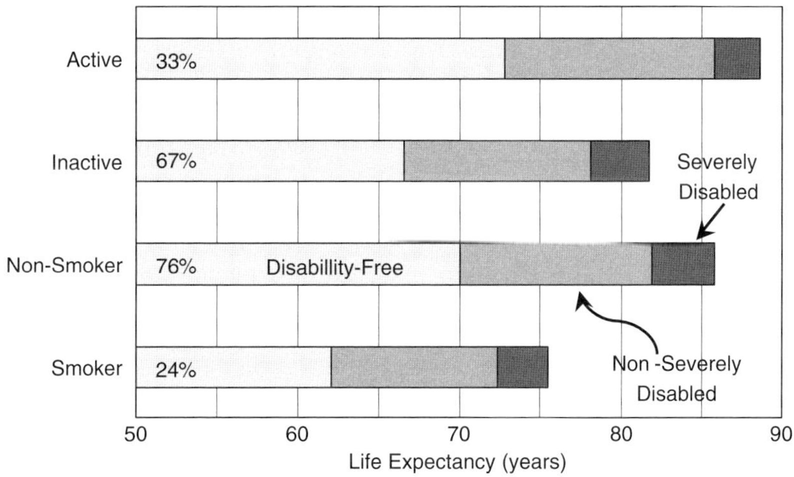

associated with drug discovery and the diffusion of new drug prescribing are likely much more important. However, the choice of whether to approve a new drug, or a new use for an existing drug, is often very difficult.

This chart in Figure 7 shows the results from the largest clinical trial of the drug Tamoxifen, used in a new way, to prevent breast cancer in otherwise healthy women, but women who are, according to specified criteria such as family history, at higher risk. The horizontal axis shows relative risks for the incidence of various diseases based on almost five years of follow-up — a relative risk less than 1 means the chances of the event happening were reduced; greater than 1 means that the drug caused an increase in the incidence of the disease. The horizontal bars show the 95% confidence intervals for the effects (the relative risks) of Tamoxifen used in this context.

As shown at the top-left, the risk of breast cancer was cut in half. However, for other clinical endpoints like the incidence of heart disease, stroke, deep-vein thrombosis, and endometrial cancer, there are highly uncertain, but often substantially adverse effects.

But these data show only disease incidence, and then only over a five-year period, and only for a population, mainly of Americans, that is not representative of Canadian women.

Figure 8 draws out the implications of the drug trial results discussed above for Canadian women, assessed not only over the initial five-year period of the clinical trial, but projected for their entire lifetimes (Will et al.,

Figure 7: Relative Risks of Preventive Tamoxifen

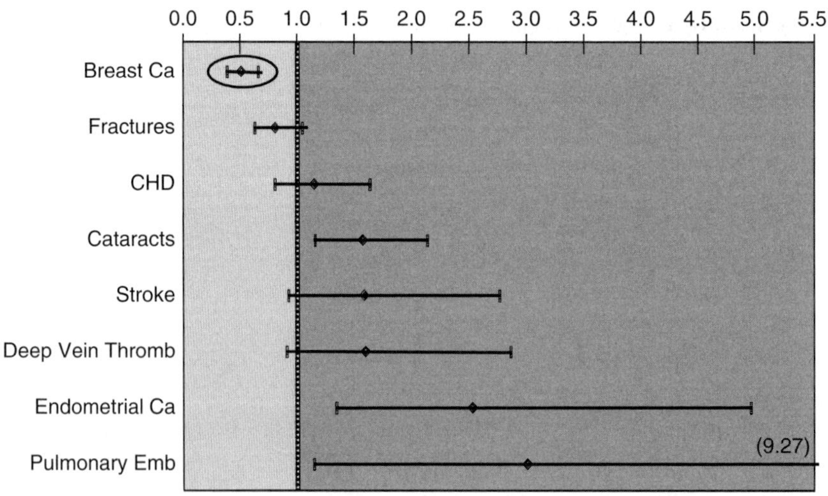

Source: Fisher et al., J National Cancer Institute, (1999)

Figure 8: Simulated Change in Life Expectancy for Canadian Women for Alternative Scenarios of Preventive Tamoxifen (95% CIs), 2001

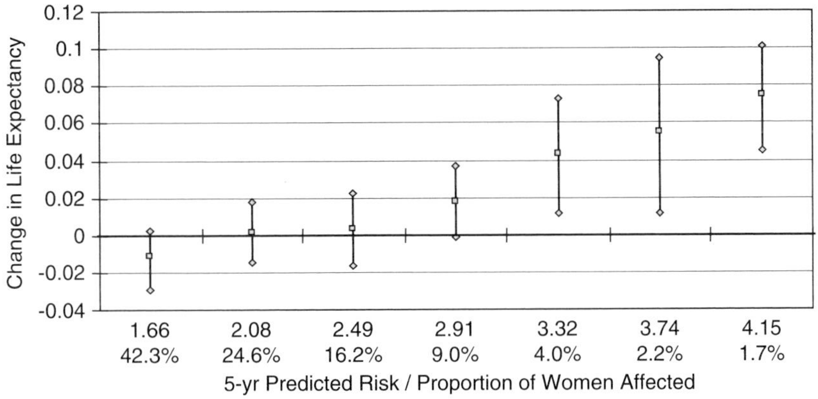

Source: Will et al., British J Cancer, (2001)

2001). The analysis used Statistics Canada's POHEM (POpulation HEalth Model, see Model 4) microsimulation model.

The scenarios along the horizontal axis range on the left from full adoption of the protocol as accepted by the U.S. FDA when it approved this use of Tamoxifen, to more targeted scenarios where a woman would have to be at a higher risk of breast cancer, so that fewer women would ever take the drug.

In each scenario, women above the specified risk threshold are assumed to take the drug as prescribed — so they will be at lower risk of breast cancer, but generally at higher albeit uncertain risks for the other diseases followed in the trial.

The results are sobering. The vertical *axis* shows expected changes in life expectancy if this drug were to be rolled out in the general Canadian population of women. The vertical *bars* represent 95% confidence intervals, based on the uncertainties in the parameter estimates from the clinical trial shown in Figure 7.

Basically, for the first four scenarios, where targeting reduces the proportion of Canadian women who would be taking the drug at some point in their lives from 42% down to 9%, there is no statistically significant improvement in life expectancy. Even in the most highly targeted scenarios, overall life expectancy improvements are less than a tenth of a year. This is in marked contrast to the smoking and physical inactivity results we showed in Figure 6, where the differences in life expectancy were measured in years.

We must emphasize here that these results are not a formal analysis of the prospective efficacy of a specific drug. Rather, they represent an exercise of taking a set of published and highly influential clinical trial results, combining them with a wide variety of data on the Canadian population, as well as a number of sometimes strong assumptions (mainly due to data limitations), and then drawing out their joint implications.

Nevertheless, these results are illustrative of a style of analysis that is often lacking in the management of the health care system. New drugs, procedures, and technologies are being introduced at substantial rates, but too often without thorough evaluation and explicit appropriateness guidelines, and virtually never with projections of their likely actual population impacts.

We close this series of examples of the role of microanalytic analysis and simulation modeling as crucial supports to effective foresight with some completely new work recently done at Statistics Canada, in partnership with colleagues at WHO, Harvard, the London School of Hygiene and Tropical Medicine, and Health Canada. In this case, we have extended our micro-simulation modeling capacity to handle co-evolving populations of individuals in order to model the transmission and spread of infectious diseases like HIV/AIDS and SARS.

In Figure 9, we have an illustration relating to the SARS epidemic, which in 2003 had a dramatic effect in Canada, as well as in many other countries. This graph shows, over a period of 200 days, what would happen to the rate of newly infected cases per day under three scenarios for public health actions to stem the spread of the disease.

The "no quarantine" scenario shows an almost invisible period of "smoldering" followed by an exponentially growing rate of new infections. This is what might have happened if there had been no public health response at all. The "quarantine" scenario traced by the line that peaks and declines

Figure 9: SARSMM: Three Sample Simulations

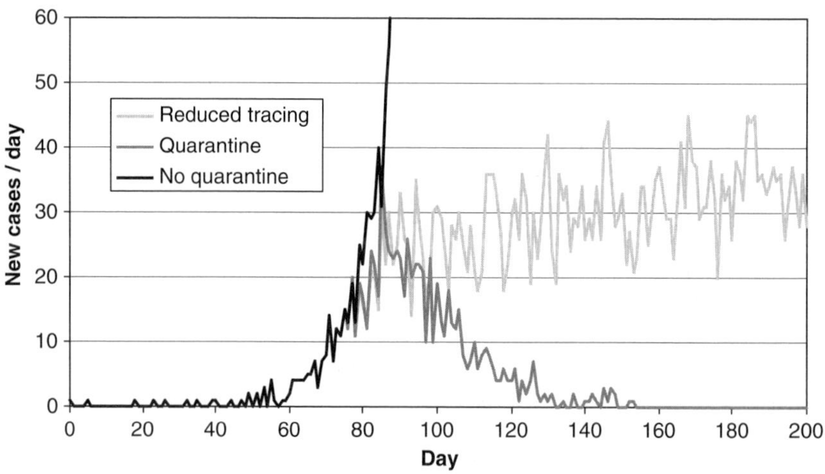

assumes that aggressive quarantine is launched at day 70, with 90% effective tracing of all contacts. The disease is wiped out by day 173. The intermediate "reduced tracing" scenario assumes contact tracing is only 50% effective. This is sufficient to contain the disease, but it remains endemic.

What is unique about this analysis is that it explicitly takes account of recent evidence from the SARS outbreak indicating that some individuals are "super-spreaders" — they are much more likely to transmit the disease than other infected individuals. Such heterogeneity within the population is usually intractable for the differential equation-based compartment models that are standard in this kind of epidemiology.

But as our data collection capabilities and epidemiological knowledge advance, being able to model infectious disease transmission in heterogeneous populations will provide much better information on the trade-offs between, or urgency of, various kinds of public health interventions.

4. Implications for Empirically Based Effective Foresight

With this brief tour of a series of empirical results and quantitative projections, we now turn to the basic question — how can such results be best produced in order to provide the empirical foundations for effective foresight. There are a number of common threads to the sampling of results presented in this chapter.

They all required a diverse range of usually rich multivariate data sets. Some results were more standard in their assembly, such as the aggregate health care costs, which build on National Accounts methods. But the others required person level micro-data, often woven together from several sources — for example household health and socio-economic surveys and censuses. In the heart attack example, linked microdata from provincial health care administrative data systems plus death certificates were essential.

The results also often required using complex data analysis tools such as multivariate hazard regressions — in order to distill key bits of empirical relationship. But the work did not stop there, merely by statistical fitting of one or another form of equation.

Numbers of such empirical results were assembled and woven together — using multi-state life tables in the earlier analyses but now using full bore microsimulation models. Computer simulation modeling is well accepted in such diverse fields as cosmology, the design of new airplane wings, macroeconomics, and tax policy. The potential power, breadth of applicability, and effectiveness of microsimulation techniques should be obvious. However, the sense is that governments today typically under-invest in these kinds of models for asking the key "what if" questions related to population ageing and health.

Of course, none of these results would be possible if it were not for the skilled and talented analysts who explore these complex data sets using increasingly sophisticated statistical software, finding patterns, and then crystallizing them quantitatively as nuggets of empirical regularity.

Not only are the results we have shown here, as well as many of the results presented in this volume, dependent directly on analysts. They are also dependent on a larger ongoing research enterprise, mostly based in universities, that gives us a continuing flow of new theories, new empirical insights, and new analytical techniques.

And finally, the policy process is a key driver of these developments. The important policy questions of the day, as in the title of this volume, and the SARS example, serve to guide and prioritize theory and tool development, as well as investments in new, and new kinds of, data, and the formation of new kinds of partnerships.

These partnership relations are summarized in the triangle shown in Figure 10. The key players are the policy process, the national statistical agencies, and the research community.

The policy process sets the agenda and determines which questions and issues have the highest priority. It also provides funding and support for new data from the statistical agencies, and to the research community. The policy process is also a consumer of the fruits of these investments in data and research.

The research community analyzes data, often from the national statistical agency, and in doing so, innovates by creating new analytical methods, and develops new theoretical insights and empirical discoveries based on the analyses carried out. Depending on how attentive the research community is to the issues of the day, it will focus on those that are more relevant to the policy process.

Statistical agencies, which can and should also contain a significant research component of their own, are the primary developers and generators

Figure 10: Core Strategy: Tripartite Collaboration

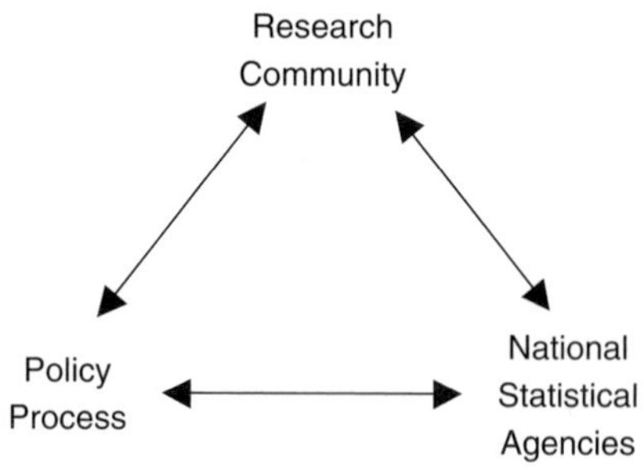

of new data. The specific character of the new data collections, ideally, is shaped both by the priorities of the policy process, and the new insights and analytical methods developed by the research community. The statistical agencies then provide the data, plus at least a first cut at the analysis, both to the policy process for its immediate use, and to the research community for more general and in-depth research purposes.

In other words, each edge of the triangle in Figure 10 represents a reciprocal relationship where there are two-way, mutually beneficial flows of data, analysis, and information.

5. Conclusions

The challenge in the context of the conference was to use what we know, and are able to know, to inform wise public policy choices with regard to population ageing and health. Meeting this challenge first requires that policy issues are clearly framed, and that key players in the policy process are supportive of and interested in foresight analysis. Not all governments are so inclined.

A second requirement is the right data — data that have been designed with the main policy issues or analytic questions in mind, are high quality, and have sufficient "multivariateness" that all the main causal factors have been covered.

Increasingly, these kinds of data are based on linked individual-level microdata originally collected for other purposes. A major example is electronic health care records from hospital and doctor visits, linked to health survey data. The public good potential of these data is enormous; so privacy and related legislation should be responsibly supportive of analytic, research, and statistical linkage and secondary uses of these kinds of very sensitive data.

Making projections into the future, exercising foresight, requires a theory of how things unfold — a network of causal stories. These should draw on the latest and best research.

Moreover, the causal stories have to be empirically grounded and represented quantitatively. This requires sophisticated analytical tools and computer simulation models, especially microanalytic models, to weave all the strands together into a coherent and comprehensive whole.

Members of the research community have to be engaged; they need to be able to access relevant data, and have the motivation to drive the analysis.

And last but by no means least, the statistical agencies should play an enabling role, which includes encouraging and facilitating access to their full range of data.

This listing is not necessarily exhaustive, but it is very difficult to imagine effective foresight without all of these key elements.

References

Assistant Treasurer (2003). Australian Treasury Speech to the 57th Congress of the International Fiscal Association, Sydney, Australia.

Bélanger, A. and Larrivée, D. (1992). New Approach for Constructing Canadian Working Life Tables, 1986–1987. *Statistical Journal of the United Nations Economic Commission for Europe*, ECE 9.

Canadian Institute for Health Information (CIHI). (2003). *Health Care in Canada,* Health Reports, Ottawa.

Gnanasekaran, K.S. and Montigny, G. (1975). *Working Life Tables for Males in Canada and Provinces, 1971.* Statistics Canada Catalogue 71-524E Occasional, Ottawa.

Johansen, H., Nair, C., Mao, L. and Wolfson, M. (2002). Revascularization and Heart Attack Outcomes. *Health Reports*, 13(2), 35–46.

Mathers, C., Vos, T. and Stevenson, C. (1999). *The Burden of Disease and Injury in Australia.* AIHW cat. no. PHE 17, Australian Institute of Health and Welfare, Canberra.

Murray, C.J.L., Lopez, A.D. (eds). (1996). The Global Burden of Disease: A Comprehensive Assessment of Mortality and Disability from Diseases, Injuries, and Risk Factors in 1990 and Projected to 2020, Vol. 1, Harvard University Press, Boston, MA.

Policy Research Initiative. (1996). www.policyresearch.gc.ca

Rowe, G. (2003). Fragments of Lives: Enabling New Policy Directions through Integrated Life-Course Data. *Horizons, Policy Research Initiative*, 6(2), 7–11.

Rowe, G. and Nguyen, H. (2004). Longitudinal Analysis of Labour Force Survey Data. *Survey Methodology*, 30(1), 105–114.

Will, B.P., Nobrega, K.M., Berthelot, J.-M., Flanagan, W., Wolfson, M.C., Logan, D.M. and Evans, W.K. (2001). First Do No Harm: Extending the Debate on the Provision of Preventive Tamoxifen. *British Journal of Cancer*, 85(9), 1280–1288.

Wolfson, M.C. and Rowe, G. (2001). Perspectives on Working Time Over the Life-Cycle, in Houseman, S. and Nakamura, A. (eds), *Working Time in Comparative Perspective: Volume II*, W.E. Upjohn Institute for Employment Research, Kalamazoo, MI.

Part I: Health Status

Chapter 3

Demographic Change, Health and Health-Risk Behaviour across Cohorts in Britain: Implications for Policy Modelling

Maria Evandrou* **and Jane Falkingham**

Centre for Research on Ageing, University of Southampton, UK

Abstract

Government projections indicate that by 2031 there will be 18.5 million people aged 60 and over living in the UK, of whom 8 million will be aged over 75. These figures have given rise to concerns over the future health and social care needs of the older population and the associated cost. Although the numbers of older people can be forecast with some certainty, less attention has been paid to the likely health and demographic characteristics of future elders and how they may differ from today's older population. This chapter analyses data over 30 years to examine trends in the patterns of family formation and dissolution, living arrangements, health and health risk behaviour amongst four different birth cohorts in Britain. Detailing how the experiences of birth cohorts differ at the same chronological point in the life course sheds light on the likely characteristics of future elders and informs the assumptions used by policy modellers.

1. Introduction

Older people are major consumers of health and social services. By 2030, it is estimated that people aged 65 and over will account for a quarter of the British population, as the large post-war baby boom cohorts enter retirement. Although the numbers of older people in the next 30 years can be forecast with some degree of certainty, less attention has been paid to the likely health and socio-economic characteristics of future generations of

*Corresponding author.

E-mail address: maria.evandrou@soton.ac.uk (*M. Evandrou*).

International Symposia in Economic Theory and Econometrics, Vol. 16

ISSN: 1571-0386 DOI: 10.1016/S1571-0386(06)16003-2

elders, and how these may differ from previous cohorts of elderly persons. Unlike Australia, Canada, and the US, Britain experienced two post-war baby booms, the first being during the mid to late 1940s and the second in the early to mid 1960s. The ageing of these two post-war baby boom cohorts, constituting over seven million people, is of great interest to policy-makers and planners.

2. Aims

This paper attempts to address these issues by looking back into the past and seeing how the experiences to date of the generations entering retirement over the next 30 years are likely to shape their future. The experiences of two cohorts that are currently retired, i.e. those born in 1916–1920 and 1931–1935, are compared with those of two younger cohorts, taken to represent those entering retirement over the next 20–30 years, i.e. those born in the late 1940s and early 1960s. Examining how experiences of birth cohorts differ at the same chronological point in the life course enables us to shed light on the likely characteristics of future elders and how they may differ from older people today. Such cohort based analysis is essential in underpinning the assumptions involved in modelling the future. Furthermore, it serves to focus attention on the life course and highlights the importance of taking a life course perspective in policy formulation. Thus, the aim of the research is to examine recent demographic change and trends in health and health risk behaviour in Britain in order to better inform future modelling for drawing out the implications of these trends for future health and social care in later life.

3. Data and Method

There is no single source of longitudinal data in Britain that currently provides demographic and socio-economic information both across an extended time-period and for a range of different birth cohorts. The British Household Panel Study at Essex University is now yielding exciting and useful data, but it is restricted in that data collection only commenced in 1991. The Office of National Statistics (ONS) Longitudinal Study covers the period since 1971, but the range of socio-economic data included is limited. This research therefore uses a pseudo-cohort approach to examine the experience of four birth cohorts at the same chronological age and to compare the differences between them.

The analysis uses data from two main sources. Firstly, vital registration data on family formation (marriages, births and divorce) is examined by birth cohort. Secondly, data from 28 years of the General Household Survey (GHS), a cross-sectional survey of individuals living in private households carried out annually by ONS, is used to generate pseudo-cohorts. The experience of representatives of each birth cohort is tracked in successive years of the GHS. For example, those respondents aged 55–59 in the 1975 GHS are taken as being representative of the birth cohort born in 1916–1920. The same birth cohort is then represented by those aged 56–60 in 1976, 57–61 in 1977, and finally those aged 81–86 in 2001. This constitutes a pseudo-cohort or quasi-cohort approach since the individuals are not the same from year to year. Rather than tracking individuals per se, it is the group means or proportions that are taken. Thus the unit of analysis is the cohort and what is measured is the *average* experience for the cohort.

The main advantages of using a pseudo-cohort approach are that it is less expensive in time and money as the data already exists, it covers a long time-period, and there is no problem of sample attrition, as with panel data. Since a fresh sample is drawn from the surviving population each year, the cohort means remain representative of that population. However there are limitations to employing such a method. Firstly, it is not possible to examine the duration of events such as marriage or unemployment for individuals, but only the *average* duration for the *cohort* as a whole. Secondly, as with any analysis of cross-sectional data over time, there may be problems with consistency of data. For example, the question on limiting long-standing illness changed in 1977 and 1978. This meant that these two years were excluded from the analysis of chronic illness in order not to jeopardise the overall findings. Thirdly, there is the problem of sampling error in the successive cross-sectional samples. The results shown do not indicate the size of the confidence intervals. However, the large sample size of the GHS means that the sample errors around the estimates are relatively small (Breeze, 1990). The middle response rate has fluctuated between 76 and 85 per cent over the period 1974–2001/2. The sample size of each five-year birth cohort varies over time as both the overall sample size of the GHS has changed and the share of the cohort in the sample population alters with age.[1] Finally, the results are affected by both age and period effects, which are often difficult to disentangle. Nevertheless, despite these limitations, pseudo-cohort analysis can provide useful insights into inter-cohort differences and help to inform policy making.

[1] The smallest sub-sample size was for men from the 1916–1920 cohort in 1998 when they were aged 78–82. By this age, their size was just 186, of which 90 were from non-manual occupational backgrounds and 96 from manual.

4. The UK Cohorts

The four cohorts selected are people born in the years 1916–1920, 1931–1935, 1946–1950, and 1961–1965. There is always debate as to the arbitrary nature of cohort boundaries. The choice here reflects a set of people born in the same five-year time period who consequently have many historical experiences in common.

- Those born in 1916–1920 represent today's 'middle aged' elderly, being aged 80–84 in 2000. Twenty-five years earlier, in 1975, they were aged 55–59 and approaching retirement.
- The cohort born in 1931–1935 are today's 'younger' elderly, aged 65–69 in 2000. In 1975 they were entering mid-life, constituting the group aged 40–44.
- The cohort born in 1946–1950 represents the 'first baby boom generation'. They were aged 25–29 in 1975. In 2000 they are aged 50–54 and starting to plan for retirement.
- The cohort born in 1961–1965 represents the 'second baby boom generation'. In 1975, aged 10–14, they were still at school. In 2000 however, they have reached their mid-to-late 30 s. Education and training has largely been completed, and occupational pathways are well established, along with family life.

Marked differences are to be expected between the cohorts, as they were born into and grew up in very different economic, technological, and social climates.The differences between the experiences of the post-war and pre-war cohorts are considerable, with neither of the 1940s and 1960s cohorts having experienced World Wars, and both growing up under the umbrella of the Welfare State, reaping the benefits of the 1944 Education Act and expecting to receive health and social care 'from the cradle to the grave' under the NHS and social services.

However, the experiences of the two post-war cohorts also differ from each other. The first baby boomers (1946–1950) were born in a period of post-war austerity, experiencing rationing and selective education. However, when they entered the labour market the economy was entering a period of relative *prosperity*. Not only was the job market buoyant, but the rapid expansion of higher education in the 1960s also meant that a growing number stayed on at school and entered university. In addition to new opportunities in education and work, the introduction of the pill heralded a new sexual freedom.

In contrast, the second baby boomers (1961–1965) were born in a period of prosperity, experiencing the consumer spending boom of the 1960s, and comprehensive secondary education. However, by the time this generation came to enter the labour market at the end of the 1970s, the economy was entering a recession, resulting in sharp rises in unemployment. Individuals born during the peak birth year of 1964 reached school-leaving age in 1980 at the depth of recession. Some may have *never* had a permanent full-time job. The spirit of radicalism and freedom, enjoyed by the preceding baby boom cohort, was missing; not only in terms of employment and income, but also in other spheres of life with 1984 seeing the first person diagnosed with AIDS. These very different economic and social environments will have affected the respective life chances of the different cohorts, as well as cohort members' expectations of employment, the welfare state, and life in general.

Figure 1 shows the number of births in England and Wales over a 60-year period. In contrast to Australia, Canada, and the US, Britain experienced two distinct post-war baby booms, with the 1946–1950 cohort being representative of the first baby boom and the 1961–1965 cohort representing the second. One of the biggest achievements of the 20th century has been the improvement in survivorship across cohorts (Figure 2a and b). Amongst women born in 1926, 50 per cent of the cohort may expect to survive to age 79 (in 2005); however, amongst those born 20 years later in 1946, half will still be alive at age 85. Similarly amongst men, half of the 1926 cohort is expected to have died by age 72; this rises to age 80 amongst the 1946 cohort. Thus not only are the baby boom cohorts larger in size than preceding cohorts, but more of them are expected to survive into old age and to live longer in retirement. The ageing of baby boom cohorts (which constitutes over 7 million people) will present a particular challenge in policy terms, both in terms of their numbers but also their diversity of experience.

Figure. 1: Average Annual Number of Births, 1916–1920 to 1976–1980 (E&W).

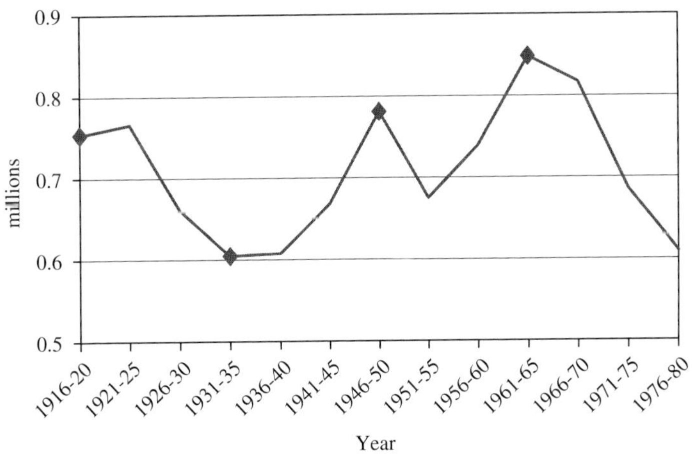

Figure 2: Proportion of (a) Women and (b) Men Surviving by Birth Cohort.

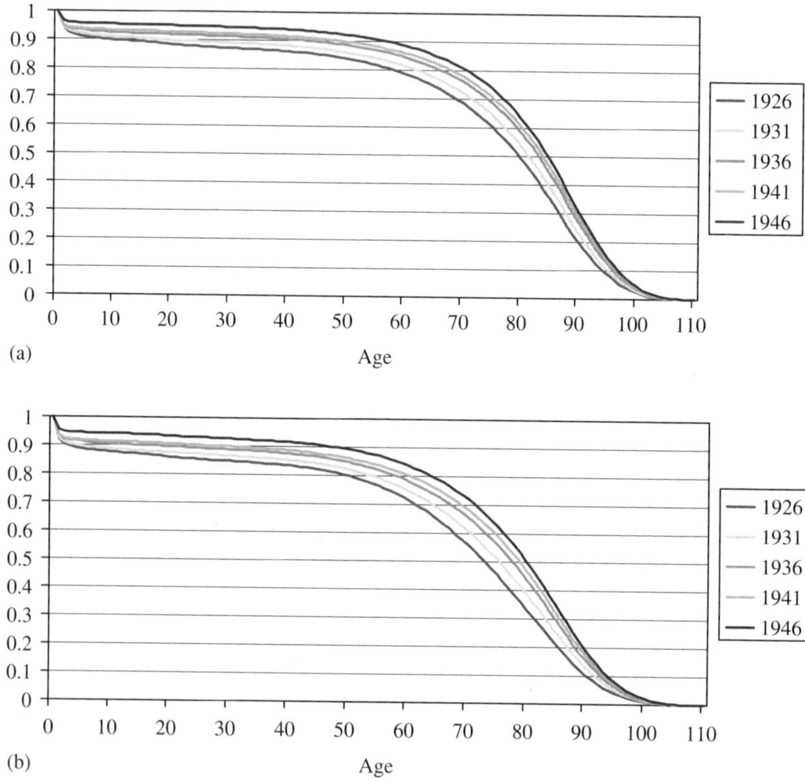

So, how will future cohorts of elders differ from previous generations of older people?

5. Changing Living Arrangements and the Potential Availability of Informal Care

The overwhelming majority of social care is provided by family members (Allen and Perkins, 1995). Current policy recognises this role and explicitly relies upon its continuance. But to what extent will it be able to continue to do so in 2020 and beyond? What are the likely changes in the family and in living arrangements?

It is likely that 'solo living' will take on greater relevance in the new millennium. A number of factors will contribute to a rise in the proportion living alone. Firstly, it is likely that fewer future elderly persons will be married or living in a co-habiting union than is the case today. Figure 3a shows the proportion of women in each birth cohort who had never married by particular ages. The likelihood of entering into a marital union increased across cohorts between those born in the 1920s and those in the 1940s. In fact, a higher proportion of the 1946 cohort have ever married than any previous cohort since vital registration data began. However, there has been a marked shift in behaviour amongst those women born in 1961, and by age 40, just under a fifth of women in this cohort remained unmarried. Similar trends are found for men; by age 40 a quarter of men born in 1961 remained unmarried compared to fewer than 10 per cent amongst those born in 1946 at the same age.

This does not necessarily mean, however, that second baby boomer men and women remain un-partnered, as, to some extent, formal marital unions have been replaced by cohabiting unions amongst younger cohorts. However, data shows that cohabiting unions are more prone to dissolution than formal unions and many are short-lived. Data from the GHS on long-term cohabitation and marital histories can be combined with vital registration

Figure 3: Percentage of (a) Women and (b) Men Remaining 'Never Married' by Birth Cohort.

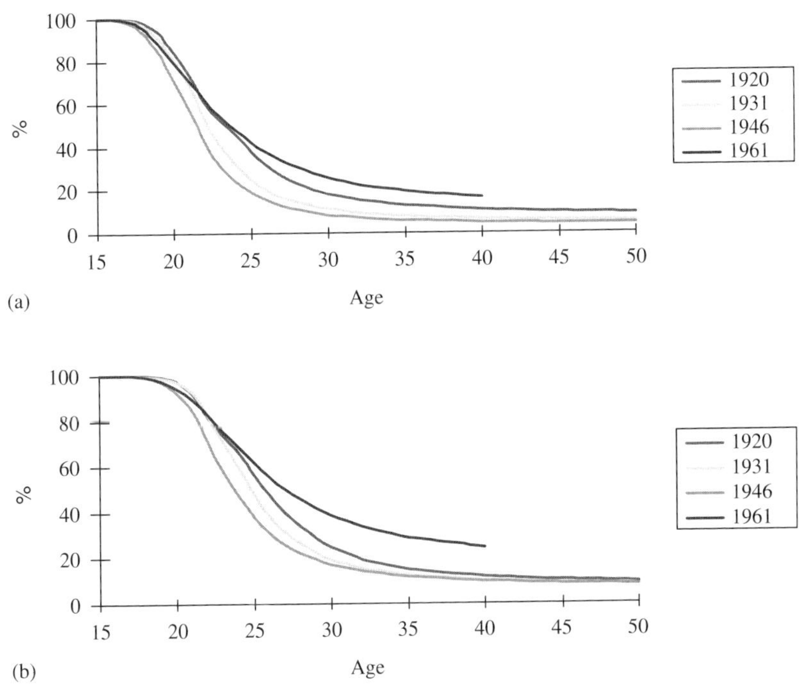

Figure 4: Percentage of Men Remaining Unmarried or in a Long-Term Cohabiting Union by Ages 30, 40, 50.

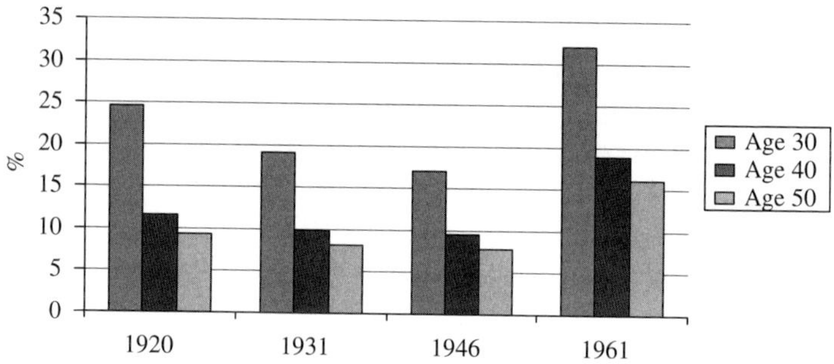

data to take cohabitation into account. If current trends continue, it is predicted that 16 per cent of men from the 1960s cohort will not have formed a marital or long-term co-habiting union by the time they reach the age of 50 (Figure 4).[2] This compares with 8 per cent of men born in 1946. The figures for women are similarly stark, with 12 per cent of women from 1960s estimated not to have formed a permanent partnership by age 50 compared to 5 per cent of women from the 1940s cohort at the same age.

Secondly, among those who have married, a greater proportion will also have experienced divorce or separation. Figure 5a and b show the rise in the proportion of women and men who have experienced divorce across the birth cohorts. Amongst those born in 1961, nearly a quarter of all women (24 per cent) and a fifth of men had undergone at least one divorce before their 40th birthday (ONS, 2006). If we take into account the significant proportion of this cohort who has never married, this means that around a third of all second baby boomer marriages had broken down by age 40. On the other hand, increasing longevity means that fewer of this cohort will experience the break-up of their union through death by the time they retire. The fall in widowhood is, however, unlikely to be sufficient to offset the rise in divorce. Thus, the marked shift to later and fewer marriages and rising divorce, coupled with the preference to live independently in one's own home, means that a greater proportion of future elders are likely to live alone.

Research estimates that 41 per cent of the 1940s cohort will be living alone by age 75 compared with 38 per cent of the 1930s cohort and 37 per cent of the 1916–1920 birth cohort (Evandrou and Falkingham, 2000). Furthermore, a quarter (26 per cent) of the 1960s cohort will already be lone

[2] These figures are derived using data from the Government Actuary's Department marital status projections.

Figure 5: Percentage of (a) Women and (b) Men Who Ever Divorced by Birth Cohort.

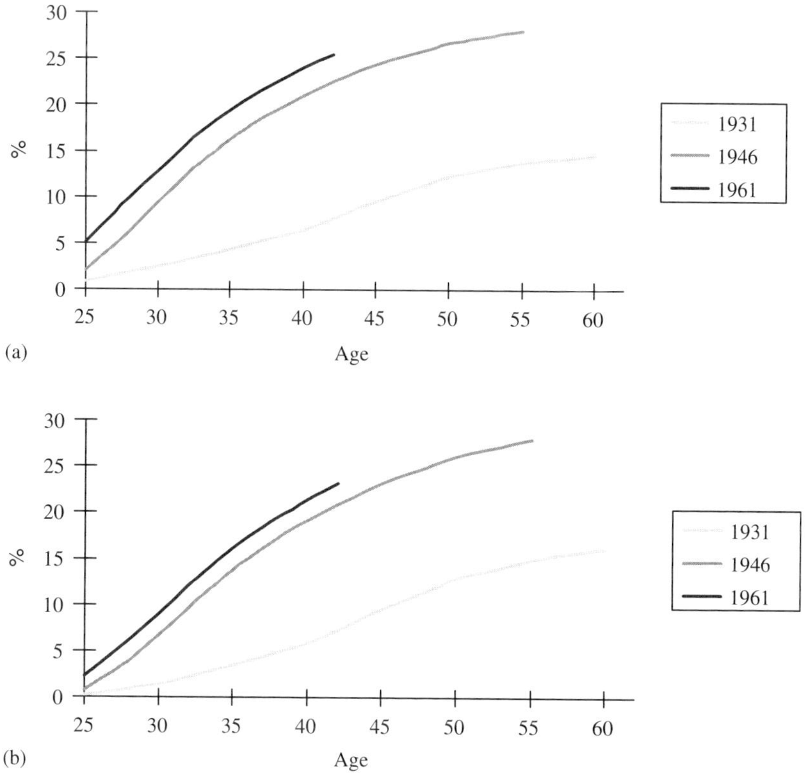

householders by age 60. As the propensity to live alone rises steeply between ages 60 and 75, it is likely that close to half of the 1960s cohort will be living alone by age 75, which is when they will be at greater risk of being in need of support. Currently, a higher proportion of older people living alone are in receipt of social care services than those living with others (Evandrou and Falkingham, 2004). Thus, the rise in solo living will have implications for the future demand for such care.

The most important source of support amongst elderly people living alone in Britain today is their adult children. Figure 6 shows that a smaller proportion of the 1946 cohort are childless than in previous generations, with just 9 per cent of women remaining childless by age 45, compared to 13 per cent of women born in 1931, and 21 per cent of those born in 1920. However, although there may be potentially more adult children to provide care for their older parents among the 1946 cohort in retirement, this doesn't automatically mean that these children will be willing or able to do so. High

Figure 6: Percentage of Women Childless at Age 30 and Age 45 by Birth Cohort.

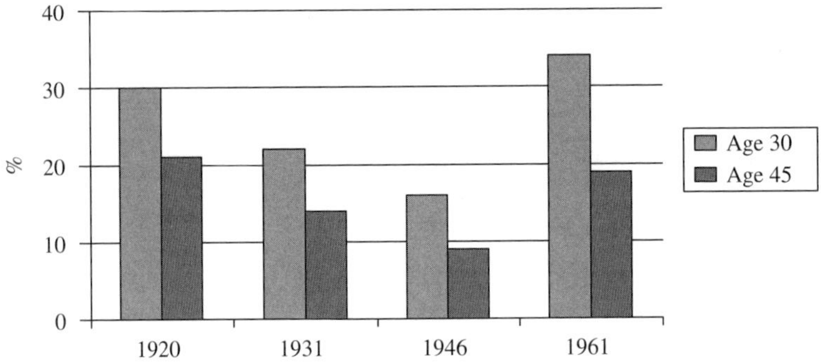

divorce rates amongst the 1940s cohort may impact upon the propensity of adult children to care for their elderly parents and parents-in-law. Little is currently known about how divorce may affect family ties and feelings of inter-generational obligation in Britain. Evidence from America found that divorced fathers were less likely to view their children as a potential source of support in later life (Goldscheider, 1994). Adult children of divorced parents were also less inclined to view co-residing with their elderly parents as an option (Goldscheider and Lawton, 1998).

Furthermore, changes in the geographical proximity of parents and adult children may also impact upon the potential of non co-residential kin to provide care. Currently 60 per cent of older people aged 70 and over living alone do not have any children or grandchildren living within a 30-min journey time (ONS, 2002). Recent research indicates that the educational and occupational status of both the older and younger generations impacts on social networks. Better educated and better off adult children tend to live further away from their family (Glaser and Tomassini, 2000) and have much lower levels of contact with their parents (Grundy and Shelton, 2001) than those with lower qualifications, reflecting longer distance migration for education and work. It is not clear whether increasing education and greater occupational mobility will mean that in future fewer adult children will live close to their elderly parents. Alternatively, more flexible working practices may result in people no longer having to move to where the work is and being able work at home, thus exercising greater choice in deciding to live near their parents. Finally the availability of care from adult children may also be affected by the increase in economic activity amongst the female children of the 1940s cohort.

Figure 6 also indicates a shift in demographic behaviour between the first and second baby boom cohort. It is estimated that a fifth (20 per cent) of women born in 1961 will remain childless at age 45. Although the rates of childlessness in this cohort are not unprecedented, being similar to those experienced by the cohort of women born in the 1920s, there are several differences between the experiences of historical and contemporary cohorts, the most important of which concerns 'choice'. In the past marriage was the gatekeeper to fertility, and the high rates of childlessness amongst English women born in the 1920s were the result of relatively low rates of marriage during a period when extra-marital births were not condoned. Today, births outside marriage are commonplace and women are increasingly *choosing* childlessness even when in a partnership (McAllister and Clarke, 1998).

Thus, it is likely that there will be a decline in the potential supply of informal care amongst the 1960s cohort from both co-residential spouses and non co-residential adult children. This challenge for policy makers will be further exacerbated by the size of the 1960s Baby Boomers cohort and their greater longevity. Although there is no doubt that there will be more persons in terms of absolute numbers, requiring support in 2030 than today, it is less clear *who* will provide it, *which* mix of care will be available, and whether this will match the preferences of older people themselves.

Demand for social care will also depend upon future trends in health and dependency, as well as people's expectations. What is the evidence on the health prospects of older people in the next two or three decades? Will younger cohorts be healthier than their parents or grandparents? What do patterns in chronic ill health, health risk behaviour, and work stress suggest? And what are the implications for demand upon health and social care?

6. Health and Dependency

It could be argued that, having benefited from the NHS and having experienced improved living conditions in their youth and middle age, the post-war baby boom cohorts will go on to 'age healthily'. Trends in mortality, morbidity, and health risk behaviour indicate that although improvements in mortality rates and increasing life expectancy suggest that we are indeed healthier (Drever and Whitehead, 1997), trends in self-reported health status suggest there is no comparable general improvement in health (Dunnell, 1997). Life expectancy in old age has risen, however the extent to which these gains are disability-free is the subject of ongoing debate (Robine et al., 1993). Research indicates that as life expectancy increases, there will be a rise in the proportion of people experiencing light to moderate disabilities, but a fall in those with severe disabilities (Bone et al., 1995). Health in later life is influenced by events throughout the life course, including quality of life during working years. Those who paid attention to health education campaigns, taking regular exercise, having a healthy diet, and who avoided smoking may escape today's major killers: strokes, lung cancer, and heart attacks (Dalley, 1997). On the other hand, new threats such as stress, pollution, and food contamination can lead to the onset of yet unknown health problems in later life.

In order to shed light on future health trends and to inform assumptions about future mortality levels, the research uses data from 28 years of the General Household Survey to examine trends in three key areas: (a) health-risk behaviour, focussing on smoking; (b) self reported morbidity, examining limiting long-standing illness; and (c) work related stress, using proxy measures such as hours of work and the experience of unemployment. The evidence on the likely health of future elders is mixed.

6.1 Health-Risk Behaviour — Smoking

The GHS has collected information on smoking in alternate years since 1974. The prevalence of cigarette smoking in Britain decreased substantially in the 1970s and early 1980s, from 45 per cent of all men and women aged 16 and over in 1974 to 35 per cent in 1982. Since then the proportion smoking decreased more gradually until the early 1990s, since when it has levelled out. In 2002, 26 per cent of people aged 16 and over were cigarette smokers (ONS, 2004). This decline in the propensity to smoke over time is reflected in the proportion of each cohort who currently smoke (Figure 7a,b) by age. Only for the youngest cohort is there any upward trend in the prevalence of smoking, as young people join the ranks of smokers during their late teens and early 20s. Moreover, the decrease in the proportion smoking by age observed *within* birth cohorts is much greater than that observed in cross-sectional data (Evandrou and Falkingham, 2002).

Although smoking is generally more common amongst men than women at young ages, men are also more likely to give up than women. Amongst the cohort born 1946–1950, at age 26, 51 per cent of men reported that they currently smoked compared to 45 of women. However, amongst the same birth cohort at age 40 the gender differential has reversed, with a slightly higher proportion of women currently smoking than men (36% vs. 34%). Similar differences in smoking behaviour by gender have been reported in birth cohort studies for other countries, such as the US (Escobedo and Peddicord, 1996), West Germany (Brenner, 1993) and Canada (Ferrence, 1988). A previous study using GHS data in Britain attributed the differentials by gender to differing responses to anti-smoking campaigns, with women being found to be less responsive to tobacco related health publicity than men (Townsend et al., 1994).

In terms of this indicator of health risk behaviour, younger cohorts show lower levels of smoking than earlier cohorts. Given that smoking is related to a wide variety of illnesses and health states, evidence of decreased prevalence amongst members of the younger cohorts in this study suggests that elderly people in 2030 will be healthier than today's generation of elders at

Figure 7: Percentage of (a) Men and (b) Women Smoking by Birth Cohort.

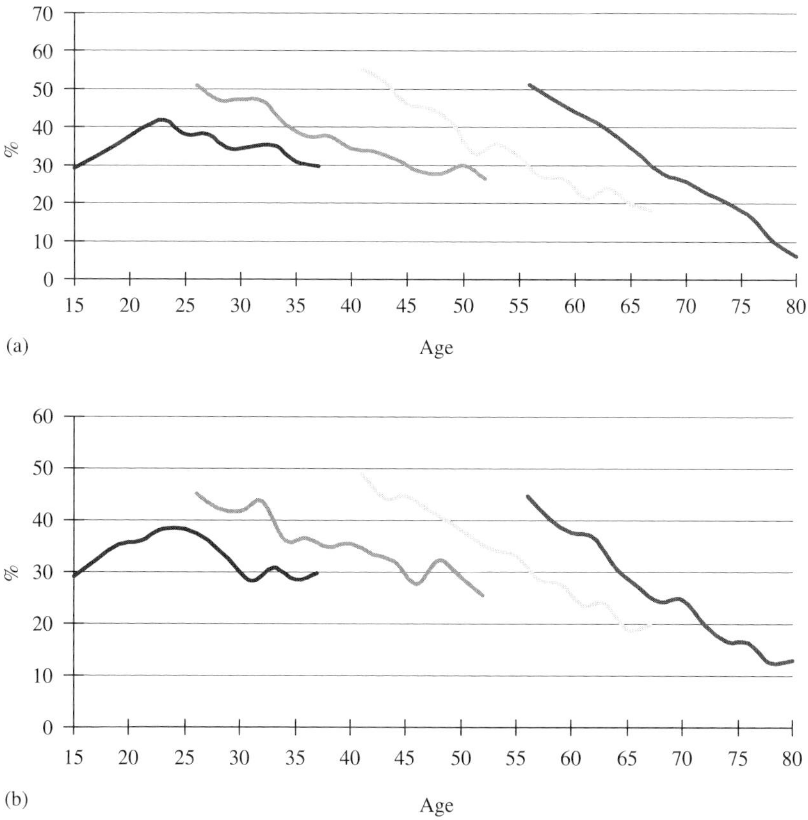

the same age. However, there is evidence that improvements in mortality from key smoking related diseases such as lung cancer are proportionately lower amongst women than men (Evandrou and Falkingham, 2002). Thus if the current UK government's targets for reducing deaths from cancer (Department of Health, 1999) are to be achieved, the gender differences in smoking behaviour need to be addressed.

There also remain significant differences in smoking behaviour by social class. Deaths from smoking related diseases vary substantially by social class and smoking is widely acknowledged as a major contributor to both the current levels of morbidity and mortality in Britain and to the persistence of health inequalities (Acheson, 1998). Figure 8a and b show the percentage of men and women who smoke at any age amongst the four birth cohorts, disaggregated by whether they work in manual or non-manual occupations. There are several points of note. First, amongst all birth cohorts, a higher

Figure 8: Percentage of (a)Men and (b) Women Currently Smoking by Social Group by Birth Cohort.

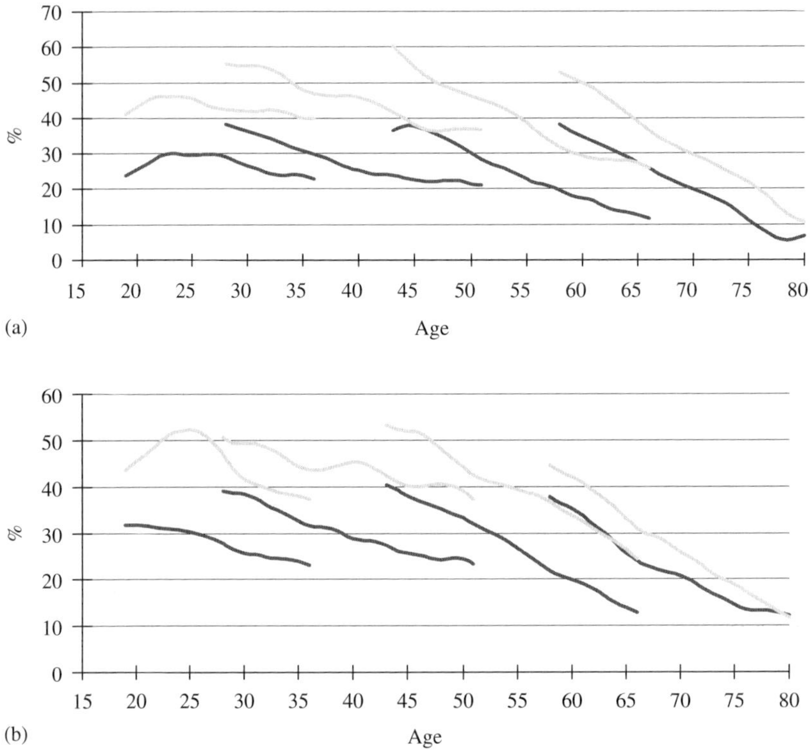

proportion of men and women working in manual occupations smoke than those working in non-manual occupations. Second, the trajectories suggest that there is a lag in smoking cessation by socio-economic group *between* birth cohorts. For example, the trajectory for manual women from the 1931 to 1935 cohort appears to be following a similar path to that of non-manual women from the 1916 to 1920 cohort. A similar pattern is found amongst men. Such patterns are consistent with diffusion theory of behaviour change, where changes in health-related behaviour are adopted first amongst the middle classes and then diffuse through the population. The most well documented example of this was the adoption of fertility regulating behaviour amongst the middle classes at the end of the 19th century (Lesthaeghe, 1983, Cleland and Wilson, 1987;). If the smoking behaviour of non-manual men and women in the *previous* birth cohort is a good guide to future behaviour amongst manual men and women, we should observe a continuation of the fall in smoking amongst manual groups.

However, the graphs also show evidence that the rate of smoking cessation is *slowing down* amongst non-manual workers in the 1940s cohort. The prevalence of smoking appears to be stabilising at around 20 per cent. Moreover, the prevalence rates amongst manual men from 1960s cohort appear to be levelling out at around 40 per cent. This has important implications for the government achieving its target of reducing the prevalence of smoking amongst all adults to 24 per cent by 2010. Finally, the gap between manual and non-manual groups is also widening both *within* birth cohorts with rising age, as non-manual groups give up smoking at a faster rate than non-manual groups (Table 1), and *between* cohorts at any given chronological age (Table 2). For example, amongst women aged 30, the odds of a woman born in 1946–1950 smoking were 1.5 greater if they were from a manual background compared to non-manual. However, amongst those women born in 1961–1965 the odds had risen to 2.06 at the same age.

Thus to summarise, the results in smoking behaviour by occupational group within birth cohorts have mixed messages. The good news is that overall prevalence of smoking at any age is lower amongst successive birth cohorts and smoking cessation is occurring at earlier ages than in previous cohorts. However, rates of giving up smoking appear to be slowing down amongst the younger cohorts. There also remain significant differences in smoking behaviour by social class with people in manual classes being more likely to smoke than non-manual. Furthermore these differentials are widening over time. This will have significant implications for the persistence of

Table 1: Prevalence of Cigarette Smoking Within Birth Cohort by Sex, Socio-Economic Group and Age

	Men			Women		
	Manual	**Non-manual**	**Odds ratio**	**Manual**	**Non-manual**	**Odds ratio**
1916–1920						
Age 60	0.50	0.35	1.86	0.42	0.34	1.41
Age 75	0.22	0.11	2.28	0.19	0.15	1.33
			Widening			Reducing
1931–1935						
Age 45	0.54	0.38	1.92	0.52	0.38	1.77
Age 60	0.29	0.17	1.99	0.35	0.20	2.15
			Widening			Widening
1946–1950						
Age 30	0.55	0.35	2.27	0.49	0.39	1.50
Age 45	0.38	0.23	2.05	0.40	0.26	1.90
			Reducing			Widening

Source: Authors' analysis of GHS 1974-2000

Table 2: Prevalence of Cigarette Smoking at Age 30, 45 and 60, by Sex, Socio-Economic Group and Birth Cohort

	Men			Women		
	Manual	**Non manual**	**Odds ratio**	**Manual**	**Non manual**	**Odds ratio**
Age 30						
1946–1950	0.55	0.35	2.27	0.49	0.39	1.50
1961–1965	0.42	0.26	2.06	0.42	0.26	2.06
			Reducing			Widening
Age 45						
1931–1935	0.54	0.38	1.92	0.52	0.38	1.77
1946–1950	0.38	0.23	2.05	0.40	0.26	1.90
			Widening			Widening
Age 60						
1916–1920	0.50	0.35	1.86	0.42	0.34	1.41
1931–1935	0.29	0.17	1.99	0.35	0.20	2.15
			Widening			Widening

Source: Authors' analysis of GHS 1974–2000

inequalities in health outcomes, given that disadvantages in health are known to be accumulated across an individuals' lifetime. There is now a 7.4 year difference in the expectation of life at birth between men in professional and managerial occupations (78.5 years) and those from unskilled manual occupations (71.1 years); and a 5.7 year differential for women (82.8 years compared with 77.1 years) (Donkin et al., 2002). This analysis suggests that unless policies are adopted that both reduce smoking overall and narrow the disparities between groups, inequalities in smoking related diseases and overall life expectancy look likely to persist well into the 21st century.

6.2 Self-Reported Morbidity

A widely used indicator of health status is long-standing illness and whether this limits people's activity. Figure 9a and b present the proportion of women and men reporting a limiting long-standing illness (LLSI) using 3 year moving averages plotted against the mid-point of the age group for the cohort. As expected, the proportion of each cohort reporting a LLSI rises with age. The shape of the trajectory for the 1916–1920 cohort peaks and troughs at older ages. This may be a selection effect, reflecting the fact that 'less healthy' people are more likely to have left the sample either through death or entry into institutional care (the GHS does not include the institutional population). More interestingly, successive younger cohorts appear to report slightly *higher* levels of LLSI than the previous cohort at the same

Figure 9: Percentage of (a) Women and (b) Men Reporting Limiting Long-Standing Illness by Birth Cohort.

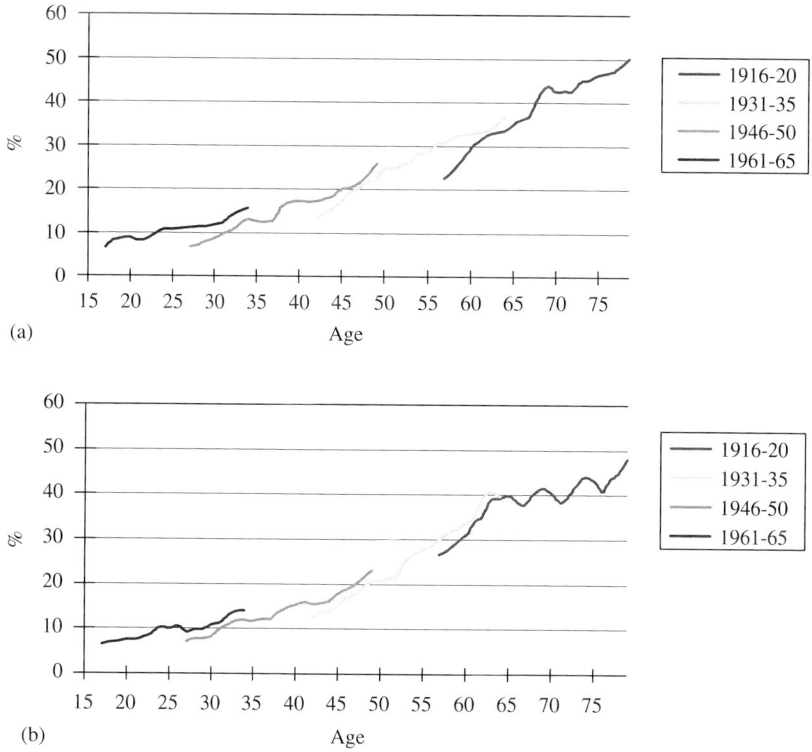

age, and women report slightly higher levels than men. For example, by age 49, 26 per cent of women in the 1940s cohort report having a LLSI compared to 22 per cent of women in the 1930s cohort at the same age. This may reflect a general increase in the propensity to report ill health regardless of age or cohort, i.e. a period effect reflecting changing perception of health and health expectations with time. Alternatively it may reflect real differences in the health status between cohorts, with younger cohorts reporting progressively worse health at the same stage in the life course. Either way, these trends have implications for the demand for health care services in the next 20–30 years.

6.3 Work Related Stress

Another potential influence upon the health of future elders may be increased levels of stress faced within the workplace. The UK's workers work amongst the longest hours in Europe and face high levels of workplace stress. In 2001, full-time employees in the EU worked on average 40 h week (European Commission, 2003). In contrast, the UK average was 44. The UK also has the highest proportion of all employees working 45 h and over a week (Bishop, 2004).

Evidence from the GHS demonstrates a general increase in the intensity of work over the last 25 years. Figure 10 shows that by age 49, 30 per cent of employed men from the 1940s cohort reported working 50 or more hours per week. This compares with just 13 per cent of men from the 1930s cohort, at the same age. If current trends continue, it is likely that an even greater proportion of the 1960s cohort will experience long working hours. Greater work intensity experienced for longer periods during working life may adversely affect health, directly or indirectly, both now and in later life (Spurgeon et al., 1997).

In addition to longer hours of work, the 1960s cohort has experienced higher levels of unemployment, at earlier stages in their life course than the 1946–1950 cohort (Figure 11). Job loss has been shown to be a highly stressful life event, affecting both physical and psychological health (Bartley, 1994). The two recessions of the early 1980s and 1990s are clearly visible in Figure 11. The unemployment rate during each recession has been greatest amongst the 1960s cohort, with 19 per cent of men being unemployed in 1983. It is also clear from Figure 11 at men from the 1930s cohort were adversely affected by the recession in the early 1980s. Unemployment rates amongst this cohort did not recover during the boom of the mid-to-late 1980s but remained relatively stable. So it appears that once out of the labour market in their 50s, men from this cohort found it particularly difficult to re-enter.

It is difficult to predict what effect unemployment and higher levels of work-related stress during working life may have on levels of physical and

Figure 10: Percentage of Employed Men Working 50 or More Hours by Birth Cohort.

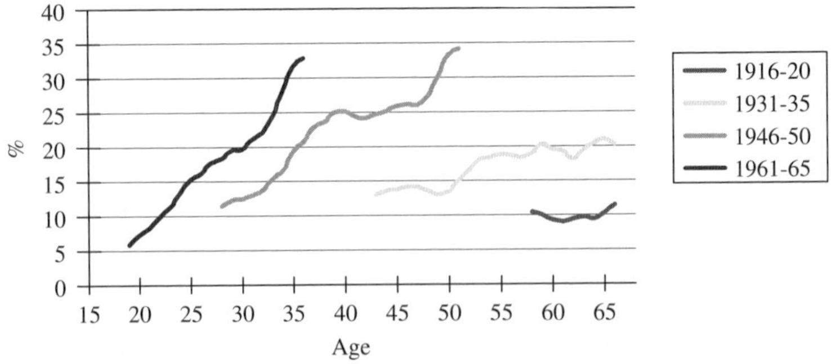

Figure 11: Percentage of Men Unemployed by Birth Cohort.

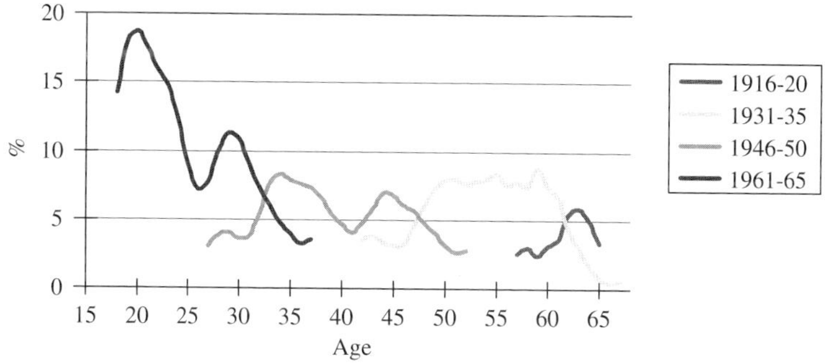

mental ill health in later life. Research using NCDS data concludes that the experience of prolonged unemployment early in the working life is likely to have a persisting effect on future health and socio-economic circumstances (Gregg and Wadsworth, 1999). Thus, the fact that members of the 1960s cohort have experienced especially high levels of unemployment early in their life course may have particular consequences for their economic and social resources, including health in old age.

7. Conclusions

The research presented above illustrates that experiences earlier in the life course impact upon resources in later life, and highlights the need for social policy to reflect life course experiences. Given this, it is essential to take account of cohort differences in projections and modelling aimed at informing policy development planning health and social care services over the next 20 years. Moreover, models need to take into account the diversity of experiences both *between* and *within* cohorts.

The key findings for planners that emerge from the research are two-fold. Firstly, there will be a rise in solo living amongst elderly people. However, this may not necessarily be accompanied by an increase in the availability of care from adult children, particularly amongst the 1960s Baby Boomers. Secondly, it may be premature to assume that tomorrow's elders will be healthier than today's. Trends in smoking provide one indication that younger generations will be healthier in later life than current generations of older people. However, the proportion reporting limiting long-standing illness suggests the opposite — with younger cohorts reporting slightly higher levels than previous cohorts at the same age. Furthermore, the 1960s cohort has experienced higher levels of unemployment, and longer working weeks for those in work, at earlier stages in their life course than the 1947 cohort.

Increased levels of work-related stress may manifest themselves in poorer health in older ages. Whether future elders will be healthier than today's elders may also depend upon the impact of factors as yet unknown. Greater use of pesticides, genetic engineering in animal farming, and advances in food technology (e.g. GM foods) may manifest themselves in better or worse health in later life. What can be said with some certainty, however, is that inequalities will remain. Thus, even if tomorrow's elders will, on average, be healthier than today's, action still needs to taken to tackle the widening inequalities in health-risk behaviour.

The pseudo-cohort analysis presented here has been useful in two main ways. Firstly, it has served to refocus attention on the life course, and to highlight the fact that economic and social experiences earlier in the life course impact upon prospects in later life. Certain characteristics are carried through time (e.g. sex), others are accumulated over time (resources), many change over time (age and health). and some are also affected by the time period in which one lives (e.g. the welfare system experienced). Secondly, the analysis has emphasised the importance of taking cohort differences into account within projections for social policy planning. In order to be better placed to plan for an ageing population in the 21st century, further research, exploiting the rich sources of birth cohort data within Britain is needed.

References

Acheson, D. (1998). *Independent Inquiry into Inequalities in Health.* TSO, London.

Allen, I. and Perkins, E. (eds). (1995). *The Future of Family Care for Older People.* HMSO, London.

Bartley, M. (1994). Unemployment and Ill Health: Understanding the Relationship. *Journal of Epidemiology and Community Health*, 48, 333–337.

Bishop, K. (2004). Working Time Patterns in the UK, France, Denmark and Sweden. *Labour Market Trends*, 112(3), 113–120.

Bone, M. R., Bebbigton, A. C., Jagger, C., Morgan, K. and Nicholaas, G. (1995). *Health Expectancy and its Uses.* HMSO, London.

Breeze, E. (1990). *Reporting on Sampling Error.* Series GHS no. 18, OPCS. HMSO, London.

Brenner, H. (1993). A Birth Cohort Analysis of the Smoking Epidemic in West Germany. *Journal of Epidemiology and Community Health*, 43, 54–58.

Cleland, J. and Wilson, C. (1987). Demand Theories of the Fertility Transition: An Iconoclastic View. *Population Studies*, 41, 5–30.

Dalley, G. (1997). Health and Health Care, in Evandrou, M. (ed), *Baby Boomers: Ageing in the 21st Century*, Age Concern, London.

Department of Health (1999). *Saving Lives: Our Healthier Nation.* TSO, London.

Donkin, A., Goldblatt, P. and Lynch, K. (2002). Trends in Life Expectancy by Social Class 1972–1999. *Health Statistics Quarterly*, 15, 5–15.

Drever, F. and Whitehead, M. (eds). TSO, Health Inequalities, London.

Dunnell, K. (1997). Are we healthier?, in Charlton, J. (ed), *The Health of Adult Britain 1841–1994, ONS Series DS nos 12 & 13*, TSO, London.

Escobedo, L. and Peddicord, J. (1996). Smoking Prevalence in US Birth Cohorts: the Influence of Gender and Education. *American Journal of Public Health*, 86, 231–236.

Evandrou, M. and Falkingham, J. (2000). Looking Back to Look Forward: Lessons from Four Birth Cohorts for Ageing in the 21st Century. *Population Trends*, 99, 21–30.

Evandrou, M. and Falkingham, J. (2002). Smoking Behaviour and Socio-Economic Status: a Cohort Analysis, 1974–1998. *Health Statistics Quarterly*, 14, 30–39.

Evandrou, M. and Falkingham, J. (2004). Demographic Change in Europe: Implications for Family Support for Older People, in Kreager, P. and Schroeder-Butterfill, E. (eds), *Elderly Without Children*, Berhahn Books, Oxford.

European Commission (2003). *Social Situation in the EU*. European Commission, Strasbourg.

Ferrence, R. (1988). Sex Differences in Cigarette Smoking in Canada, 1900–1978: a Reconstructed Cohort Study. *Canadian Journal of Public Health*, 79, 160–165.

Glaser, K. and Tomassini, C. (2000). Proximity of Older Women to Their Children: A Comparison of Britain and Italy. *The Gerontologist*, 40, 729–737.

Goldscheider, F. (1994). Divorce and Remarriage: Effects on the Elderly Population. *Reviews in Clinical Gerontology*, 4, 253–259.

Goldscheider, F. and Lawton, L. (1998). Family Experiences and the Erosion of Support for Intergenerational Coresidence. *Journal of Marriage and the Family*, 60, 623–632.

Gregg, P. and Wadsworth, M. (1999). *The Scarring Effects of Unemployment*. Manchester University Press, Manchester.

Grundy, E. and Shelton, N. (2001). Contact Between Adult Children and Their Parents in Great Britain 1986–1999. *Environment and Planning A*, 33, 685–698.

Lesthaeghe, R. (1983). A Century of Demographic and Cultural Change in Western Europe. An Exploration of Underlying Dimensions. *Population and Development Review*, 9(3), 411–435.

McAllister, F. with Clarke, L. (1998). Choosing Childlessness. London: Family Policy Studies Centre.

ONS (2002). *ONS Omnibus Survey, Non-Resident Parental Contact Module*. ESDS, Manchester.

ONS (2004). *Living in Britain. Results from the 2002 General Household Survey*. TSO, London.

ONS (2006). *Marriage and Divorce Statistics, Series FM2 no. 31*. TSO, London.

Robine, J.M., Mathers, C., Bone, M. and Romieu, I. (1993). Calculation of Health Expectancies: Harmonisation, Consensus Achieved and Future Perspectives. Colloque INSERM/ John Libbey Eurotext Ltd.

Spurgeon, A., Harrington, J. and Cooper, C. (1997). Health and Safety Problems Associated with Long Working Hours: A Review of the Current Position. *Occupational and Environmental Medicine*, 54, 375–376.

Townsend, J., Roderick, P. and Cooper, J. (1994). Cigarette Smoking by Socio-Economic Group, Sex and Age: Effects of Price, Income and Health Publicity. *British Medical Journal*, 309, 923–927.

Chapter 4

Measures of Dependency among Older People in Community and Residential Settings in Scotland — Their Development and Application in Resource Forecasting

Adam Redpath

Information and Statistics Division, NHSScotland, UK

Abstract

The provision of government-funded health and social care for older people in Scotland depends on the professional assessment of clients' needs, carried out by a multi-disciplinary team — the Single Shared Assessment (SSA). The Scottish Executive wished to develop an iso-resource classification[1] *— the Resource Use Measure (RUM) — derived from the SSA process which would form the basis for a standard dataset describing the characteristics of elderly people, their needs and service provision in a variety of care settings across Scotland.*

This study had three objectives:

1. *To develop an RUM which allowed care professionals to categorise their elderly service users (over age 65) into a limited number of relative need groups.*
2. *To develop a related set of data.*
3. *To explore the application of such data in stock and flow models.*

Data on care costs and needs characteristics were gathered on two samples of elderly service users. The RUM was developed using a combination of statistical analysis (AID/CART methods) and input from care professionals. The Ithink modelling tool was used to explore the dynamics of the care system for the 65–74 age group.

[1] Iso-resource — i.e. cases in each group would be similar in terms of the level of resources required to meet their needs.

International Symposia in Economic Theory and Econometrics, Vol. 16

ISSN: 1571-0386 DOI: 10.1016/S1571-0386(06)16004-4

The final RUM grouping, with nine relative need groups (labelled A–I), explained 30 per cent of variation in resource use and was accepted by practitioners as a reliable and easy-to-use tool. Modelling showed the relative impact of rehabilitation and quality of care on residential populations.

In conclusion, the RUM can be a vital tool in service planning for the elderly.

1. Introduction

1.1 Policy Background

The establishment of the Scottish Parliament in 1999, with devolved powers in health and social care, allowed the development of a distinct approach to the provision of care in Scotland. The Sutherland Report (The Royal Commission on Long Term Care, 1999) recommended that nursing care be provided free of charge to all people over 65 in need of it. Prior to this, nursing care was provided for free to people in community and in-patient settings, whereas the provision of nursing care in nursing homes was subject to a means test. The policy of free nursing care was adopted by the Scottish Executive (and subsequently by Department of Health in England), and this policy was later expanded to include free personal care as well. The implementation of this policy began in Scotland in July 2002.

One of the key drivers for development of the assessment process for older people is the Scottish Executive's Joint Future agenda. The aim of Joint Future is to improve partnership workings between agencies (through joint resourcing and joint management) and to secure better outcomes for service users and their carers. A key element of Joint Future is the establishment of locally agreed, single shared assessment (SSA) procedures for all groups within the remit of community care. According to the Scottish Executive, the benefits of SSA are as follows:

- a single point of entry to community care services;
- a holistic, structured approach to the assessment;
- less bureaucracy, duplication and delay;
- information shared between professionals and agencies appropriately; and
- outcomes accepted by fellow professionals (Scottish Executive, 2003b).

The development of a standard tool to measure need across different care settings, based on information collected by the SSA process, would provide valuable information to monitor equity of access to services across the country. The development of the Resource Use Measure (RUM) was funded by the Scottish Executive for this reason.

1.2 Balance of Care

The provision of care for older people in Scotland occurs in three main types of settings:

- in the individual's home in the community;
- in a residential setting — nursing or residential (providing social care) home; and
- in a hospital setting (long stay or acute).

Over the last 20 years Scotland has seen a marked decline in the number of long-stay geriatric hospital beds and an increase in the number of nursing home and special housing places. However, the number of community care clients declined, and the packages supplied became more intensive (Joint Future Group, 2000) (Figure 1).

Table 1 presents data from the 2001 UK census on the numbers of people over 65 living in communal establishments, and residency rate per 1000, by age group. Not surprisingly, the rates are heavily age dependent.

Figure 1: Balance of Care for Older People, Scotland 1980–2001 (Scottish Executive, 2002b)

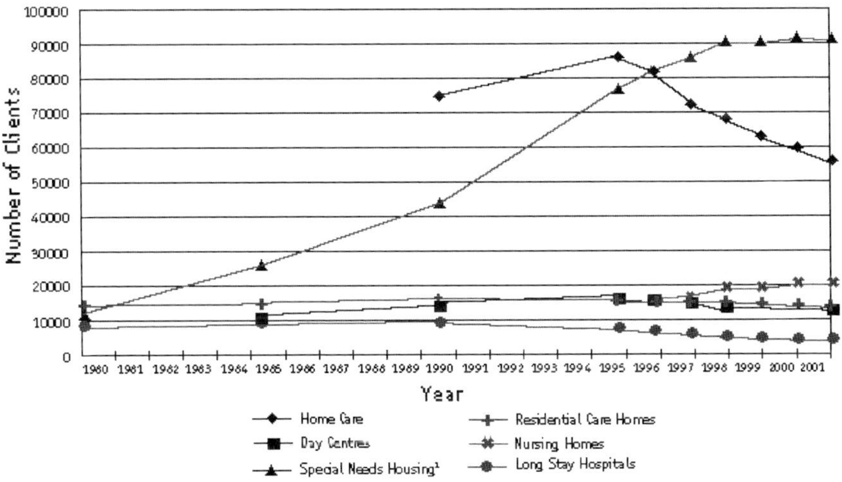

¹Indicates number of dwellings rather than clients.

Source: Scottish Executive, Scottish Community Care Statistics 2001, Edinburgh, Scottish Executive (2002, *p. 1*)

Table 1: Persons Over 65 in Communal Establishments by Age Group 2001 — Numbers and Percentage of Population (GRO Scotland, 2003)

Age group	Hospital	Nursing and residential home	Other	Total	% of total population 2001
65–74	1,166	4,010	461	5,637	1.26
75–84	2,048	11,239	470	13,757	5.06
85+	1,907	16,286	311	18,504	20.84
Total	5,121	31,535	1,242	37,898	4.7

Source: General Register Office (Scotland), Scottish Census Results online (SCROL), http://www.scrol.gov.uk/scrol/common/home.jsp, Edinburgh, GRO(S), Table S232 (2003)

Table 2: Projected Population of Scotland, by Sex and Age: 2001–2026 ('000s)

Age	Estimated population	Projected population at 30th June/year					% Increase 2001–2026
	30th June 2001	2006	2011	2016	2021	2026	
65–69	239	241	255	301	288	320	33.9
70–74	207	210	214	228	270	260	25.6
65–74	446	451	469	529	558	580	30.0
75–79	166	167	173	179	192	228	37.3
80–84	106	117	121	130	136	147	38.7
75–84	272	284	294	309	328	375	37.9
85–89	59	61	68	73	81	87	47.5
90+	29	30	31	36	41	48	65.5
85+	88	91	99	109	122	135	53.4

Source: © *General Register Office for Scotland (2003)*

The Joint Future report (Joint Future Group, 2000) argued that the balance of care in Scotland was too skewed towards residential care. Elderly people, and the public at large, wanted care provided at home.

Demographic Trends

Population projections for Scotland show a growth in the population over 65, especially for those over 85 (see Table 2).

The increase in the number of elderly people applied to the existing residency rates leads to projected increases in the numbers in hospital and care homes as set out in Table 3.

Table 3: Number of Residents in Communal Establishments, Projected 2001–2026

Age	Population (2001 census)	Projected population/year					% Increase 2001–2026
		2006	2011	2016	2021	2026	
65–69	239	241	255	301	288	320	33.9
70–74	207	210	214	228	270	260	25.6
Hospitals	5,121	5,289	5,585	6,072	6,572	7,265	41.9
75–79	166	167	173	179	192	228	37.3
80–84	106	117	121	130	136	147	38.7
Care homes	31,535	32,631	34,687	37,697	41,148	45,694	44.9
85–89	59	61	68	73	81	87	47.5
90+	29	30	31	36	41	48	65.5

Source: © *General Register Office for Scotland (2003)*

1.4 Effective Use of Resources

The growth in demand for residential care facilities for the over-65s will put pressure on resources and makes it vital that they are used appropriately. Figures from NHSScotland routine surveys of elderly people in residential care settings showed that 10 per cent of long-stay NHS hospital residents, 29 per cent of nursing home residents and 71 per cent of people in residential homes were in low-dependency groups in 2001–2002 (ISD Scotland, 2003). According to the Scottish Executive, as many as 20 per cent of residents in nursing homes would be capable of being cared for in a community setting (Joint Future Group, 2000, p. 11).

There may be several reasons for the use of such facilities by people in low-dependency groups:

1. Historic reasons — the growth in nursing home places during the 1990s (Joint Future Group, 2000, p. 10).
2. The impact of behavioural and other problems necessitating residential care may be underestimated by the measures used[2] (ISD Scotland, 2004).
3. Self-referral by self-funded elderly people.
4. A lack of more appropriate care arrangements — e.g. sheltered housing or care at home

[2] Scottish Health Resource Groups (SHRUGS), used in long-stay geriatric hospitals, and Scottish Care Resource Utilisation Groups (SCRUGS) used nursing and care homes — see below.

5. Perverse incentives in the system — hospital care is expensive, but has always been free. Referral to a nursing home by local government providers could in the past result in an individual's care costs being entirely met by the sale of the person's home.

Some health authorities in Scotland have reviewed the balance of care between residential, nursing and hospital settings, and have decreased the proportion of low-dependency patients in long-stay hospital and nursing home accommodation, thus ensuring a more efficient use of scarce resources.

Existing measures of dependency[3] provide useful information to care managers about the balance of care between different types of residential facilities, but they were not designed to measure relative need across residential and non-residential settings. The RUM was developed to measure relative need across a range of community and residential care settings, allowing comparisons to be made in the balance of care provided for older people across Scotland.

2. Objective

The RUM was developed to summarise the relative level of needs of service users — including service users who needed both residential and non-residential care, based on information collected as part of the SSA process.

There is not a standard assessment tool used across Scotland. Each local area has developed its own tool(s), and some items are free text. The RUM was conceived as an instrument comprised of closed, tick box questions, with comprehensive guidance and training backup designed to give a standardised score for relative need. It is *not* designed to be an assessment tool, linking specific client characteristics to needs for particular services, but a tool to measure the relative overall need of groups of service users.

The RUM instrument was to be capable of completion within five minutes, given the necessary information being available, and was not to impose significant burdens of extra work on staff.

Information gathered by the RUM would allow inter-area comparisons of service provision between groups with similar levels of need, and highlight differences between areas in terms of how needs are met and how different types of care settings are utilised. Such information would serve to promote equity of access to care across Scotland.

[3] SCRUGS and SHRUGS.

3. Methods

The approach adopted by the RUM development team (Scottish Executive, 2002a) was to combine statistical analysis of data on resource use with information about client characteristics obtained from practitioners in order to arrive at an algorithm that used key characteristics to classify service users into iso-resource groups. The RUM was to classify clients into groups with similar levels of need, as measured by the weekly cost of meeting their needs (including unpaid care input, unmet need and equipment costs). The RUM would be validated both by empirical evidence and by expert opinion, and, as it would have been developed in co-operation with practitioners themselves, would have a much greater chance of widespread acceptance by those working in direct patient and client care.

3.1 RUM Development

The RUM was developed to cover clients in a variety of care settings — i.e. those being cared for in their own homes, and those in residential care facilities and nursing homes. The initial development, Phase 1, focused on an evaluation of two rather different tools for measuring need:

1. Scottish Health Resource Utilisation Groups (SHRUGS) and Scottish Care Resource Utilisation Groups (SCRUGS), derived from the American RUGS system (Urquhart et al., 1999). SHRUGS and SCRUGS were developed for application in hospital and residential care settings, respectively.
2. The Interval Need (IN) measure, developed by Isaacs and Neville (1975), which classified people according to the length of time which elapsed between necessary interventions. The IN approach had been applied in a population study of older people in a variety of care settings in a small local authority in central Scotland (Bond and Carstairs, 1982).

The merits of the two methods were evaluated in Phase 1 of the RUM development, and it was expected that one would be chosen and adapted to form the final RUM.

Shrugs and Scrugs

ISD Scotland developed measures of need for nursing care and social care that adapted RUGS to Scottish circumstances (Urquhart et al., 1999). The resulting instrument, called SHRUGS, classified patients in long-stay geriatric wards into groups with similar levels of need for care and dependency. An additional tool, SCRUGS, was developed for use in residential and nursing homes, where clients' needs were less than those of residents in long-stay hospitals. Both SHRUGS and SCRUGS are classification trees designed to predict need for staff resources.

The primary, and most important variable in the SHRUGS and SCRUGS classifications is the Activities of Daily Living (ADL) score — a summary variable derived from the residents' ability to perform basic functions such as eating, using the toilet and transferring position, with or without assistance. SHRUGS uses additional classification variables relating to behavioural needs, clinical and special care needs (e.g. feeding by tube, pressure sores); SCRUGS uses variables relating to problem behaviour, reflecting the different problems of less-dependent residents in nursing homes. The SHRUGS and SCRUGS instruments are used by trained interviewers, who collect data annually from staff in long-stay hospitals and care homes across Scotland.

Interval Need

The IN measure classifies people according to the length of time that can reasonably be allowed to elapse between necessary interventions. The group with the lowest needs were classified as independent. The next groups were classified as having 'long-interval' needs (requiring irregular interventions), 'short-interval' needs (requiring regular interventions — e.g. for dressing) and 'critical interval' needs (e.g. requiring frequent interventions for immobility and incontinence).

Two questionnaires were developed — one based on the IN approach and the second based on the existing SCRUGS approach. Questionnaires were completed by local assessment teams (comprising NHS, local authority social work and housing staff) for a representative sample of 197 older people from six areas across Scotland. Training in the use of the questionnaire was provided by the RUM development team, to ensure accurate data recording. The actual instruments used to measure IN were not available and the RUM development team, working in collaboration with colleagues and practitioners, developed a set of questions to measure IN for the study. The existing SCRUGS tool required little adaptation.

The questionnaire included a section on resource use, which recorded a wide range of social care and nursing staff inputs. These inputs were then costed using standard unit cost figures from the Personal Social Services Research Unit at the University of Kent (Netten et al., 2001). Practitioners were also asked to record the number of hours of 'informal' or unpaid care supplied by family members (and others), and this was costed at the rate of a social care worker. The logic was to record the number of hours that would have had to be supplied to the client if an unpaid carer had not been available. Just as inputs from some types of staff can substitute for inputs from other types (e.g. nursing staff can supply social care inputs), so special equipment can meet a range of needs for an older client, and minimise the need for human intervention. Capital costs for special equipment and adaptations were estimated from standard costings (Netten and Curtis, 2002), converted to weekly costs and added to weekly staff costs to arrive at a total cost estimate per week for each service user.

The six areas that participated in Phase 1 of the RUM development ranged from urban to rural and reflected a mix of socio-economic circumstances. Costings were derived for each of the cases and the relative merits of each approach (SHRUGS and IN) compared in terms of which best predicted resource use. The method chosen was a combination of the two — using the SCRUGS classification tree method (as opposed to a regression model) incorporating items from both the IN and SCRUGS sets of questions.

It was agreed in advance that the final RUM would need to explain at least 30 per cent of the variation[4] in the dependent variable — i.e. cost — in order to be considered a valid and statistically effective tool. The use of an AID (Morgan and Sonquist, 1963) or regression tree approach was preferred to multiple regression (MR) as the data were known to have interactions — e.g. in low-dependency groups, behavioural problems had a large impact on resource use and the need for care, whereas in high-dependency groups, clinical needs had more impact. The AID tree, as opposed to MR, was more suited to classifying cases into groups, as opposed to a continuous score, and yielded a simpler method for practitioners to use in practice. Although we suspected the AID model would be more suitable, we nevertheless compared the proportion of variation in cost explained between MR and AID to allow for the possibility that MR might be a more suitable method.

The software used for the AID analysis was PC-Group, used to develop the RUGS-III classification (Austin Data Management Associates, 1992). For the MR analysis, SPSS's multiple stepwise regression was used (SPSS, 2001). The PC-Group software allows the user to specify the splits required for tree building rather than the process being automatic. This facilitated the incorporation of the views of practitioners into the development of the regression trees. A similar approach has been used previously in the development of iso-resource groups in acute patient care — Diagnosis Related Groups (DRGs) (Bardsley et al., 1987).

[4] Proportion measured by η-squared or r-squared statistic.

3.2 Phase 2 of the RUM Development

The aim of Phase 2 was to arrive at a final version of the RUM, based on a larger study involving a larger number of areas across Scotland. Data were collected on 890 clients receiving care in their own homes. The extension of the RUM to care homes is currently under development. A collaborative approach was again the key to development since the RUM not only had to be a good predictor statistically, but it also had to reflect the views and experience of practitioners involved in planning and delivering care.

Feedback from practitioners indicated that the RUM questions in Phase 1 had to be augmented to better measure the behavioural and mental health issues relevant to a client's need for care. A set of 'mental health and behaviour' questions was developed, while the questions shown to add little to the RUM's ability to predict resource use in Phase 1 were dropped.

The development of an RUM instrument required that only questions yielding reliable and accurate information be included. All the questionnaire items that were candidates for inclusion in the RUM in Phase 2 were assessed for both inter-rater and test-retest reliability.

Once an initial RUM classification had been derived, client rankings were produced and the results discussed with the practitioners who had completed the questionnaires. This allowed the identification of any systematic misclassification of clients' need rankings. Suggestions from practitioners could also be taken back to the statistical analysis and the classification algorithm modified accordingly. Final client rankings were then re-checked for validity.

The validity of the RUM model was checked by splitting the Phase 2 sample into two roughly equal halves, by randomly allocating areas to two sub-samples. Only those variables, which predicted resource use in both sub-samples, were included in the final model.

RUM Data Development

The dataset specification was discussed with practitioners as the study progressed. Practitioners, including front line staff and managers, were asked to describe their information needs. We also consulted senior staff and central government to ascertain their information requirements. The contents of the proposed dataset are outlined in the results and discussion section below.

Model Development

Building statistical models of flows of service users into the care system, and from one dependency state to another allows (a) the information requirements for effective planning to be identified, and (b) the impact of particular sets of assumptions on the system dynamics to be roughly quantified.

The model is not intended as a forecasting tool but a method of exploring some of the system dynamics affected by quality of assessment, provision and rehabilitation. Forecasting models, e.g. Wittenberg (1998), use estimates of static populations from surveys and censuses, together with estimates of need to arrive at demand forecasts. Our model tracks groups of clients through a simple model of a care system to estimate the effect of variations in some key parameters, whose initial values we have had to guesstimate. Changes in the numbers of elderly people in different age groups and trends in the levels of dependency are not investigated.

The model shows the flows of clients into the system and their flow into low and then high dependency and consequently into home or residential care. The model allows for the following factors that may cause inappropriate or inefficient use of resources:

1. low-dependency clients allocated to residential care;
2. residential care causing loss of independence in the less-dependent service user; and
3. there are low rates of recovery for clients moving into higher dependency states.

A basic outline of the model is shown with four stocks — low- and high-dependency receiving care at home (left-hand side of figure A and B) and low- and high-dependency receiving care in a residential setting (mostly residential and nursing homes — known collectively as 'care homes' since April 2003). The model has been developed for the 65–74 age group — a group that should, almost exclusively, be cared for in their own homes.

The rate at which low-dependency clients move into residential care[5] is a function of the effectiveness of support services not only to the client or service user, but also of the presence or absence of a carer and the extent to which they are given adequate backup. The RUM-ICADS dataset is designed to gather limited data on the carer — age, sex, relationship, whether or not they live with the service user (and if not the distance) and the numbers of hours of care provided. The model allows the effect of variations in the size of this flow to be quantified.

We have seen for (1) that this is the case in Scotland.

For assumption (2) that residential care causing loss of independence is difficult to ascertain — there does not seem to be any published literature. The problem is that elderly people are admitted to residential care because of loss of function following illness or injury. It is therefore difficult to

[5] Residential care — for the purposes of this model includes long-stay hospital care, which has, to a large extent, been replaced by nursing home care.

disentangle any loss of function caused by the placement in residential care from the loss of function caused by the incident precipitating the placement. It does seem reasonable to assume that, for the client in the early stages of dementia, the move from home to residential accommodation might result in disorientation, increased likelihood of falls and depression.

The Royal College of Physicians report 'The health and care of older people in care homes' concluded that "the current health and personal care to older people in care homes is unsatisfactory" (Royal College of Physicians, 2000, p. 23). Particular criticisms were directed at inadequate and inconsistent assessment, the provision of health care (surprisingly), and, of relevance to the hypothesised (factor 3), "widespread restrictions on the availability of professional rehabilitative support" (Royal College of Physicians, 2000, para. 2.12). Although this report applied to England, its authors specifically stated its relevance to Scotland (Royal College of Physicians, 2000, para. 1.7), although no Scottish evidence was cited.

There is literature showing that hospitalisation has a negative impact on the functional status of elderly people (Creditor, 1993; Covinsky et al., 2002), although in the 65–74 age group there are very few residents in long-stay hospital accommodation.

The published information allowing the parameterisation and construction of a flow model is inadequate. There is no published information or known national datasets in Scotland which

- describe the dependency of need status of the elderly by age group for residential care settings;
- describe the chance of an elderly person of moving from one dependency status to another within a specified time period in different settings;
- describe the chance of people in different dependency/need groups being admitted to residential care; and
- record mortality by dependency or need group.

An initial model was set up for the 65–74 age group — shown in Appendix 2. The model shows the following stocks and flows:

- Flow 1 (into stock A) — the number of clients becoming dependent in any year — it is assumed that they are initially cared for at home.
- Stock A — number of clients cared for at home with low dependency.
- Flow 2 (from stock A) — the number of low-dependency clients becoming independent — this is partly a function of the effectiveness of rehabilitation services and of client characteristics.
- Stock B — high dependency and care at home.

- Flow 3a & 3b — the number from stock A to stock B — becoming high dependency at home and the reverse flow.
- Flow 4 — from stock A to stock C — low-dependency transfer to long-stay residential care — it is assumed that this is a one-way flow — i.e. that few clients transfer back to their own homes from long-stay residential care.
- Stock C — low dependency in residential care.
- Stock D — high dependency in residential care.
- Flow 5 — from stock B to stock D — high-dependency transfer to residential care. As for flow 4, this is assumed to be a one-way flow.
- Flow 6a & 6b — the number from stock C to stock D — becoming high dependency in residential care, and the reverse flow.
- Each stock has an associated flow for (a) mortality and (b) to allow 65–74 year olds to move to the 75+ age group.
- The unit of time adopted was a year — i.e. the model cycles through on an annual basis.
- Flows are generated by the product of an annual probability and the numbers in the stock from which the flow originates.

The approach adopted was to set up an initial run using any existing data to estimate flows and start values for stocks — see Appendix 3. A set up of the model was sought which, as far as possible, was in stasis for the main stocks — A, B, C and D. The model has several parameters, which could then be varied to judge the effects on the stocks:

- *Transfer gearing* describes the extent to which the flow from low to high dependency (from A to B and from C to D) is higher than the reverse flows. The value of this figure reflects, for a given case mix of low-dependency clients, the effectiveness of rehabilitation arrangements. The initial steady-state model value was set at 0.55 — i.e. the probability of moving from high to low dependency was 55 per cent of the low to high move in any year.
- *Dep factor* — or dependency factor — reflects the extent to which the chance of moving from low to high dependency may be higher in residential settings — see above.
- *Lodeptoindeppropn* — the chance of moving from low dependency to independence. *Dep factor* reduces this for clients in residential care. This proportion reflects the case mix of clients and the effectiveness of rehabilitation.
- *Restransferlodep6574* — the chance of those in stock A — low-dependency home care — moving to residential care. This was set at a low value of 0.06 per cent per annum — largely reflecting severe constraints of provision and the absence of public funding for this option.

4. Results and Discussion

4.1 RUM Development

The AID method was tested for ability to predict resource use compared to the MR method — in the whole study population they were similar in that they both explained 30 per cent of the variation in resource use. However, an analysis splitting the Phase 2 study sample into two groups showed that the MR model variables, except ADL, were different in each sub-sample — i.e. that the MR model was overfitted and idiosyncratic. The RUM model had better split-half reliability. The ADL model showed that there were interactions in the data — different variables explained variation within the three primary ADL groups identified by PC-Group (see below and Appendix 1), and, given the poor split-half reliability and the interactions, the AID model was preferred. Only those variables shown to be predictors of resource use in both sub-samples were used in the RUM tree.

The final RUM tree is shown in Appendix 1. The most important predictor was the ADL score, which was a summary of three questions on — eating, moving position and using the toilet. The ADL score was used to split the sample into three groups — low, medium and high ADL groups. The low ADL group split on a personal care score — developed to measure ability to perform basic self-care tasks, the medium ADL group split on a mental health and behaviour scale and the high ADL group (the most dependent) split on a question on whether help was required to maintain bowel function — shown to be a marker for a range of other clinically related needs.

Discussions with local assessment teams of the initial RUM algorithm revealed some problems with how it classified clients with low physical dependency, who also had cognitive and behavioural problems. Following amendments to the RUM (to make sure cognitive difficulties in performing ADL tasks were taken into account), final client rankings were checked with the professionals in each local assessment team. The number of clients whose relative (to other clients covered by the assessment team) need ranking was erroneous, was minimal — the validity of the RUM was confirmed by the practising professional assessors of client needs.

Data quality was generally good. The percentage agreement between raters was 70 per cent or better on items included in the RUM. The percentage agreement on test retest was slightly higher, in general better than 75 per cent. One question relating to emotional and psychological needs had a low reliability — possibly due to its subjective nature — and was excluded from the analysis.

The use of the AID approach allowed the final RUM instrument to be pared down to the bare minimum of questions (only 12 were included in the final version) as only those variables adding to the explanatory power of the 'tree' were included. This allowed our target of the 5 min completion time to be easily achieved, many practitioners reporting completion in substantially less time once they had become accustomed to it.

4.2 Development of an Integrated Information System for Care of the Elderly

In order for information to support the modelling of care patterns and the forecasting of demand for services, it has to describe the pathways of care rather than simple counts at census points. Data have to be person-based and be capable of being linked both through time and across service boundaries. In order to fulfil this requirement, the information must

- be person based;
- match need to service provision;
- be based on common definitions of person characteristics (age, sex, level of need, geography, etc.), circumstances (e.g. lives alone, with carer, etc.) and service use (often defined differently in different areas); and
- use a common identification number/ID to allow the linkage of person-based information across service boundaries, between areas and over time.

The Scottish Executive has circulated a discussion document concerning the development of such a person-based data set (Scottish Executive, 2003a). This document proposes that the 'Resource Use Measure Integrated Care Assessment Data Summary' (RUM-ICADS) should record demographic details, services used (both NHS and local authority), RUM score and carer details (including carer workload). It is envisaged that the use of a common identifier would facilitate linkage of hospital episodes and NHS primary care data. The development of common data standards will allow the collection and collation of standardised client history data across service boundaries.

NHSScotland has developed the Community Health Index (CHI) system to give all patients a common ID number for use across primary, community and hospital care settings. The CHI numbers function as a unique patient identifier (UPI) for the Scottish population as a whole. However, local authority service user identifiers are still allocated locally. In some areas of Scotland, common IT systems have been set up to allow a translation between local authority service user identifiers and the NHS CHI to allow information sharing.

The Social Care Data Standards Project was set up by the Scottish Executive to provide a common set of definitions and standards to enable the collection and sharing of data across Scotland between NHS and local government — i.e. social work and housing departments (Scottish Social Care Data Standards Project, 2003).

The RUM-ICADS information and associated systems could support the delivery of integrated care to clients and patients and answer the following key questions:

- Can care resources across the domestic, residential and hospital sectors be more appropriately and effectively utilised?
- Are there systematic inequities in access to services by area, sex, ethnic group and socio-economic group?
- What are the care pathways in the elderly care sector and the flows associated with them — e.g. from care at home, to acute hospital, to residential setting?
- What are the outcomes associated with different types of care for clients with differing types of dependency and socio-economic circumstances?

4.3 Models

Steady state — the models were run for a period of 14 years. Many attempts, using Ithink, were made to find a perfect steady-state model, but none were entirely successful. The one given represents the best model resulting in a largely steady state for residential populations.

Steady-State Model

	Home		Residential					
	High Dependency	Low Dependency	High Dependency	Low Dependency	Home Total	Residential Total	High Dependency Total	Low Dependency Total
Initial	21,000	88,000	7,453	2,763	109,000	10,216	28,453	90,763
Year 14	20,401	82,733	7,617	2,732	103,134	10,349	28,018	85,465
% change	−2.85	−5.99	2.20	−1.12	−5.38	1.30	−1.53	−5.84

Note: Variable settings: transfer gearing = 0.55 per cent, dep factor = 1.5 per cent, and lodeptoindeppropn = 8.8 per cent.

Neutral dep factor — the model was then rerun to see the effect of a neutral 'dep factor' — i.e. that the chance of moving from (a) low dependency to high dependency and (b) low dependency to independence is the same for home-based care and residential care.

Neutral 'Dep Factor'

	Home		Residential					
	High Dependency	Low Dependency	High Dependency	Low Dependency	Home Total	Residential Total	High Dependency Total	Low Dependency Total
Initial	21,000	88,000	7,453	2,763	109,000	10,216	28,453	90,763
Year 14	20,401	82,733	6,982	2,810	103,134	9,792	27,383	85,543
% change	−2.85	−5.98	−6.32	1.68	−5.38	−4.15	−3.76	−5.75

A small to moderate change can be seen in the numbers of high-dependency residents.

Improvement in rehabilitation — the proportion of low-dependency service users returned to independence was changed from 8.8 per cent in the steady-state model to 15 per cent. There are no published data allowing an estimate to be made for this parameter. However, a Finnish study of rehabilitation of elderly patients with dementia following hip fracture (Huusko et al., 2000) — a very dependent group — reported the proportion of the intervention group who received 'active' rehabilitation, 'living independently'[6] after 3 months were: (a) 91 per cent of those with moderate dementia, and (b) 63 per cent of those with moderate dementia. Although the numbers in the study were small, it does not seem reasonable to hope that 15 per cent of those clients in the low-dependency group receiving home care might be restored to functional independence in a period of a year.

The model shows not only that the balance of need/dependency in residential care swings towards the high-dependency group, i.e. better use is made of this scarce resource, but also that the numbers in the high-dependency group declines. There is an argument to be made in many health and social care settings that early intervention may avoid deterioration of the patient or client's ability to function.

Rehabilitation Percentage at 15 per cent

	Home		Residential					
	High Dependency	Low Dependency	High Dependency	Low Dependency	Home Total	Residential Total	High Dependency Total	Low Dependency Total
Initial	21,000	88,000	7,453	2,763	109,000	10,216	28,453	90,763
Year 14	17,110	67,121	6,015	1,991	84,231	8,006	23,125	69,112
% change	−18.52	−23.73	−19.30	−27.94	−22.72	−21.64	−18.73	−23.85

[6] 'Living independently' was not defined clearly in terms of level of social care at home.

5. Conclusions

The collection of reliable person-based service use and dependency data is (a) possible, and (b) can be a vital tool in service planning for the elderly.

The RUM tool can be used to place elderly service users in relative need groups quickly and the classification is fully endorsed by practitioners as a valid tool. It can form part of an information set that could provide valuable person-based care histories, linking need to service use through time.

The construction of flow models linking levels of need and service use requires data to estimate initial stock levels and rates of flow. Published statistics in Scotland provide some data on populations in residential accommodation but few data are available on levels of need for different groups of service user in the community, or on people's care pathways. The UK Treasury's Wanless report on the long-term future of health care in the UK "considered it vital to extend its terms of reference to begin to consider social ca*re" but reported that it did not have the information to allow it (Wanless, 2002, p. 120). The development of improved integrated information systems is essential to allow monitoring of equity and efficiency, best use of scarce resources, and planning for future needs.

The models showed potential in allowing the impact of differences in rehabilitation and effectiveness of care for the less dependent to be seen. The impact of a relatively small improvement in levels of rehabilitation had a significant impact on numbers in residential care and their level of dependency.

References

Austin Data Management Associates. (1992). *PC-Group User's Guide, Version 3.01*, Austin.

Bardsley, M., Coles, J. and Jenkins, L. (eds). (1987). *DRGs and Health Care: The Management of Case Mix*, King Edward's Hospital Fund for London, London.

Bond, J. and Carstairs, V. (1982). *Services for the Elderly.* Scottish Health Service studies, no. 42, Scottish Home and Health Department, Edinburgh.

Covinsky, K., Palmer, R., Fortinsky, R., Counsell, S., Stewart, A., Kresevic, D., Burant, C. and Landefeld, C. (2002). Loss of Independence in Activities of Daily Living in Older Adults Hospitalised with Medical Illnesses: Increased Vulnerability with Age. *Journal of the American Geriatrics Society*, 51, 1451–1458.

Creditor, M.C. (1993). Hazards of Hospitalisation of the Elderly. *Annals of Internal Medicine*, 118, 219–223.

General Register Office (Scotland). (2003). *Scottish Census Results on Line (SCROL).* <http://www.scrol.gov.uk/scrol/common/home.jsp>, GRO(S), Table S232, Edinburgh.

Huusko, T.M., Karrpi, P., Avikaineen, V., Kautiainen, H. and Sulkava, R. (2000). Randomised, Clinically Controlled Trial of Intensive Geriatric Rehabilitation in Patients with Hip Fracture: Subgroup Analysis of Patients with Dementia. *BMJ*, 321, 1107–1111.

Isaacs, B. and Neville, Y. (1975). *The Measurement of Need in Old People.* Scottish Health Service Studies, no. 34, Scottish Home and Health Department, Edinburgh.

ISD Scotland. (2003). *Scottish Health Resource Utilisation Groups and Scottish Care Resource Utilisation Groups — Statistical Report 2001—02.* <http://www.show.scot.nhs.uk/isd/joint_futures/shrugs/shrugs_report_contents.htm>, ISD Scotland, Edinburgh.

ISD Scotland. (2004). *Scottish Health Resource Utilisation Groups and Scottish Care Resource Utilisation Groups — Statistical Report 2002–03*, forthcoming, ISD Scotland, Edinburgh.

Joint Future Group. (2000). *Report of the Joint Future Group*, Scottish Executive, Edinburgh.

Morgan, J.N. and Sonquist, J.A. (1963). Problems in the Analysis of Survey Data, and a Proposal. *Journal of the American Statistical Association*, 58, 415–434.

Netten, A. and Curtis, L. (2002). *Unit Costs of Health and Social Care 2002.* Personal and Social Services Research Unit, University of Kent at Canterbury.

Netten, A., Rees, A. and Harrison, G. (2001). *Unit Costs of Health and Social Care 2001.* Personal and Social Services Research Unit, University of Kent at Canterbury.

Richmond, B. (2001). *An Introduction to Systems Thinking.* High Performance Systems Inc., Hanover (NH,USA).

Royal College of Physicians. (2000). *The Health and Care of Older People in Care Homes*, Royal College of Physicians, London.

Scottish Executive. (2002a). *A Report on the Development of a Resource Use Measure for Scotland*, Scottish Executive, Edinburgh.

Scottish Executive. (2002b). *Scottish Community Care Statistics 2001*, Scottish Executive, Edinburgh, p. 1.

Scottish Executive. (2003a). *Joint Future: Data Strategy Resource Use Measure (RUM) and the Integrated Care Assessment Data Summary* (*RUM-ICADS*) <http://www.scotland.gov.uk/consultations/health/rumc-01.asp>, Scottish Executive, Edinburgh.

Scottish Executive. (2003b). *Joint Future Website.* <http://www.scotland.gov.uk/health/jointfutureunit/singshareass.asp>, Scottish Executive, Edinburgh.

Scottish Social Care Data Standards Project. (2003). Home page, http://www.show.scot.nhs.uk/scds/.

SPSS (2001). *SPSS for Windows Version 10.1.* SPSS Inc., Chicago.

The Royal Commission on Long Term Care. (1999). *With Respect to Old Age: Long Term Care — Rights and Responsibilities — A Report by The Royal Commission on Long Term Care*, Cm 4192, TSO, London.

Urquhart, J., Kennie, D., Murdoch, P.S., Smith, R. and Lennox, I. (1999). Costing for Long Term Care: The Development of Scottish Health Service Resource Utilization Groups as a Case Mix Instrument. *Age and Ageing*, 28, 187–192.

Wanless, D. (2002). *Securing Our Future Health: Taking a Long Term View*, HM Treasury, London.

Wittenberg, R. (1998). *Demand for Long-Term Care: Projections of Long-Term Finance for Elderly People.* Personal and Social Services Research Unit, University of Kent at Canterbury, Canterbury.

Appendix 1: RUM Classification Tree

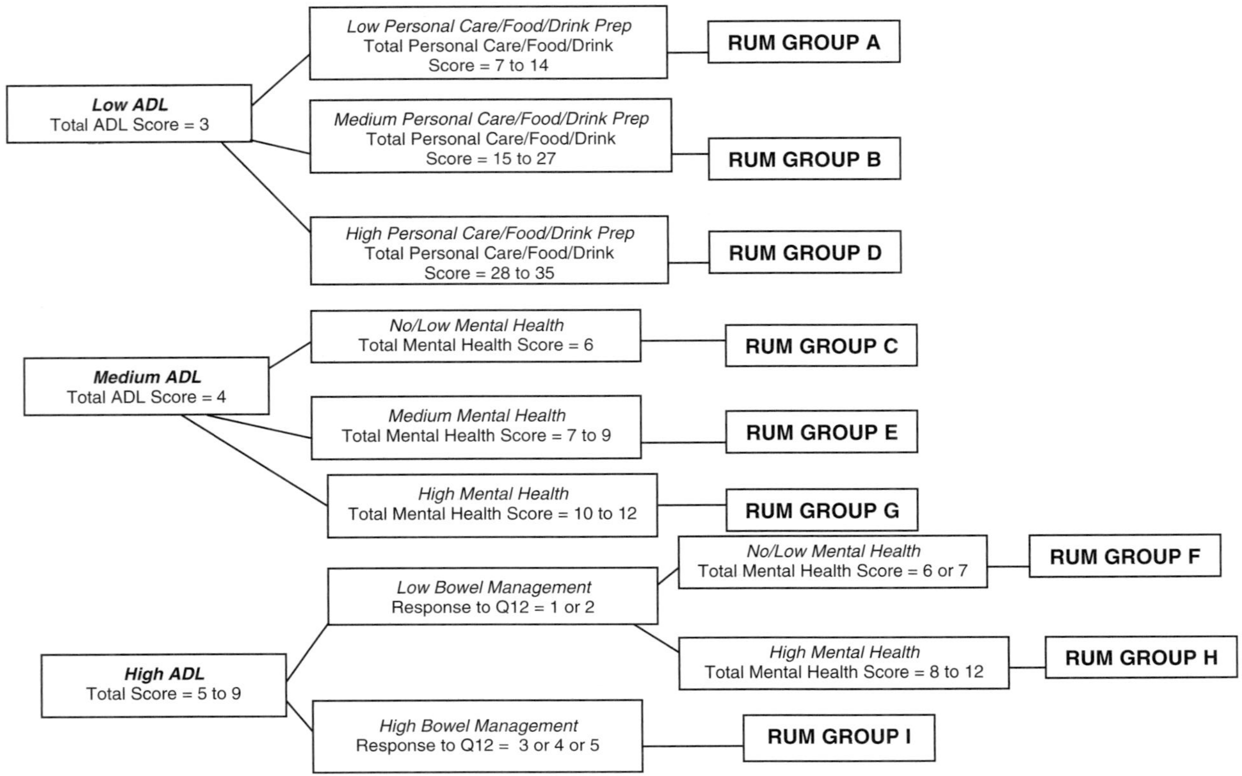

Appendix 2: Care Model Ages 65–74

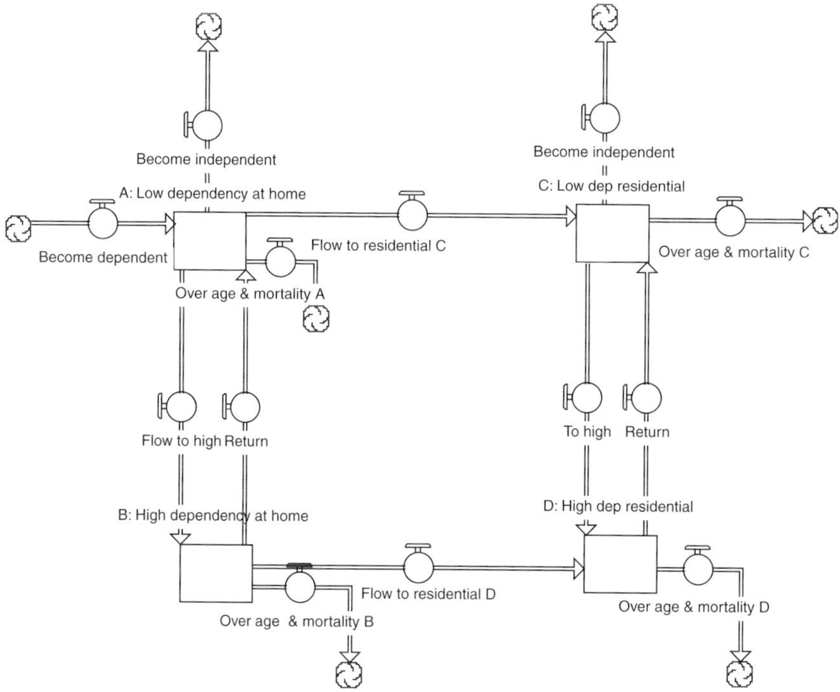

Figure 1: Outline model

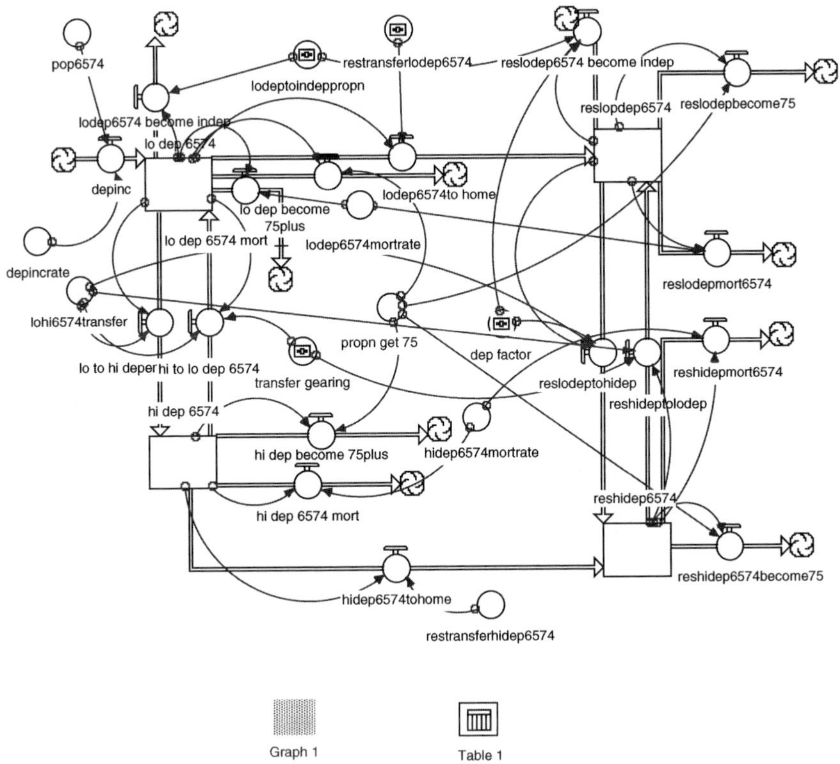

Figure 2: Detail model

Appendix 3: Parameters for Model

The model was developed using ***Ithink*** software (Richmond, 2001).

Flow 1 — the number of clients becoming dependent in any year (**depinc**): the flow is the product of the population as at 2001 (left constant) and the incidence rate — set at 2.5 per cent per annum. In England, the proportion of those aged 65–74 assessed in 2001–2002 and receiving new services was approximately 2.5 per cent of the age group.[7] If we assume that 50 per cent

[7] Department of Health. (2002). *Community Care Statistics 2001–02: Referrals, Assessments and Packages of Care for Adults — Report of findings from the second year of RAP*, <http://www.doh.gov.uk/public/comcare2002/ccstats2002.htm#key>, DoH, London.

of those needing services do not apply and receive services from family or privately, then we have 5 per cent incidence per year.

Stock A — number of clients cared for at home with low dependency (**lodep6574**): the proportion of 'not good health and limiting long-term illness' of the 2001 census for 60–64 was similar to that for 65–84 (in households) at around 20 per cent.[8] The Clackmannan study long-interval dependency for 65–69s was 30 per cent — including some in residential care.[9] The initial value was set at 20 per cent of the 2001 population.

Flow 2 — the number of low-dependency clients — stock A — becoming independent (**lodep6574 become indep**) — this is partly a function of the effectiveness of rehabilitation services and of client characteristics. The proportion of stock A becoming independent (**lodeptoindeppropn**) per annum was set to 8.8 per cent in the steady-state model.

Stock B — high dependency and care at home (**hidep6574**): the initial value was based on numbers in the short and critical dependency categories from the Clackmannan study, i.e. 4.7 per cent of the population = 20,680.

Flow 3a & 3b — the number from stock A to stock B becoming high dependency at home and the reverse flow (**lo to hi dependency 6574 hi to lo dep 6574**). No satisfactory estimates could be found for these flows. The model assumes that 15 per cent of those in low-dependency move into the high-dependency group in any year. The literature puts the average survival from the onset of dementia at around 5 years — which seems a good marker condition. The setting of the transfer proportion (**lohi6574transfer**) at 10 per cent assumes around 50 per cent of those in the group will become high dependency within a 5-year period. The flow in the reverse order is reduced by a variable factor — the transfer gearing; 55 per cent of flow 3a was the setting for the steady-state model. This factor will vary according to the efficacy of rehabilitation. Rehabilitation will be more effective following dependency due to trauma than where it is due to dementia or stroke.

Flow 4 — from stock A to stock C — low-dependency transfer to residential care (**lodep6574tohome**). The overall rate of transfer (numbers per year) to residential care is severely constrained by the availability of beds, and, in the system overall, may largely be a function of resident mortality. The proportion transferring in one year (**restransferlodep6574**) was set to 0.6 per cent in the steady state and other models.

Stock C — low dependency in residential care (**reslodep6574**) — the numbers in low-dependency groups in hospital care are low but numbers in

[8] General Register Office (Scotland). (2002). *SCROL Census 2001 Website*, <http://www.scrol.gov.uk/scrol/common/home.jsp>, Table CAS019, GRO(S), Edinburgh.

[9] Bond, J. and Carstairs, V. (1982). *Services for the Elderly*, Scottish Health Service studies, No. 42, Scottish Home and Health Department, 32 Edinburgh.

nursing and residential homes[10] are substantial. ISD Scotland SCRUGS and SHRUGS data estimate 27 per cent of nursing home residents and 72 per cent aged 65–74 are in low-dependency groups. Applied to 2001 census data this would mean that 1,763 clients were in this group in 2001.

Stock D — high dependency in residential care (**reshidep6574**) — defined as non-low dependency SCRUGS/SHRUGS groups. The numbers are therefore those in residential care less stock C — 7,453 patients and residents.

Flow 5 — high dependency at home transferring to residential care (**hidep6574tohome**). As for flow 4, this flow is heavily constrained by the availability of places in residential care. The chance of moving from care at home to residential care (**restransferhidep6574**) for this group was set at a very conservative 5 per cent per annum in all models.

Flow 6a & 6b — the number from stock C to stock D — becoming high dependency in residential care, and the reverse flow (**reslodeptohidep, reshideptolodep**). The proportion flowing from C to D is a product of the low- to high-dependency proportion used for the A–B flow, increased by the '*dep factor*' — to account for the hypothesised increased chance of becoming high dependency in residential settings. The flow from D to C is the flow from C to D reduced by the '*transfer gearing*'.

Each stock has an associated flow for (a) mortality and (b) to allow 65–74 year olds to move to the 75+ age group. The mortality level for the low-dependency groups was set at the 2002 Scottish figure for 65–74 year olds, and that for high-dependency clients who are likely to have significant co-morbidities, 50 per cent higher. The figure of 50 per cent may be an underestimate.

[10] Nursing and residential homes are designated 'care homes' — in Scotland.

Chapter 5

Health Status, Health Inequalities and the Ability of Older Australians to Stay in the Labour Force

Agnes Walker[☆]

Australian National University (ANU), Australia

Abstract

This contribution describes one of the few research projects that include health status within a dynamic microsimulation model. It illustrates the usefulness of such an approach through application of that model to the topical issue of longer working lives. First, construction and validation of a new 'health state transition' module are described, together with the way that module has been embedded into a population-wide dynamic microsimulation model. Second, illustrative simulations are carried out assessing the impact on individuals and governments of longer working lives. If, in 1998, 65–70 year olds had the same employment patterns as 45–64 year olds, they would have benefited from additional earnings (wages or salaries) totalling around A$15 billion (A$28 billion in 2018). Also, government expenditures on the age pension would have been around A$2 billion lower (A$4 billion in 2018).

1. Introduction

An issue of concern throughout the developed world is the ageing of populations and the consequent shrinking of the proportion of the 'working-age'

[☆] This paper was prepared as part of the author's PhD project for the National Centre for Epidemiology and Population Health, Australian National University (degree awarded in 2005). Valuable contributions by Professor Niels Becker to the methodologies used in modelling health state transitions are gratefully acknowledged. The author wishes to thank the National Centre for Social and Economic Modelling for making its dynamic microsimulation model, DYNAMOD, available for this PhD project.

International Symposia in Economic Theory and Econometrics, Vol. 16

ISSN: 1571-0386 DOI: 10.1016/S1571-0386(06)16005-6

population. In Australia, the Prime Minister recently called for increases in workforce participation rates, in particular at the mature age end of the population — 55 years and over (Howard, 2003).

Policies to facilitate greater mature age workforce participation have been considered in several developed countries, and in some the official pension age is currently above that in Australia (that is above 65 years). For example, in Norway the official age of retirement is 67 years (Frederiksen and Stolen, 2003). Initiatives in Australia include the gradual alignment of the pension age for men and women to 65 years and the increasing of the vesting age to superannuation, so that the related pension can no longer be accessed at age 55.

In the public debate there seems to be an assumption that if employers needed more workers and the incentives were 'right', then all those currently retired would be able to take on a job. However, over 80 percent of Australians aged 65 years or more have at least one long-term chronic disease (Walker et al., 2003). It is thus likely that, for health reasons, many in that age group will not be able to remain in the workforce.

The key issue addressed in this paper is how health impacts on the ability of older Australians to remain in the labour force. Since presentation of this paper at the 2003 Conference the author carried out further studies on this topic. These are mentioned in later sections, together with references to the related publications.

1.1 Aims

The main aim of this paper is to provide preliminary estimates of the proportion of older Australians, aged 65 to 70, with sufficiently good health to allow them to remain in the workforce. Using these predicted proportions by health status, and under an illustrative scenario, the aim is to estimate:

- How many are likely to work more than 15 h per week under more favourable labour market conditions and/or greater incentives to remain in the workforce;
- What their extra earnings would amount to; and
- What implications this would have for government expenditures on the age pension.

The illustrative scenario is described in Section 7.

1.2 About the Study

We focussed on the 65 to 70 age group because this group is the one expected to have significant employment opportunities as the proportion of the 'younger workforce' in the population declines. For this 65 to 70 age group we defined 'work' as having a paid job for 15 h or more per week.

In this study we made use of a dynamic microsimulation model, DYNAMOD, to which the author had previously added a health-socio-economic status Module (Walker, 2002, 2003). To be able to carry out the analyses planned for this paper, a 'health state transition' Module has also been added (Sections 3 and 4). Addition of that Module allowed the linking of people's ability to work to the severity of their illness.

2. Overview of the Dynamic Microsimulation Model

2.1 The Original Model

The dynamic microsimulation model DYNAMOD[1] to which a health SES module has been added is a model able to project the entire Australian population forward. In the application reported in this paper the model simulates individuals' life cycles from 1986 onwards, with findings reported for 1998, the year for which model results can be compared with official statistics, and a date 20 years later (i.e. 2018).

The model is based on a 1 per cent representative sample of the Australian population (around 150,000 persons) extracted by the Australian Bureau of Statistics (ABS) from its 1986 Census.[2] It was developed over the past decade by the National Centre for Social and Economic Modelling, University of Canberra.

The simulations account for future events occurring in the lives of persons' in the model's Base year population such as: couple formation, birth of a child, education, leaving home, migration, divorce, being employed, income from work and government, wealth accumulation, becoming disabled (0,1 variable), recovering from disability,[3] and death. In recognition of the strong links between disability (which mainly arises from disabling chronic

[1] The basic modules constructed during the initial stage of DYNAMOD's development are described in Antcliff et al. (1996). King et al. (1999a) provide an overview of stage 2 of DYNAMOD's development, with details in King et al. (1999b), Abello et al. (2002), King et al. (2002), Robinson and Bækgaard (2002) and Bækgaard (2002 a and b). Stage 3 is described in Kelly (2002, 2003).

[2] With the complete 1 per cent sample the weight for each DYNAMOD person, when estimating total population results, would be 100. However, because some records had been deleted in the model's Base dataset — e.g. in cases of 'non-response' — the weight attached to each person in the model is 103.

[3] For definition of disability see Section 3.

illnesses) and mortality, these two variables are linked in DYNAMOD through a complex set of equations (Walker, 2002).

2.2 The Socioeconomic Status Module

Socioeconomic Status

In the version used in this paper an indicator of socioeconomic status (SES) has been added to the original model. This SES measure was developed so that the two health status indicators already in the model — mortality and disability — could be differentiated by SES. Thus in that version the mortality and disability (0,1 variable) statistics in the input data to DYNAMOD reflected the well-known pattern of poorer Australians becoming disabled and dying at younger ages than better off Australians. Walker (2005a) describes the way SES was accounted for in DYNAMOD's input data, imputed to its Base population and incorporated into its simulation phase. In the enhanced model SES can be accounted for in three different ways:

- Income = Family income (earned + government benefits); or
- Income_Wealth = Family income (earned + government benefits) + annualised wealth); or
- Equivalent Income_Wealth = family income (earned + government benefits) + annualised family wealth)/(equivalence scale factor).[4]

In each simulated year the SES indicator is computed for each family, the population is sorted by that indicator and then divided into five equal parts — the 20 per cent poorest group being labelled SES quintile 1 and the richest 20 per cent SES quintile 5.

In this paper we used the SES indicator based on family income, because at the time of its preparation, the indicators accounting for wealth have not as yet been validated. For older age groups the most appropriate indicator is Equivalent Income_Wealth. This is because this measure accounts for the 'cash poor but asset rich' status of many older Australians, as well as for their smaller family sizes. Relative to use of the 'Income' measure, use of the 'Equivalent Income_Wealth' measure would have resulted in more older people being allocated to the higher quintiles of the income distribution.

[4] The equivalence scale factor equals the sum of 1.0 for the first adult, 0.5 for the second adult and 0.3 for each dependent child.

2.3 The New 'Health State Transition' Module

In the version of DYNAMOD described in Walker (2003) health was indicated by disability — '1' if the person was disabled and '0' otherwise. However, as will be seen in Section 6, many mildly disabled persons are able to have jobs which severely disabled persons can no longer hold. So, to study the employment consequences of ill health we needed to adopt a more complex indicator of health than what was available in the original version of DYNAMOD. In essence, we needed a measure of health status that was also an indicator of functionality — such as ability to cope with work or to live independently.

Section 3 describes the new 'health state transition' Module developed for this paper in which the original (0,1) 'disability' variable was disaggregated into a (0,1,2,3) 'health state' variable, allowing for progression of diseases to more severe stages. This introduced considerable complications into the modelling process. In addition, it required realigning the model to published aggregate statistics by 'health states' (Section 4).

3. Modelling Health State Transitions

3.1 The Available Data

In microsimulation models such as DYNAMOD, changes in individuals' status are usually estimated either through hazard functions or transition probabilities. In the case of 'health states' there are no Australian longitudinal data suitable for estimation of hazard functions that would yield 'duration' till a change of status occurs (from, for example, mild disability to severe disability). Because the ABS only conducts disability surveys at 5-year intervals, matching across individuals over time — as was done when estimating DYNAMOD's labour force transitions using the ABS's monthly labour force surveys — was not possible in our case. Also, while use of multi-decrements technique was possible with the (0,1) specification of disability (and death) in the original model (Antcliff et al., 1996), there was insufficient data for adopting a similar approach at the several 'health state' levels required for our new module. Therefore, the only option for our purposes seems to have been to assign plausible values to health transition probabilities at the multi-health-state level that were consistent with the cross-sectional data embedded in the ABS's 1998 Disability survey. Details of how this was done can be found in Sections 3 and 4.

In the 1998 survey disability is defined as a limitation, restriction or impairment which has lasted or is likely to last for at least six months and restricts every day 'core activities'. These core activities are grouped under the headings of communication, mobility and self care (ABS, 1999b). Each person is classified into one of eight health classes (ABS, 1999a):

1. has disability and is *profoundly* restricted in core activities;
2. has disability and is *severely* restricted in core activities;
3. has disability and is *moderately* restricted in core activities;
4. has disability and is *mildly* restricted in core activities;
5. has disability, *not restricted* in core activities but restricted in schooling or employment;
6. has disability and is *not restricted* in core activities, schooling or employment;
7. has a long-term health condition without disability; and
8. has no long-term health condition.

It is worth noting that, in every day life, even a mild disability will have a highly restricting effect on a person's functionality. Examples of mild disability are an inability to easily walk 200 metres, walk up and down stairs without a handrail, or use public transport.

3.2 The Health States Modelled

In order to limit the complexity of the computation of health status transition probabilities, some grouping of the above eight health classes in the 1998 Disability survey was required. There was also a need to bear in mind the fact that there will be a limit to the degree of disaggregation possible, due to the data being drawn from a sample survey.

Because we expected that estimation of the effects of disability on 'functionality' — that is the ability to cope with work, and/or live independently — will be an important application of DYNAMOD, we chose the following groupings for modelling purposes:

- health_status = 0: 'has no long-term health condition' (Survey class 8);
- health_status = 1: 'has a long-term health condition' and disability with 'no impact on core activities' (classes 5,6,7);
- health_status = 2: 'mild/moderate impact on core activities' (classes 3,4)
- health_status = 3: 'severe/profound impact on core activities' (classes 1,2).

3.3 Methodology for Estimating Transition Probabilities

To estimate transition matrices from the cross-sectional data embedded in the ABS's 1998 Disability survey (ABS, 1999a) we needed to make a few simplifying assumptions. We also needed to show that these assumptions were supported by the available evidence.

Assumption 1: *Age is the key driver of disability*

This assumption is based on the observation that age is the key driver of disability. Evidence for this is presented in Figure 2, Section 5.

Assumption 2: *Steady progression towards severe disability*

Although we only have cross-sectional data, the proportions in Figure 2 (Section 5) present striking evidence that age is the key driver of not only disability but also of its severity. A steady progression from mild versions of a disease to more severe forms as people age has also been demonstrated by longitudinal data collected in some developed countries (such as the extensive longitudinal data on diabetes collected and analysed at the Diabetes Trial Unit, Oxford University, UK).

In developing the new Health Status and Disease Progression Module we assumed that progression of health states always goes from a better health state to a worse one — that is, 'recovery' is not possible. While this assumption is clearly not always correct, 'recovery' at the levels of aggregation we are concerned with is a very rare event.

3.4 Computing Health Transition Probabilities

The four health state classes were disaggregated by age groups: 0–14, 15–24, 25–44; 45–54; 55–64; 65–69; 70–74 and 75+(8 classes)[5]; gender (2 classes) and quintiles SES (5 classes). These levels of disaggregation meant that transition probabilities had to be estimated for $8*5*2 = 80$ groupings (or cells).

Equation (1) illustrates how transition probabilities can be estimated for one particular 'cell': (a) = 45–54 years males in SES quintile 1, moving to the (a + 1) = 55–64 age group.

[5] The age groups were selected so that they matched the groups used in DYNAMOD's Labour force Module (i.e. 15–24, 25–44 and 45+); that they covered all ages (so we added the 0–14 group); and that they were more disaggregated the older people were (since severity of disability increased considerably in older age groups).

The matrix equation for each 'cell' is described in equations (1) and (2).
General Notation, without Assumptions

$$\begin{bmatrix} P[D_{0(a+1)}] \\ P[D_{1(a+1)}] \\ P[D_{2(a+1)}] \\ P[D_{3(a+1)}] \end{bmatrix} \begin{matrix} = \\ = \\ = \\ = \end{matrix} \begin{bmatrix} P[D_{0(a+1)}|D_{0(a)}] & P[D_{0(a+1)}|D_{1(a)}] & P[D_{0(a+1)}|D_{2(a)}] & P[D_{0(a+1)}|D_{3(a)}] \\ P[D_{1(a+1)}|D_{0(a)}] & P[D_{1(a+1)}|D_{1(a)}] & P[D_{1(a+1)}|D_{2(a)}] & P[D_{1(a+1)}|D_{3(a)}] \\ P[D_{2(a+1)}|D_{0(a)}] & P[D_{2(a+1)}|D_{1(a)}] & P[D_{2(a+1)}|D_{2(a)}] & P[D_{2(a+1)}|D_{3(a)}] \\ P[D_{3(a+1)}|D_{0(a)}] & P[D_{3(a+1)}|D_{1(a)}] & P[D_{3(a+5)}|D_{2(a)}] & P[D_{3(a+1)}|D_{3(a)}] \end{bmatrix} \begin{bmatrix} P[D_{0(a)}] \\ P[D_{1(a)}] \\ P[D_{2(a)}] \\ P[D_{3(a)}] \end{bmatrix} \tag{1}$$

Let $P[D_{o(a)}]$ be the probability that a 45–54 years male has no illness/disability, with subscripts 1 … 3 referring to the long-term illness/disabled categories.
$P[D_{o(a+1)}/D_{o(a)}]$ indicate the probability that, when that man progresses to the next age group, he will remain in the no illness/disability class.
$P[D_{1(a+1)}/D_{o(a)}]$ indicate the probability that, when that man progresses to the next age group, he will move to the 'Long-term illness' class, etc.

General Notation, with Assumption that People's Health can only get Worse

$$\begin{bmatrix} P[D_{0(a+1)}] \\ P[D_{1(a+1)}] \\ P[D_{2(a+1)}] \\ P[D_{3(a+1)}] \end{bmatrix} \begin{matrix} = \\ = \\ = \\ = \end{matrix} \begin{bmatrix} P[D_{0(a+1)}|D_{0(a)}] & 0 & 0 & 0 \\ P[D_{1(a+1)}|D_{0(a)}] & P[D_{1(a+1)}|D_{1(a)}] & 0 & 0 \\ P[D_{2(a+1)}|D_{0(a)}] & P[D_{2(a+1)}|D_{1(a)}] & P[D_{2(a+1)}|D_{2(a)}] & 0 \\ P[D_{3(a+1)}|D_{0(a)}] & P[D_{3(a+1)}|D_{1(a)}] & P[D_{3(a+1)}|D_{2(a)}] & P[D_{3(a+1)}|D_{3(a)}] \end{bmatrix} \begin{bmatrix} P[D_{0(a)}] \\ P[D_{1(a)}] \\ P[D_{2(a)}] \\ P[D_{3(a)}] \end{bmatrix} \tag{2}$$

Our assumption that people's health state can only get worse led to many of the conditional probabilities being zeros (equation (2)). Estimation of the probabilities in the first and the last columns of equation (2) could be done using data from the 1998 Disability survey. To obtain estimates of the conditional probabilities in the middle columns, we first used the multiplication theorem of matrix algebra and then assigned plausible values to these probabilities that were consistent with Disability survey statistics. The matrix algebra multiplication equations are:

(i) $P[D_{0(a+1)}] = P[D_{0(a+1)}|D_{0(a)}] * P[D_{0(a)}]$
which can be solved uniquely for $P[D_{0(a+1)}|D_{0(a)}]$

(ii) $P[D_{1(a+1)}] = P[D_{1(a+1)}|D_{0(a)}]*P[D_{0(a)}] + P[D_{1(a+1)}|D_{1(a)}]*P[D_{1(a)}]$

(iii) $P[D_{2(a+1)}] = P[D_{2(a+1)}|D_{0(a)}]*P[D_{0(a)}] + P[D_{2(a+1)}|D_{1(a)}]*P[D_{1(a)}] + P[D_{2(a+1)}|D_{2(a)}]*P[D_{2(a)}]$

(iv) $P[D_{3(a+1)}] = P[D_{3(a+1)}|D_{0(a)}]*P[D_{0(a)}] + P[D_{3(a+1)}|D_{1(a)}]*P[D_{1(a)}] + P[D_{3(a+1)}|D_{2(a)}]*P[D_{2(a)}] + P[D_{3(a+1)}|D_{3(a)}]*P[D_{3(a)}]$

The non-zero transition probability values — obtained partly through the above equations — were estimated using 'trial and error' techniques

Table 1: Example of Transition Probability Matrix: From 45–54 to 55–64 Year Olds

	55–64 YO						45–54 YO
Health states			$\mid D_{0(a)}$	$\mid D_{1(a)}$	$\mid D_{2(a)}$	$\mid D_{3(a)}$	
No illness	0.201	0.201	0.634	0.000	0.000	0.000	0.317
LT illness	0.310	0.310	0.327	0.950	0.000	0.000	0.218
Mild disability	0.309	0.309	0.030	0.030	0.980	0.000	0.299
Severe disability	0.180	0.180	0.009	0.020	0.020	1.000	0.167
Sum	1.000	1.000	1.000	1.000	1.000	1.000	1.000

ensuring that the transition probabilities for each 'transition' column summed to 1.00. Results for one of the 80 tables — males in quintile 1 moving from the 45–54 year age group to the 55–64 age group — are in Table 1.

The first and last shaded columns contain actual probabilities (i.e. population proportions from the 1998 Disability survey — e.g. 20.1 per cent of 55–64 year olds had no long-term illness or disability), while the second shaded column contains the estimated 'matrix algebra' products based on the 45–54 age group's actual probabilities (last shaded column). We estimated the non-zero conditional probabilities so that their 'matrix algebra' product with the 45–54 (a) age group's probabilities (second shaded column) amounted to a value close to the known 55–64 (a + 1) probabilities (first shaded column). The fact that the numbers in the first and second shaded columns are equal thus means that, in this example, our matrix algebra estimates exactly matched the actual 55–64 age group's probabilities.[6]

3.5 Implementation in the Model

Input Data

An additional input dataset has been added to DYNAMOD which contains the transition probabilities from the 80 tables (example given in Table 1). In that input dataset the probabilities have been arranged in a cumulative format. For example, considering the |D0(a) column of Table 1, the

[6] While close to exact matches were obtained for most of the tables, in some instances this was not possible. This occurred in particular in the younger low disability groups — e.g. when moving from the higher severe disability state of 0–14 year olds to a lesser disability state in the 15–24 age group — e.g. due to children outgrowing disabilities such as those due to asthma.

probabilities are presented as 0.634, then $(0.634+0.327)=0.961$, then $(0.961+0.03)=0.991$ and $(0.991+0.009)=1.000$.

Implementation in the Base Data of the Model

To the Base data of the model — based on the 1986 Census — we needed to impute the health states from the 1998 Disability survey (ABS, 1999a) by age, sex and SES. That provided each person in the Base dataset with a starting health status. At this stage new born babies and immigrants entering Australia were allocated a health status of '0' (i.e. 'No illness or disability').

Implementation in the Simulation Part of the Model

In each simulation year DYNAMOD was re-programmed to assess, using random numbers within set limits, whether the health state of each person entering the next health transition age group would change or not. The eight age groups used for these computations were listed in Section 3.

Using the example in Table 1 and the related cumulative probabilities, a man without illness who just reached age 55 would be studied in DYNAMOD by comparing a (0 to 1) random number to the cumulative brackets specified in the input data. Thus, if the random number fell below 0.634, then there would be no change in that man's health state. If however it fell between 0.634 and 0.961 then there would be a change in his health state to having at least one long-term illness — and so on.

4. Calibration of the Health State Transition Module

DYNAMOD has been calibrated in a number of respects by earlier researches— see footnote 1 and Walker (2003). In this section, we describe calibration of the new work carried out for this paper.

Calibration of the model by health status involved a set of complex processes. First, the 'health states' imputed to the 1986 base population of DYNAMOD had to be calibrated, so that in 1998 the simulated distribution of 'health states' broadly matched the actual distribution in the 1998 Disability survey (ABS, 1999a).

Second, the transitions in the simulation phase of the model from one health state to the next had to be calibrated, so that progression of health states from one severity level to another were broadly in line with observed trends.

The trend across four disability surveys (1981, 1988, 1993 and 1998) indicated steadily *increasing* disability rates — from 14.6 per cent in 1981 to 18.8 per cent in 1998 (ABS, 1999c). The ABS reported that the greater part of the increase between 1993 (from 17.2 per cent) and 1998 (to 18.8 per cent) was for people with severe and profound restrictions (ABS, 1999c). At a later date the Australian Institute of Health and Welfare examined the trends across the ABS's 1993 and 1998 Disability surveys. It noted that, while the surveys showed an increase in disability prevalence rates between 1993 and 1998, much of that increase was due to changes in the design and methods of the 1998 survey. It also noted that prevalence rates of severe or profound restriction were relatively stable during the 1980s and early 1990s (AIHW, 2001).

On the basis of the above, we calibrated DYNAMOD so that its simulated 1998 disability rates, which were broadly in line with data in ABS (1999a), remained virtually unchanged throughout each year of the simulation period. The implication of this is that in our simulations we have essentially assumed that disability rates changed very little over time. Should there be interest at a later date in studying scenarios in which disability rates drifted either upward (e.g. through the impact of higher obesity rates), or downward (e.g. through slower progression to higher severity states due to earlier detection and better management of chronic diseases, or improved medical technology), then the model would need to be re-calibrated.

Comparisons of the simulated distributions of the population in 1998 by health status with published ABS statistics for the same year are in Figure 1. These indicate that the calibration process achieved a reasonable match.

5. Australians' Health Status by Age and Socioeconomic Status

In this section we examine data from the 1998 Disability survey to provide a background for the scenario analysed later in the paper. The survey data show that the vast majority of disability is caused by illness (ABS, 1999a). Out of the 3.6 million persons disabled in 1998, only 245,000 arose from 'Injury/poisoning/other external causes'. Some 3 million were due to physical illnesses — e.g. 1.2 million to musculo-skeletal diseases (of which half a million was due to arthritis); a quarter of a million to respiratory diseases (of which 170,000 was due to asthma); and to diseases of the eye (180,000). In addition there were some 600,000 persons with 'mental and behavioural diseases' as their 'main disabling condition'. Overall, in 1998, 78 per cent of people with a severe or profound core activity restriction had a physical disorder as their main disabling condition (ABS, 1999c).

5.1 Health by Age

The Disability survey data show that in 1998 the vast majority of Australians were healthy, not having either a long-term condition or a disability (12 million out a total of 18.7 million); that around 3 million had at least one

Figure 1: Proportion of the Australian Population by Health Status, ABS Survey and DYNAMOD, 1998

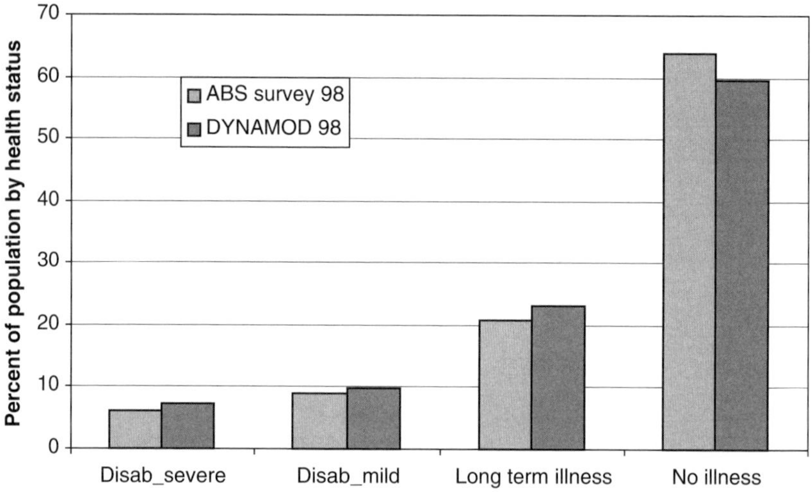

Sources: 1998 Disability survey (ABS, 1999a) and simulations with DYNAMOD
Note: The 'No illness' health state comprises people with neither long-term illness nor disability — see Section 3.

long-term condition without disability; and that 3.6 million were disabled, representing 19 per cent of the Australian population (ABS, 1999a). Among the latter around 800,000 were not restricted in everyday activities, one million were moderately or mildly restricted, and the remainder were severely or profoundly restricted.

Unlike in the rest of this paper, in Figure 2 we grouped the various health states available from the 1998 Disability survey into five categories: survey classes (1,2) for the disabled with severe restrictions; classes (3,4) for the disabled with mild restrictions; classes (5,6) for the disabled with no restrictions; class (7) for those with long-term illness; and class (8) for people with no long-term illness or disability. The only difference here is that we separately identified those disabled who did not experience any restrictions in core activities. Using this classification allowed us to ascertain that the vast majority of people classified as disabled in the survey have also experienced restrictions to some extent.

Figure 2 graphically illustrates that age is the key determinant of the health of Australians, as well as of the degree of severity of their illnesses. It shows that up to age 50 over half of Australians have no long-term illnesses or disability. Between 50 and 85 years, however, the proportions with long-term illness and with disability increase rapidly. Severity of disability also

Figure 2: Proportion of the population by age and health status, 1998

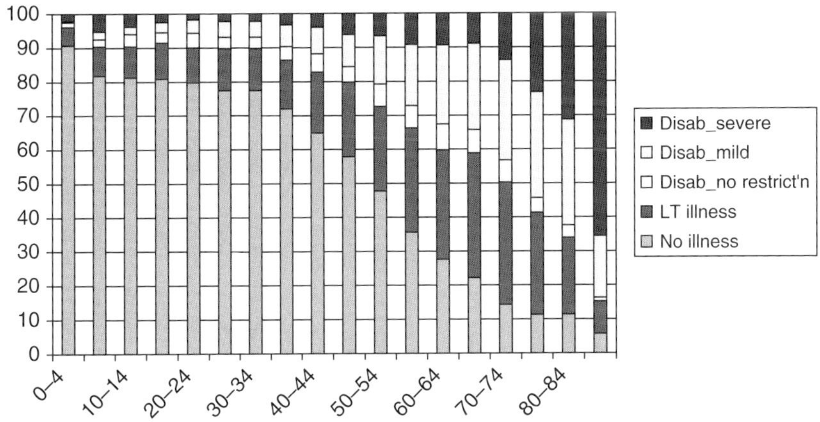

Source: Author's computations using unit record survey data in ABS (1999a)
Note: The severity groupings are survey classes (1,2) for Disab_severe; (3,4) for Disab_mild; (5,6) for Disab_no restriction; (7) for long-term illness; and (8) for no illness — see Section 3.

clearly increases with age since, by age 85 or above, the majority (65 per cent) in that group were severely disabled — up from 30 per cent for the previous age group (80–84). An important feature of the pattern in Figure 2 is that, for the 85+ age group, most of the dramatic increase in the proportion of severely disabled arose from considerable declines in the proportion of those mildly disabled and those with long-term health conditions.

6. Australians' Health and Employment

There is considerable international literature — summarised by Bradbury et al. (2001) — on the correlation between severe disability and low labour force participation, low employment rates, low income and poverty.

We examined the 1998 Disability survey and found that virtually no 65–70 year olds worked more than 15 h per week (Table 2). Next, we studied the relationship in 1998 between the health of 45–64 year olds, their SES, and whether they worked more than 15 h per week (Figure 3).

A striking feature of Figure 3 is that, regardless of their health status, only a very small proportion of 45–64 year olds in the lowest SES quintile worked more than 15 h per week. By comparison well over 80 per cent of people in the top SES quintile worked more than 15 h per week, most of them with either no illnesses, or with at least one long-term illness. The differences

Table 2: Proportion of 45–64 Year Olds by Health Status and SES and whether Working for more than 15 H per week, 1998

	Disability severe[a]			Disability mild[a]			Long–term illness[a]			No illness[a]		
	Work (%)	No work (%)	All (%)	Work (%)	No work (%)	All (%)	Work (%)	No work (%)	All (%)	Work (%)	No work (%)	All (%)
SES quintiles												
INC_Q1	2.6	97.4	100	7.3	92.7	100	15.1	84.9	100	19.8	80.2	100
INC_Q2	8.8	91.2	100	23.3	76.7	100	38.5	61.5	100	47.0	53.0	100
INC_Q3	35.5	64.5	100	56.3	43.7	100	64.9	35.1	100	74.2	25.8	100
INC_Q4	60.1	39.9	100	73.0	27.0	100	78.5	21.5	100	83.5	16.5	100
INC_Q5	64.7	35.3	100	76.6	23.4	100	87.4	12.6	100	90.9	9.1	100
All quints	18.0	82.0	100	31.8	68.2	100	58.0	42.0	100	70.1	29.9	100

Source: Author's computations from the unit record files of the 1998 Disability survey — ABS 1999a

[a] *The groupings are: Disability severe and profound restriction; Disability mild and moderate restriction; Long-term illness and disability without restriction; No illness or disability — see definitions in Section 3.*

Figure 3: Proportion of 45–64 Year Olds Working (0–15 h/wk), and not Working (16 h/wk or more) by SES (%)

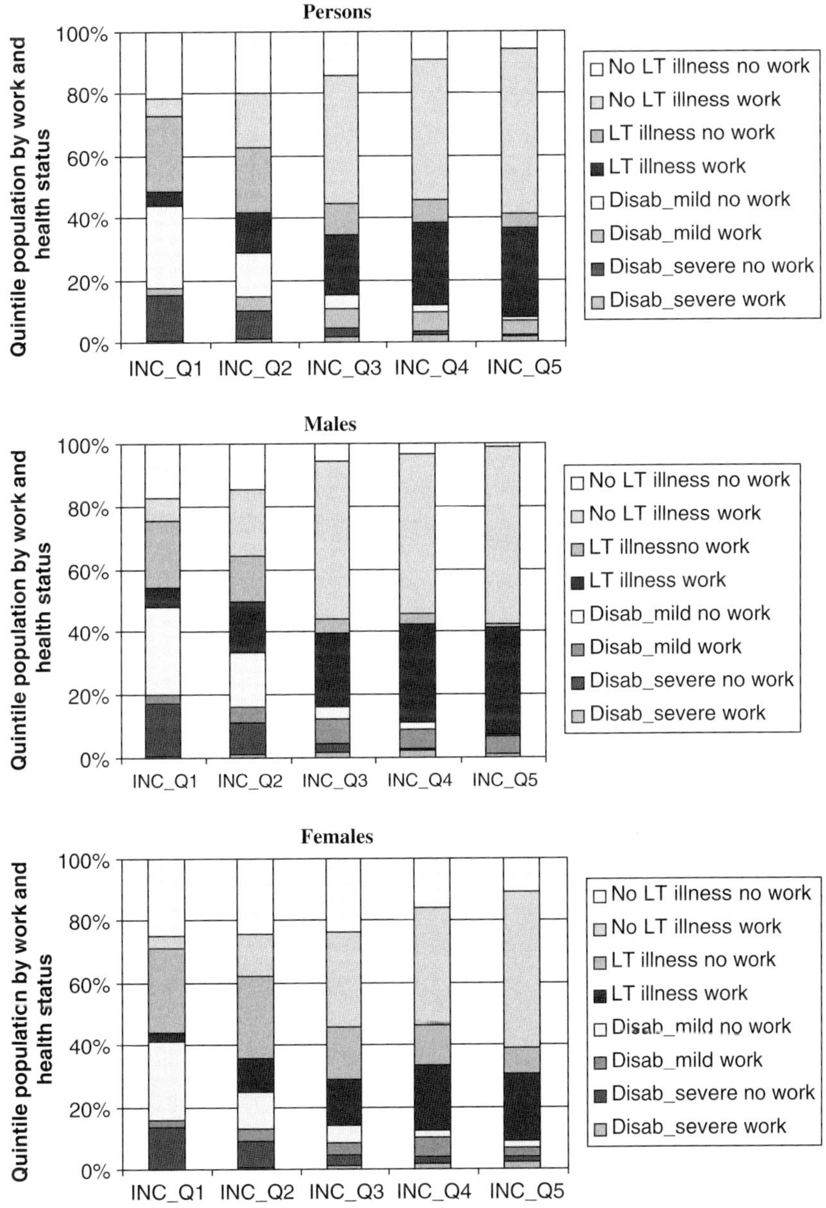

between men and women were also striking, with a significantly higher proportion of men 'working' in that age group (especially those with no illness or with at least one long-term illness).

7. Results: Illustrative Scenario

Projections of health status, which are rarely reported in the literature, were carried out for this application through simulations by DYNAMOD. An advantage of using a health-status-enhanced dynamic microsimulation model was that projections of health status could be carried out at the level of the individual, and in a manner consistent with projections of other personal characteristics that people and families consider when making work–retirement choices.

In this section we distinguish between people aged 65–70 who are able to continue to work, and people who are not able to do so due to ill health. We do this through simulations of the illustrative 'Improved Employment Access' scenario. Under this scenario 65–70 year olds are assumed to have the same employment patterns in 1998 as 45–64 year olds within the same health-SES group. These patterns were presented in Table 2. A more sophisticated way of predicting an individual's work status was developed *after* presentation of this paper. It used logistic regressions to account for own health, sex, SES, and whether had spouse and/or dependents played a role in the decision of whether to remain in the workforce (Walker, 2004, 2005a).

The first two subsections below report on the numbers projected by health state for the Australian population, and for 65–70 year olds. Further subsections provide estimates of the additional earnings of 65–70 year olds under the scenario and of the consequent savings by government on state pension expenditures.

7.1 Actual and Predicted Distribution of the Australian Population by Health Status

Figure 4 shows that while the simulation results exhibit a broadly similar pattern to that evident in the ABS (1999a) survey, they reallocate a small proportion of people from the 'No illness' category to the 'Long-term illness' grouping.

The proportions of the groups with disability remain stable over time — very close to the proportions in the survey. Although it would have been possible to refine the calibration of the model to more closely match the non-disabled proportions to those in the survey, it was not considered necessary to do so. This was partly because our analyses focussed on the disabled and partly because the pattern in Figure 4 was close to expectations. Basically

Figure 4: Proportion of the Population by Health Status, ABS Survey for 1998 and Scenario Simulations for 1998 and 2018

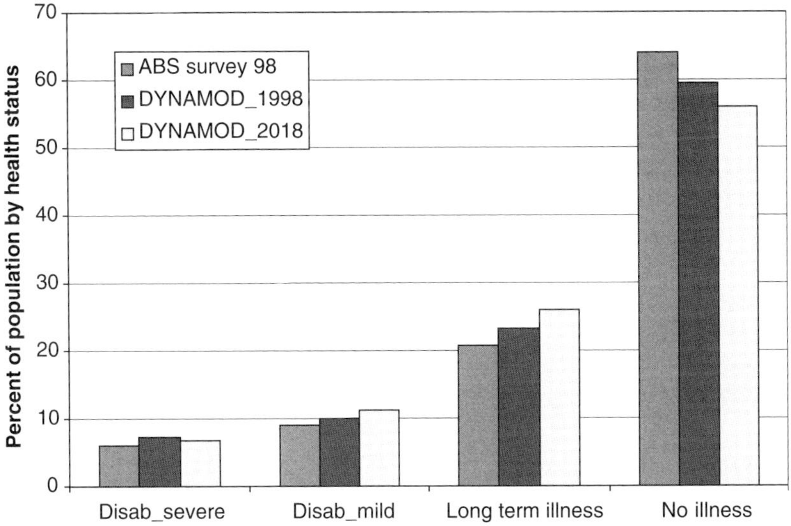

Sources: 1998 Disability survey (ABS, 1999a) and simulations with DYNAMOD
Note: The 'No illness' health state comprises people with neither long-term illness nor disability — see Section 3.

that pattern is consistent with a future in which lifestyle related risk factors, such as obesity, lead to a higher proportion of Australians having long-term illness(es), but in which progression of the ensuing chronic illnesses is slowed through early detection and more effective management of such illnesses (e.g. due to more effective screening processes and improvements in medical technology). The drift towards a somewhat higher proportion of the population being in the 'long-term illness' group in future is realistic in view of obesity becoming such a problem in Australia.[7]

As noted in Section 7, in subsequent research we used logistic regressions to estimate, within the dynamic microsimulation model itself, the numbers of older persons 'working' (Walker, 2004). Simulations with that further-enhanced model indicated that, due to uniquely poorer health, around 7 per

[7] It is well known that obesity is a risk factor for most chronic diseases, which are mainly the ones comprising the 'long term illness' category — see, for example, National Health and Medical Research Council (2002) and World Health Organisation (2003).

Table 3: Persons Aged 65–70 years by Health Status 1998 and 2018

	65–67 year olds		68–70 year olds		65–70 year olds	
	('000)	(%)	('000)	(%)	('000)	(%)
1998						
No illness or disability	145	32.7	123	29.2	268	31.0
Long-term illness	165	37.2	155	36.9	320	37.1
Disabled, mild restr'n	82	18.5	79	18.7	161	18.6
Disabled, severe restr'n	51	11.6	64	15.2	115	13.3
Total	443	100	421	100	864	100
2018						
No illness or disability	241	31.4	206	27.8	446	29.6
Long-term illness	316	41.2	314	42.5	630	41.8
Disabled, mild restr'n	134	17.5	138	18.6	272	18.0
Disabled, severe restr'n	77	10.0	82	11.2	159	10.6
Total	767	100	740	100	1507	100

Source: DYNAMOD simulations

cent less of the 65–70 year old population were 'working' in 1998 than in the ABS survey's 45–54 year old population.

7.2 Predicted Numbers of 65–70 Year Olds by Health Status

In our illustrative application we aim to quantify the impact of a greater proportion of older Australians — aged 65–70 years — working more than 15 h per week (Section 1). The first step is to estimate how many older people will be healthy enough to be able to take on or maintain a job with 15 h or more per week. We used DYNAMOD to simulate, under the scenario, the numbers of 65–70 year olds in each health state in 1998 and in 2018 (Table 3).

Table 3 shows that, out of the 864,000 65–70 year olds in 1998, 31 per cent had no illness or disability, 37 per cent had at least one long-term illness, and the remainder were disabled (19 per cent with mild restrictions in daily activities and 13 per cent with severe restrictions).[8] For 2018 the estimated number of 65–70 years olds was nearly twice as high (1.5 million), with 30 per cent having no illness or disability, 42 per cent having at least one long-term illness, and the remainder being disabled.

[8] Owing to small numbers of observations, we were not able to disaggregate the data by socioeconomic status as well as by health state, either when computing earnings statistics or when estimating numbers of persons through the simulations.

7.3 Predicted Earnings of 65–70 Year Olds (if their employment pattern was the same as that of 45–64 year olds)

To estimate the likely magnitude of the earnings that the new 65–70 year old workers' families may get, we assumed that their earnings would be the same as what 55–64 year olds had in the 1998 Disability survey (Table 4). Although the earnings of 60–64 year olds would have been more appropriate, there were too few respondents in the 1998 Disability survey in that age group who reported wages or salaries as their main source of income. Table 4 shows that the mean weekly cash income of 55–64 year olds from wages or salaries was, in 1998, A$685. If repeated 52 times, then this mean amounts to around A$35,000 a year. This was above the average earnings of the population as a whole (as indicated in the 1998 Disability survey (ABS, 1999a).

It is worth noting that in both the 55–59 and 60–64 age groups the earned incomes of the disabled were well above the age pension (A$9,289.80 a year for singles and A$7,750.60 each for couples in 1998, Department of Family and Community Services, 2004). However, they were significantly lower than the earned incomes of the rest of the population. Also, Table 4 shows that the earned incomes of 60–64 year olds were generally lower than those of the 55–59 age group.

Using the DYNAMOD generated population estimates by age and health status (Table 3), individuals' earnings (Table 4), and the proportions working more than 15 h per week (Table 2), we present estimates in Table 5 for total earnings in 1998 and 2018.

The estimates had been computed under the assumptions that those aged 65–70 years had the same employment patterns as 45–64 year olds the same average earnings as 55–64 year olds, and that the weekly earnings reported in the 1998 survey were repeated 52 times in the year.

Table 4: Mean Weekly Cash Incomes of 55–64 Year Olds Who worked more than 15 h per week and whose Main Source of Income was from Wages and Salaries (1998 dollars)

Age	55–59($)	60–64($)	55–64($)
1998			
Disab_Severe restr'n	600	565	587
Disab_Mild restr'n	606	617	610
Long-term illness	707	657	693
No illness/disability	719	636	700
All health states	702	641	685

Source: Author's computations from the unit record files of the 1998 Disability survey — ABS, 1999a

Table 5: Annual Earnings[a] of 65–70 Year Olds Under the Scenario (1998 dollars)

Age	65–67 ($ million)	68–70 ($ million)	65–70 ($ million)
1998			
Disab_Severe restr'n	286	338	625
Disab_Mild restr'n	822	806	1,628
Long-term illness	3,518	3,071	6,590
No illness/disability	3,800	2,852	6,652
Total	8,427	7,067	15,494
2018			
Disab_Severe restr'n	432	434	866
Disab_Mild restr'n	1,343	1,408	2,751
Long-term illness	6,738	6,222	12,960
No illness/disability	6,316	4,776	11,092
Total	14,830	12,839	27,669

Sources: Table 3 for the populations by age group by health status; Table 2 for the proportions assumed to be working more than 15 h per week; and Table 4 for the person level estimates of earnings

[a]*Total earnings assume that the weekly earnings reported in the survey were repeated 52 times in the year.*

Under these assumptions, Table 5 indicates that the combined earnings of 65–70 year olds in 1998 would have been A$15.5 billion and A$27.7 billion in 2018 (both in constant 1998 dollars). These earnings can be considered additional to what 65–70 year olds actually earned in 1998, since less than 50 respondents in the Disability survey[9] were aged 65–70 and with main source of income from a paid job.

Table 5 is set out so that the reader can easily check what the results would have been under certain alternative assumptions. For example, had the greater job opportunities (or lesser preference for younger people by employers) only impacted on 65–67 year olds,[10] then the additional earnings would have been A$8.4 billion in 1998 and A$14.8 billion in 2018. Or, had 65–67 year olds only worked on average six months in a year, say by taking on contract or casual jobs, then the additional earnings would have been halved (A$4.2 billion in 1998 and A$7.4 billion in 2018).

[9] The full sample in the 1998 survey included 37,580 persons from households and 5,761 from cared accommodation establishments (ABS, 1999b).

[10] This possibility is considered because it seems quite realistic, since in some countries the state pension qualifying age is already 67 years (Section 1). Once the pension age is 65 years for both men and women in Australia, the next step might be to increase this to age 66 or 67.

7.4 Predicted Expenditures on the Age Pension for 65–70 Year Olds (if their employment pattern was the same as that of 45–64 year olds)

As seen earlier, in 1998 the age pension was A$9,289.80 a year for singles and A$7,750.60 each for couples. As more 65–70 year old Australians worked under the scenario, and virtually none worked 15 h or more per week in 1998, for every person working under the scenario the government is likely to save on the age pension. Table 6 shows that disaggregating by family size when estimating 'age pension' savings — i.e. whether couple or single — is important, since the average family size of 55–64 year olds declines steadily as their health worsens. In 1998, family size was close to two persons on average for the healthiest 55–64 year olds, but was only 1.8 persons for the disabled with severe restrictions.

On the basis of statistics from Department of Family and Community Services (1999), we assumed for both 1998 and 2018 that 70 per cent of 65–70 year old Australians received the age pension. Of these, 47.3 per cent received the single rate, and 52.7 per cent the couple rate, with 8.2 per cent receiving the full pension and 31.8 per cent a part pension. On the basis of the same document, we also assumed that the ratio of part pension to full pension was 0.5.

Assuming that all those aged 65–70 years who continued working in the more favourable environment earned the average incomes listed in Table 5 — and thus were no longer eligible for the age pension — Table 7 shows the estimated savings to government in terms of pension expenditures to be A$2.1 billion in 1998 and A$4.0 billion in 2018 (both in constant 1998 dollars). Once again such estimates should be seen as an upper limit. If, for example, only the 65–67 year olds remained in the workforce, then the estimated saving would be around $1.2 billion, and if 65–67 year olds only worked for 6 months in the year, then this estimate would fall to $0.6 billion.

Table 6: Average Family Size of 55–64 Year Olds whose main Source of Income was from Wages/Salaries, by Health State, 1998

Age	55–59 (no.)	60–64 (no.)	55 64 (no.)
Severe restriction	1.77	1.88	1.80
Mild restriction	1.79	1.88	1.83
Long-term illness	1.93	1.88	1.91
No illness/disability	2.01	1.91	1.99

Source: Author's computations from the unit record files of the 1998 Disability survey — ABS, 1999a

Table 7: Potential Savings on the Age Pension[a] of 65–70 Year Olds under the Scenario (1998 dollars)

Age	65–67 ($ million)	68–70 ($ million)	65–70 ($ million)
1998			
Disability Severe restrictionn	507	430	938
Disability Mild restriction	478	289	767
Long–term illness	130	159	289
No illness/disability	46	90	136
Total	1,161	968	2,129
2018			
DisabilitySevere restriction	69	74	143
Disability Mild restriction	213	219	432
Long-term illness	915	909	1,824
No illness/disability	843	721	1,564
Total	2,040	1,923	3,962

Sources: Table 3 for the populations by age group by health status; Table 2 for the proportions assumed to work more than 15 h per week; and Table 4 for the person level estimates of earnings
[a] *The age pension was the rate applied as on 20 September 1998, assuming that 65–70 year olds worked 52 weeks in the year.*

8. Conclusions

At this stage, the analyses presented in this paper are only illustrative. However, they are part of the building of a dynamic microsimulation capacity in Australia. Dynamic microsimulation models are now being routinely used by government departments, universities, and other organisations throughout the developed world.

While the illustrative application reported in this paper could have been analysed using a complex spreadsheet model, use of a dynamic microsimulation model had the advantage of opening up the possibility for a whole range of more complex and more varied applications. One advantage that dynamic microsimulation models have over traditional methods is that they allow a greater number of variables to be incorporated in the model, with minimum expansion in size and complexity. In macrosimulation models each additional variable produces an exponential increase in the number of transitions to be modelled. But the size of a microsimulation model is not affected by additional variables, provided that these are part of the initial microdata set (see, for example, Walker (1997) and Department of Housing and RegionalDevelopment (1995).

More recent examples of possible applications of the enhanced dynamic microsimulation model include consideration of the impact of improved population health (Walker, 2005b) and a joint simulation of such health improvements with a 'longer working lives' scenario (Walker, 2004) similar to that described in this paper.

Possible future extensions include:

- using logistic regressions to determine who will work (or not work) as a function of own health, spouse's health, after tax family income and wealth, and whether there are dependents (with initial work on this having been reported in Walker, 2004);
- improving the coverage and complexity of the costing exercises presented in this paper — e.g. by considering the vast amount of unpaid caring and voluntary work currently done by older Australians (Vaus et al., 2003) that would no longer take place if older people continued to have paid jobs;
- accounting in the model for differentials by SES for factors other than health (e.g. employment, education, profession);
- carrying out analyses under a broader range of possible visions for the future (e.g. different disease progression scenarios, due either to changes in lifestyle patterns or improvements in medical technologies; different policy settings, focus on different age groups; intergenerational issues); and
- when suitable longitudinal data becomes available, re-building the model using such data.

References

Abello, A., Kelly, S. and King, A. (2002). *Demographic projections with DYNAMOD-2,* Technical Paper No. 21, National Centre for Social and Economic Modelling, University of Canberra.

ABS (Australian Bureau of Statistics). (1999a). *Disability Ageing and Carers, 1998*, Confidentialised Unit Record Files.

ABS (Australian Bureau of Statistics). (1999b). *Disability Ageing and Carers, 1998, User Guide*, Cat no. 4431.0, Canberra.

ABS (Australian Bureau of Statistics). (1999c). *Disability Ageing and Carers 1998: Summary of Findings*, Cat no. 4430.0, Canberra.

AIHW (Australian Institute of Health and Welfare). (2001). *Australia's welfare 2001*, Canberra.

Antcliff, S., Bracher, M., Gruskin, A., Hardin, A. and Kapuscinski, C. (1996). *Development of DYNAMOD: 1993 and 1994*, Technical Paper No. 1, National Centre for Social and Economic Modelling, University of Canberra.

Bækgaard, H. (2002a). *Micro-macro Linkage and the Alignment of Transition Processes,* Technical Paper No. 25, National Centre for Social and Economic Modelling, University of Canberra.

Bækgaard, H. (2002b). *Modelling the Dynamics of the Distribution of Earned Income*, Technical Paper No. 24, National Centre for Social and Economic Modelling, University of Canberra.

Bradbury, B., Norris, K. and Abello, D. (2001). *Socioeconomic Disadvantage and the Prevalence of Disability*, Social Policy Research Centre, SPRC Report 1/01 prepared for the Victorian Department of Human Services, University of New South Wales, Sydney.

Department of Family and Community Services. (1999). *Income Support Customers: A Statistical Overview*, Canberra.

Department of Family and Community Services. (2004). *Rates of Pension*, Accessed from http://www.facs.gov.au/guide/ssguide/52210.htm on 14 March 2004.

Department of Housing and Regional Development. (1995). *Household and Family Forecasting Models — A Review*. AGPS, Canberra.

Frederiksen, D. and Stolen, M. (2003). *Possible Ways to Moderate Future Pension Burden in Norway*, 7th Nordic Conference on Microsimulation Models, 12–13 June, Helsinki, Finland.

Howard, J., Prime Minister. (2003). *Address to Symposium on Mature Age Employment*, Sydney, 27 August.

Kelly, S. (2002). *Simulating Future Trends in Wealth Inequality*, Australian Conference of Economists, 3 October, Adelaide, Australia.

Kelly, S. (2003). *Estimating the Wealth of Australians: A New Approach Using Microsimulation*, PhD Thesis, University of Canberra, unpublished.

King, A., Bækgaard, H. and Robinson, M. (1999a). *Dynamod-2: An Overview,* Technical Paper No. 19, National Centre for Social and Economic Modelling, University of Canberra.

King, A., Bækgaard, H. and Robinson, M. (1999b). *The Base Data for Dynamod-2*, Technical Paper No. 20 National Centre for Social and Economic Modelling, University of Canberra.

King, A., Walker, A. and Bækgaard, H. (2002). *Modelling Overseas Migration in DYNAMOD-2*, Technical Paper No. 22, National Centre for Social and Economic Modelling, University of Canberra.

National Health and Medical Research Council. (2002). Acting on Australia's Weight: A Strategic Plan for the Prevention of Overweight and Obesity, Canberra.

Robinson, M. and Bækgaard, H. (2002). *Modelling Students in DYNAMOD-2*, Technical Paper No. 23 National Centre for Social and Economic Modelling, University of Canberra.

Vaus, D., Gray, M. and Stanton, D. (2003). *Measuring the Value of Unpaid Household, Caring and Voluntary Work of Older Australians*, Research Paper No. 34, Australian Institute of Family Studies, Melbourne.

Walker, A. (1997), Australia's Ageing Population: How Important are Family Structures?, Discussion Paper no. 19, National Centre for Social and Economic Modelling, University of Canberra.

Walker, A. (2002). Modeling Health Inequalities Using Dynamic Microsimulation: Statistical Issues and Future Scope, in Gulati, C., Lin, Y., Mishra, S. and Rayner, J. (eds), *Advances in Statistics, Combinatorics and Related Areas*, World Scientific, Singapore, pp. 332–348.

Walker, A. (2003). *Narrower Health Inequalities in Australia: Impacts Simulated Using a Dynamic Microsimulation Model*, 7th Nordic Conference on Microsimulation Models, 12–13 June, Helsinki, Finland.

Walker, A. (2004). Impact of Health on the Ability of Older Australians to Stay in the Workforce — with Possible Contributions to Economic Sustainability,

Refereed Proceedings of the Conference: 'A Future that Works — Economics, Employment and the Environment', University of Newcastle, 8–10 December.

Walker, A. (2005a). *Modelling the Links between Socioeconomic Status and Health in Australia: A Dynamic Microsimulation Approach*, PhD Thesis, available at http://thesis.anu.edu.au/browse.html.

Walker, A. (2005b). Economic and Health Impacts of Narrower Health Inequalities in Australia, in Yfantopoulos, J. (ed), *The Economics of Health Reforms*, Atiner, Athens.

Walker, A., Kelly, S., Harding, A. and Abello, A. (2003). *Does Your Wealth Depend on Good Health?* AMP-NATSEM Income and Wealth Report, National Centre for Social and Economic Modelling, University of Canberra, March.

World Health Organisation. (2003). Controlling the Global Obesity Epidemic, http://www.who.int/nut/obs.htm.

Part II: Pharmacare and Health Expenditure Issues

Chapter 6

Evaluating Catastrophic Drug Expenditure Plans

Michael McCracken and Bert Waslander

Informetrica Limited, Ottawa, Canada

Abstract

Protecting the population against catastrophic health expenditures is a high priority of health policy in Canada. Several proposals for prescription drugs are on the table. We review studies of the policy challenge and proposed solutions that use various tools of analysis, including micromodels. We report some results and key strengths and limitations of the various approaches, and suggest extensions and improvements. On the basis of this review we conclude with some observations on the use and utility of micromodels.

1. Introduction

Basic health care — physicians' care and hospital care — is 100% publicly funded in Canada. Prescription drugs, services by other health care providers, medical equipment and supplies, and dental care are not so covered.

Many of these other services are insured through private and public plans. Private plans tend to be employer-paid, as employer premiums are recognized as costs of doing business by the tax system, and benefits to participants are not included in income. Public plans cover social assistance recipients, drug expenses of senior citizens, certain drugs (e.g., AIDS treatments), and catastrophic expenses. These plans vary by province and territory. The federal government covers First Nation and Inuit people, the armed forces and veterans, and inmates of federal penitentiaries. Of the total outlays for prescription drugs, private plans cover 34%, public plans 44%, and individuals pay 22%.[1]

[1] Data for the year 1999, as reported in "The Romanow Report, November 2002", p. 195.

International Symposia in Economic Theory and Econometrics, Vol. 16

ISSN: 1571-0386 DOI: 10.1016/S1571-0386(06)16006-8

The system has been under strain as costs rise and governments have tackled fiscal deficits and the public debt through restraint on health outlays. Waiting times for many procedures are long; facilities and equipment are not updated as needed.

Two major inquiries have been held by:

- *Roy Romanow*, a former Premier of Saskatchewan, at the request of the federal government (The Romanow Report, 2002),
- *Senator Michael Kirby, Chair*, Standing Senate Committee on Social Affairs, Science and Technology (The Kirby Report, 2002).

Both reports have called for infusion of more federal cash, reform of primary care, support for home care, greater protection against catastrophically high drug expenses, and improved reporting and accountability.

The federal, provincial, and territorial governments responded in February 2003 with a Health Care Renewal Accord. It reforms federal transfers to provinces and territories and establishes a Health Reform Fund (sic) for primary care, home care, and catastrophic drug coverage; a Diagnostic/Medical Equipment Fund to improve access to diagnostic services; and a national system of electronic health records. It also promises improved reporting to the public on use of funds and health care system performance. Governments also made new commitments regarding funding.

Protection against catastrophic drug expenses is clearly a health policy priority in Canada in the early 21st century. Because of the existing intricate patchwork of private and public plans, determining the incidence and cost of various designs for catastrophic drug coverage that leave this patchwork intact is a major challenge. In this paper, we review five studies, including those included in the Romanow and Kirby reports and two by our company. We hope that our findings are of interest to an international audience concerned with policy analysis and micromodelling.

2. The Romanow Report

Romanow proposes a Catastrophic Drug Transfer to offset the cost of provincial and territorial drug plans and reduce disparities in coverage across the country. The federal government would reimburse 50% of the cost of provincial and territorial drug insurance plans above $1,500 per person per year (the point at which expenses would be considered catastrophic). Federal–provincial agreements would ensure that provinces limit deductibles and co-payments and expand coverage and the drug formulary of their plans.[2]

To estimate the cost of the transfer, microdata on drug expenses of Manitoba's Pharmacare programme were extrapolated to the Canadian population. Of 1.2 million Manitobans, 40,000 (3.3%) had drug expenses in excess of $1,500 in the year 2002, and the expenses above $1,500 cost the Manitoba Treasury $52 million. The Transfer would be one-half of this amount, scaled to the population of Canada, plus a margin of error of 15%, which works out to between $750 million and $1 billion.

2.1 Comments

Romanow fixes the federal contribution at 50% of provincial cost above a threshold, but does not define the provincial costs. Manitoba's Pharmacare plan, according to Romanow, is fairly generous and provides complete coverage of the population on a voluntary basis. By basing his estimates on that plan he implies that he expects other provinces to adopt similar plans, something he also says would be the purpose of the federal transfer. All this needs to be worked out through federal–provincial negotiations. Romanow's plan does not guarantee that no Canadian has out-of-pocket expenses of more than $1,500. So Romanow offers only a partial plan, and analysis of costs and distributional impact thus can proceed only with further assumptions about the features of the plan. It also seems that the proposed transfer would not change coverage for residents of Manitoba, but only pass some of the cost of the pharmacare programme to the federal government.

Romanow only considers provincial and territorial drug plans, and does not discuss expenditures covered by private insurance. It is not clear whether drug expenditures in excess of $1,500 per person in Manitoba include the amount covered by private insurance or not.

3. The Kirby Proposal

Kirby aims to ensure that no Canadian individual or family has out-of-pocket expenses of more than 3% of total family income. Total annual drug expenses in excess of $5,000 are considered catastrophic, and the federal government would pay 90% of the expenses above $5,000, provided that:

---

[2] Romanow does not go as far as Kirby in guaranteeing coverage of the population against catastrophic expenditures. He does not say that provinces have to limit out-of-pocket expenditures to $1,500 per person or that coverage has to be comprehensive.

- the province reimburses families for any out-of-pocket expenses in excess of 3% of family income;
- private plans agree to limit out-of-pocket expenses to $1,500 per individual plan member.

This plan seems rather complex administratively and requires redesign of private and provincial insurance schemes. The plan is estimated to cost $500 million per year.

Kirby used a dedicated micromodel to calculate the cost of his catastrophic drug coverage plan.

The study by Fraser Group/Tristat Resources: "Drug Expense Coverage in the Canadian Population: Protection from Severe Drug Expenses" gives a description of the model and findings as to the coverage of the Canadian population (Fraser Group/Tristat Resources, 2002). The documentation of the model is found on pages 17–24 of this study.

The data sources are:

- The 1998 Survey of Labour and Income Dynamics (SLID), 79,000 individuals in 40,000 families. The sample weights are adjusted to population in the year 2000. Underreporting of social assistance (SA) is corrected (presumably to get a better fix on coverage of medical expenses through SA).
- The Survey of Work Arrangements.
- Government economic statistics.
- Analysis of public drug plan features.
- A proprietary database of private sector drug plans containing records of drug expenses of 80,000 persons.

Coverage by public plans is imputed based on province of residence, age, income, and family status. Potential coverage of the entire population under 65 by Alberta Blue Cross (ABC) and coverage by Ontario's Trillium plan (maximum of 4% of income) is imputed, i.e., it is assumed that people will apply to these plans when this is to their advantage. The three-month waiting time for ABC is treated as a deductible.

Individual private insurance policies (~1% of the population) are imputed, as well as coverage of university students and of retirees by former employers.

Further assumptions are:

- People enroll in every drug plan for which they are eligible, but avoid duplicate coverage: every individual is covered by a maximum of one private and one public plan.
- Average dispensing fees are the same in 2000 as in 1998.

3.1 Comments

Fraser/Tristat comment that protection from private plans may be understated, as the model does not recognize a situation where both spouses are in employer-sponsored plans. We wonder if coverage is overstated because of the assumption that each family has only a single private plan (this would be the case if total membership in private plans is spread over all families, assuming no double coverage, while in reality double coverage does occur).

The study does not detail the features of private plans: the deductible, co-payment, restricted formularies, maximum payments, and caps on out-of-pocket expenses. Hence we cannot comment on the information content of this micromodel.

4. Crossley et al: Analysis of Household Expenditure Data

Recently, Crossley, Grootendorst, and Veall, three Canadian economists, used the Survey of Household Spending (SHS) to examine the Kirby plan for catastrophic drug expenditure coverage (The Kirby Report, (2002); Crossley et al., 2003). The survey contains 14,087 household records suitable for analysis, with sample weights that reflect the entire population. For each household, expenditures on prescription drugs are given as one of nine health-related categories of expenditure. Income by source, household structure, and characteristics of household members are also available, but the file contains no information about public or private medical insurance and use of tax facilities for medical expenses and disability.

Crossley et al. estimate equations for probability of drug expenses and for the amount spent. Their stated intent is to examine distributional effects across households while controlling for household characteristics, a familiar and valid rationale for regression analysis. The characteristics they include in their equations are age of head, marital status, number of children, number of adults other than spouse, number of full-time earners, household income quintiles, and province of residence. They provide separate estimates for households of seniors as seniors tend to be covered by provincial drug plans. Using a bootstrap technique, they develop confidence intervals for their estimates.

The authors introduce a regional variable, with each province representing a separate category, and they assume that the distribution of the error terms varies systematically by province. This may be intended to reflect the difference in coverage by public (i.e., provincial government) plans as well as the difference in private plan coverage related to differences in industrial structure, as most private plans are employer plans.

Apart from these two regional features, the model applies to the country as a whole. Thus, the relationship between income, family characteristics, and other independent variables on the one hand, and the probability of receiving a transfer under the Kirby plan and the amount of the transfer on the other, is the same in all provinces.

The main dimension of interest to the authors was income. They show that, even though under the Kirby plan the transfer per receiving household increases with income, more money is received by low-income households on average because of greater incidence of high prescription drug expenditures among low-income households.

4.1 Comments

In this study, statistical methods take the place of information about private and public insurance coverage for drug expenses. Differences in drug expense coverage across the country appear as regional dummy variables and province-specific variances of error terms. The data permit analysis of the main features of the Kirby plan: capping drug expenses per individual and expenses as a share of income for families. But the effect of the plan on insurers cannot be examined.

The finding about the distributional effect of the Kirby plan derives from the distribution of high drug expenditures among households by income class. The regression-based estimates of the Kirby transfers by income quintile capture a pure relationship between drug expense and household income, separate from differences in family characteristics among income quintiles. Micromodels do not pursue this type of analysis aimed at causal relationships — estimating the pure effect of individual factors — but aim to describe the attributes of programme clients in full detail.

5. Analysis with a General-Purpose Micromodel

5.1 SPSD/M: The Database and Model

Informetrica Limited has examined variants to Canada's Medical Expenses Tax Credit (METC) using the Social Policy Simulation Database and Model (SPSD/M) (Informetrica Limited (2002)). This is a static annual micromodel intended to simulate income and sales taxes and income transfer programmes. The model was developed and is maintained by Statistics Canada for use by the public.

The database is drawn from several different sources:

- The Survey of Consumer Finances (SCF) is the host database. The high-income group is expanded using income tax data. Employment Insurance

(EI) histories are imputed. The data are corrected for underreporting of social assistance and other transfers.

- A fairly large sample (400,000) of income tax records is used to impute income taxes. The imputation involves some averaging to maintain confidentiality, and grouping by family type, income, and region. A few tax credits are allocated according to characteristics identified in the host dataset (for tuition, attendance at a post-secondary institution), but the METC is not so treated. Only the amounts claimed and the value of the METC credit are given for each taxpayer, without any modelling of expenses or the credit.
- The SHS is imputed based on region, tenure, family type and size, and income. The roughly 15,000 records of the SHS are expanded to 90,000 needed for SPSD/M by duplication. Some categories of expenditures (e.g., mortgage interest payments) are allocated according to characteristics available in the host dataset (home owner with mortgage), but health expenditures are not so treated.
- There is no link between income tax and SHS imputations, hence no correspondence at the microlevel between household medical expenditures from the SHS and the METC from tax records.

The model comprises a detailed federal and provincial income tax calculator, and an equally detailed description of EI and income transfer programmes for seniors. Social Assistance, the Canada Pension Plan, and provincial programmes are not simulated but benefit amounts are included in the database for the individuals and families concerned.

In 1999, there were 1.7 million taxable returns — 11.6% of all taxable returns — with an "allowable portion of medical expenses" (expenses in excess of 3% of income), with an average amount of $1,518, for a total of $2.6 billion. There were 2.1 million taxable and non-taxable returns — 9.5% of all returns — with an average allowable portion of medical expenses of $1,736, for a total of $3.6 billion. The average federal tax reduction for medical expenses per taxable return was $257.

Households spend far more on health care than is reported in income tax returns. According to the 1998 SHS, 98% of Canada's 11.7 million households had some expenses for health care, for a total of $13.6 billion. There were 4.6 million households in which at least one person had taxable income (income >$7,000) and medical expenses (other than insurance premiums and non-prescription drugs) in excess of 3% of the taxable income of the spouse with the lower taxable income. The total allowable amount was $4.6 billion. By contrast, as shown above, the Canada Custom and Revenue Agency (CCRA) reported 1.7 million taxable returns with $2.6 billion in allowable expenses for the year 1999.

Not all household expenditures on health care reported in the SHS are eligible for the METC. In contrast, certain other expenditures like medically necessary transportation and home renovations related to disability are eligible for the credit but are not included in household spending on health care as reported in the SHS. Without more detail about expenses incurred and expenses claimed it is impossible to reconcile the SHS and tax credit numbers, but the comparison suggests there is potential for greater use of the credit. There may be up to several million households that could, under present rules, claim the credit but do not, or are close to being able to claim the credit. Changes to the credit (e.g., reducing the threshold, increasing the tax credit rate, or refundability) may make these households alert to the opportunity for tax savings, with potentially substantial effects on federal and provincial revenues.

In our 2002 paper we treated expenses above a fixed amount of $10,000 or a level of 20% of a household's net income as catastrophic.[3] According to SPSD/M, there were 46,800 households, or 0.4% of the nearly 12 million households in Canada, that had catastrophic medical expenses measured as expenses in excess of $10,000, and 59,200 households or 0.5% of households, when we use the threshold of 20%. Using the latter definition, we find many households with low incomes, almost all single persons, mostly older and female. Almost one-half of such households (48%) had disposable incomes of <$15,000, with medical expenses amounting to 108% of that income. Another 41% have between $15,000 and $30,000, with medical expenses making up 57% of income (Table 1).

One option for assisting those with such high medical bills would be to apply the highest federal income tax rate of 29% to medical expenses above 20% of net income, and to make this portion of the credit fully refundable. This change would cost a total of $81.4 million, of which $26 million (31%) would go to households with disposable incomes below $15,000, and $43 million (51%) to those in the $15,000–$30,000 range. On average, the medical expenses credit would increase by $1,375 for each household (Table 1).[4]

This estimate of revenue forgone is too low. While there are probably no households with taxable income and catastrophic medical expenses who fail to report these expenses, households without taxable income have no reason

[3] These are very high thresholds compared to those proposed by Kirby and Romanow. Our study was conducted before these two reports were issued.

[4] This model simulation is based on data for 1997 to which overall growth rates for population and income were applied. Thus, the number of tax filers using the METC, the total allowable expenses claimed, and the amount of the credit are understated in 1999 compared to actual numbers. This means that the impacts of policy changes are also understated. Precisely by how much the impacts are understated is impossible to say. Impacts also do not include tax filers who did not report medical expenses but begin to do so in response to a policy change.

Table 1: Simulation of a 29% Federal Income Tax Credit for Households with Medical Expenses in Excess of 20% of Net Income, 1999

	Household with medical expense above 20% of net Income					Simulation: refundable 29% credit	
Income group ($'000)	Number of households (thousands)	Average age of eldest	Average medical expenses allowed	Medical expenses allowed as % of total income	Average medical tax credit currently	Average increase in medical tax credit	Cost of program alteration ($M)
0–15	28.9	67	4300.6	107.7	731.1	887.9	25.5
15–30	24.2	73.8	9128.9	56.8	1551.9	1779.3	43.1
30–50	4.7	70.4	16424.6	38.1	2792.2	2219.7	10.4
50–70	1.3	75.2	18345.5	29.1	3118.7	1792.3	2.4
> 70	0	0	0	0	0	0	0
All	59.2	70.1	7536.7	79.2	1281.2	1374.7	81.4

to report their medical expenses. Refundability would give them such a reason, and the take-up rate for the METC would therefore increase. Furthermore, enhanced support for very high medical expenditures might encourage provinces to off-load medical expenses onto individuals, and thus shift some of the cost of health care from the provinces to the federal government and Canadian families.

5.2 Comments

The simulations could have been performed on tax data only. Use of SPSD/M made it easy to perform the simulations, and gave us information about households using the credit, information that might not have been fully available in tax data only. So we did gain something from the merging of data of different sources, but the quality of the information gained of course depends on the quality of the data-merging process. Without going into detail, we may say that the process of pasting tax data onto SPSD/M did not ensure that high medical expenses were allocated precisely to families and households with the right characteristics.

In these simulations we did not in any way benefit from the household expenditure data in the SPSD/M model. As noted above, the SHS records all expenditures, irrespective of how they are treated by the tax system. The SHS distinguishes nine categories of health-related spending, but this is insufficient to isolate spending eligible for the tax credit. For the METC we only know the amount claimed, not the uses of the funds. Thus, we were not able to simulate a catastrophic drug expense plan, only a plan for catastrophic medical expenses. Further, the SHS data were merged into SPSD/M without considering the relationship between health expenditures as per the SHS and the METC amount.

SPSD/M could be made more useful in several ways:

- By imputing household expenditure data to conform better with METC microdata, by matching households on the basis of the level of health expenditures and METC expenditures.
- By obtaining detail from Canada Revenue Agency (CRA) on the type of expenses claimed under METC, and the person or persons for whom the expenditures were incurred, and imputing this to the model.
- By imputing client data of private and public plans or household survey data on insurance coverage and use.

In other words, SPSD/M can be made more useful by turning it into a medical expense microsimulation model. The more the expenditure detail from the different sources is cast in the same categories, the more useful the merged database would be. If the SHS supplied the information about medical expenses needed to claim a tax credit for all households including households that do not claim the credit, then analysis of the likely effects of expansion of the credit would be facilitated.

6. Analysis with Semi-Aggregate Programme Data

In 2003, Informetrica Limited estimated the costs and distribution of hypothetical catastrophic drug programmes in a Canadian province (Informetrica Limited (2003)). We received data on membership and claims from a general, voluntary provincial drug coverage plan for 34 ranges of total expenditures on prescription drugs for a recent year. The first seven categories were collapsed into Category 1($0–$1,000) and the next two categories became Category 2($1,001–$2,000). This resulted in 26 categories, each with a range of $1,000 and an open-ended category for over $26,000 for analytical purposes. The data consisted of the number of claims (individual prescriptions), number of claimants, total cost and shares of the individual, the province's drug plan, and other insurance. The data were provided for four segments of the population: seniors, widows of seniors, and non-seniors subdivided as to whether their premiums were subsidized. Finally, the number of singles, families and persons in those families that belong to the plan and paid monthly fees was also given for the four segments.

The plan covers all of the drug costs, except for a 30% co-payment, limited to a maximum of $25 per prescription. Payments by other insurers cover only a minor part of total expenditures. As the plan is voluntary, one expects members to be in need of prescription drugs on a regular basis, and indeed, the number of claimants in the year for which data were provided ranges from 79% to 95% of the number of members among the four groups.

With this information we developed a calculator for catastrophic drug expense coverage that takes account of the full detail in the programme data. Various ceilings, co-payments, deductibles, maximum out-of-pocket expenses per prescription can be specified, and the cost and incidence of the programme examined. This is possible because the programme data includes number of prescriptions.

6.1 Comments

These data reveal some aspects of the pattern of drug expenses that are not covered in the expenditure and tax data reviewed earlier.

Per member, the average annual expenditure (out-of-pocket plus drug plans) for prescription drugs is ~$1,092. However, the distribution is a Pareto or power function, with a few people having large expenditures, and many having relatively small expenses (Chart 1). Over 60% would incur

Chart 1: Number of Claimants by Expenditure Class

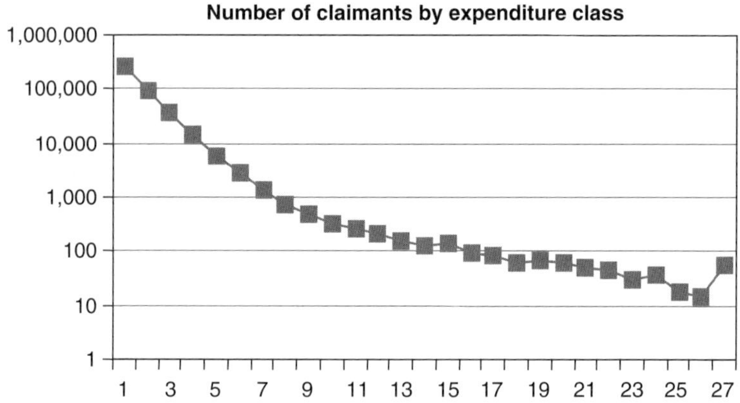

<$1,000, with a few requiring in excess of $5,000 (~3.3%) and very few in excess of $25,000 (0.02%).

The average claimant obtains about 21 prescriptions per year. However, when the data are arranged by expenditure class, both the average cost per prescription and the total number of prescriptions per year rise. That is, people in higher expenditure classes have more prescriptions (Chart 2). They also have a higher cost per prescription (Chart 3). Examination of a file of 1,500,000 prescriptions shows a distribution of prices with a median value of about $26, a mean of $62, and a mode of $14. The low to high values are $1 to $5,500.

No information was provided on personal and family characteristics of members including age, sex and income, and the breakdown of members and claimants into four groups provides the only detail in this regard. This lack of data makes it impossible to build more than the most rudimentary linkages to other information. By combining the income distribution for each of the four groups with the programme data for each group we can calculate drug expenses and programme benefits by income decile for the province as a whole, but this is a crude approximation since within each group drug expenses are independent of the income distribution.

We can define catastrophic drug expenditures in different ways and deal with them in various ways (lower co-payment, caps on out-of-pocket expenses). We have introduced an annual deductible amount as a way of defraying some of the cost of coverage of catastrophic expenses. These calculations are not very precise, but they are detailed enough. We can also apply different fees, but of course, without knowing how participation in the plan may be affected.

Chart 2: Number of Prescriptions by Expenditure Class

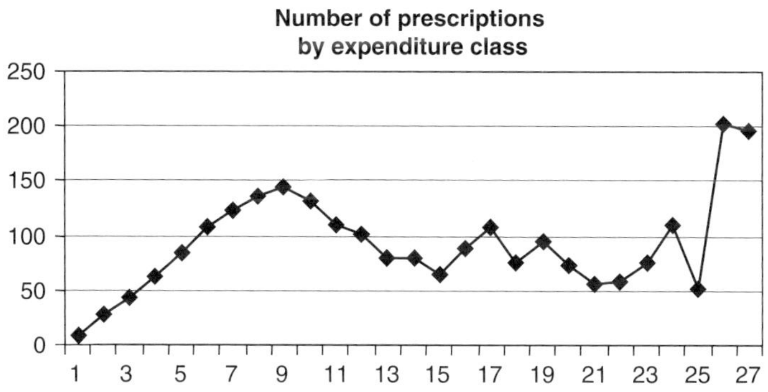

Chart 3: Price Per Prescription by Expenditure Class

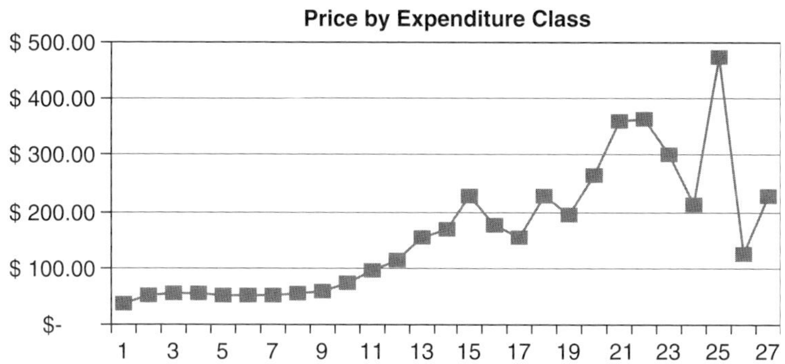

We can examine a cap on out-of-pocket expenses in relation to income, as both Romanow and Kirby have proposed. This is restricted, however, to assuming the same prescription drug use across income classes. We cannot examine a cap at the *family* level, as we have no information on the family ties of claimants. And we do not know to what extent the METC assists those with high drug expenses, as we have no information on their income, that of family members, and the taxes they all pay.

Finally, we cannot estimate to what extent catastrophic drug expense coverage may increase expenditures on drugs and increase the cost of the plan through changes in behaviour. Nor can we estimate what savings are possible in other areas of health care if the use of prescription drugs is no longer subject to household income constraints. Rather different data are required to get at such effects.

7. Conclusions

In reviewing the various studies, what have we learned of interest to others who might be considering microsimulation as an approach for evaluating drug expenditures?

Undertaking microsimulation exercises based on household expenditure files or tax records is not enough for examining many interesting issues about prescription drugs. The drug histories (number of prescriptions and their prices) need to be known to explore various charging schemes (caps, deductibles, maximum per prescription, etc.).

Further, one needs to be able to link costs and preferably drug histories to the individuals. In turn, the individuals need to be joined into families, so that rules can be applied both to the individuals and to the pooled experience of the family unit. The ability to move back and forth between claims, claimants, and families is an important aspect of modelling drug programmes in Canada. Public and private plans have many details such as deductibles and caps per person or per family, and the METC operates at the level of the extended family.

Data from private and public drug insurance plans have been largely unavailable for analysis to date. The Fraser/Tristat model constitutes a first step in this regard.

Provincial programmes that provide coverage against high drug expenditures on a voluntary basis are a useful source for examining catastrophic expenditure plans, as we have demonstrated in our work. Romanow and Kirby have also made use of data from such plans.

Detail on the expenditures claimed under the METC and the persons for whom the expenses are claimed would be an important step forward. At this point we know only the total amount claimed, and do not know how much is claimed for prescription drugs. The METC already provides some protection against high expenses by reducing the tax burden of those affected, and this needs to be taken into account as an offset to the cost of a catastrophic drug expenditure plan.

The METC covers a wide range of health-related expenditures and can therefore be used to examine how drug expenses interact with other expenses for health care. Interestingly, monitoring of expenditures claimed under METC could provide important signals for health care policy. Changes in coverage by private and public plans, changes in drug formularies, advances in medical treatment, changing incidence of various diseases — all these would show up in the METC claims. This is not a comment on micromodelling but rather a comment on use of information for policy purposes, but one that we feel is worth making.

General-purpose models like SPSD/M are useful in that they describe family and household structures in the population along with economic circumstances of individuals and the basic social units. Such models will be more useful for analysis of health expenditures when more data from donor databases with health care and health expenditure data are exploited. SPSD/M would be a more powerful tool for analysis of catastrophic drug expenses coverage if detailed health-related expenditures contained in tax and household spending data were imputed in a way that takes account of health attributes of units in the host database, and links between the two donor bases. SPSD/M was not designed to do this, and what we suggest here comes close to asking for a health expenditure micromodel.

As long as Canada has a patchwork of private and public insurance for drugs and a range of other expenditures, and governments are very concerned about limiting their share of health expenditures, the patchwork is likely to continue. The system may become even more complicated as both Romanow and Kirby are proposing. Analytical tools that capture this complexity will be needed.

By contrast, if there were a universal drug plan providing full coverage, microsimulation efforts could be directed to other interesting questions. In particular, linking drug use histories with other interventions and their outcomes would allow a better understanding of the ways in which drugs may substitute for other medical interventions or complement other interventions to reach improved health outcomes.

References

Crossley, T.F., Grootendorst, P.V. and Veall, M.R. (2003). *National Catastrophic Drug Insurance Revisited: Who Would Benefit from Senator Kirby's Recommendations?*, SEDAP (A Program for Research on Social and Economic Dimensions of an Aging Population). Research Paper 105, McMaster University.

Fraser Group/Tristat Resources (2002). *Drug Expense Coverage in the Canadian Population: Protection from Severe Drug Expenses.* Canadian Life and Health Insurance Association website.

Informetrica Limited (2002). *The Medical Expenses Tax Credit: Background and Options for Change.*

Informetrica Limited (2003). *Catastrophic Drug Expenditure: How Much Should A Person Spend?*

The Kirby Report (2002). *The Health of Canadians — The Federal Role. Final Report on state of the health care system in Canada.* Standing Senate Committee on Social Affairs, Science and Technology. Chair: The Honourable Michael J.L. Kirby.

The Romanow Report (2002). *Building on Values. The Future of Health Care in Canada.* Commission on the Future of Health Care in Canada. Roy J. Romanow, Q.C. Commissioner.

Chapter 7

Projections of Commonwealth Health Expenditure in Australia's First Intergenerational Report

Deborah Schofield and George Rothman

University of Sydney (Northern Rivers University Department of Rural Health, School of Public Health) and Department of the Treasury, Australia

Abstract

Australia's first Intergenerational Report 2002–2003 (The Department of the Treasury, 2002) provides a basis for considering the Commonwealth's fiscal outlook over the long term and identifies emerging pressures. Health expenditure was projected to be a source of very significant future spending pressure, with spending on health projected to increase from about 4 per cent of GDP in 2001–2002 to about 8 per cent in 2041–2042. The pharmaceutical benefits scheme was projected to be the fastest growing component, increasing about five-fold as a percentage of GDP. Technological change and increased use and cost of services were found to be the main drivers of Commonwealth health spending, with population growth and ageing being much less significant drivers of growth. Projections are presented for the main components of health spending and the sensitivity of the projections to demographic and other assumptions is assessed.

1. Background

Australia's first Intergenerational Report (IGR, The Department of the Treasury, 2002) was published in May 2002 as part of the 2002–2003 Commonwealth Budget. The report provides a basis for considering the Commonwealth's fiscal outlook over the long term (40 years), and for identifying emerging issues associated with an ageing population. Preparation of the Report was required by the *Charter of Budget Honesty Act 1998*.

The projections were prepared against a background of strong Commonwealth government finances. The Commonwealth Budget recorded an

International Symposia in Economic Theory and Econometrics, Vol. 16

ISSN: 1571-0386 DOI: 10.1016/S1571-0386(06)16007-X

accumulated cash surplus of $23.7 billion from 1997–1998 to 2000–2001. During this period, Commonwealth government net debt, already one of the lowest among the industrialised economies, has fallen from $82.9 to $39.3 billion.

A steadily ageing population is likely to continue to place significant pressure on Commonwealth government finances. But, Australia is well placed to meet the challenges. Australia's superannuation system generates private saving for retirement, complementing an age pension system that is better targeted and more affordable than in many other industrialised countries. In addition, Australia's health system is very efficient by international standards. Further, Australia's social welfare payments are well targeted and government debt is low.

The projections in the IGR suggest that, if trends continue and policies are not adjusted, the current generation of taxpayers is likely to impose a higher tax burden on the next generation. The required adjustment in taxes and spending is about 5.0 per cent of GDP by 2041–2042, or $87 billion in today's dollars (Figure 1). Governments will need to exercise sound policy management to minimise the tax burden transferred to the next generation.

Although the ageing impact on the Commonwealth's budget is not a major one for at least 15 years (Figure 1), forward planning is important, to ensure that governments will be well placed to meet emerging policy challenges in a timely and effective manner.

The publication of the IGR has been well received. It has already stimulated relevant policy debate and some policy changes and continues to be influential.

Figure 1: Projection of Fiscal Pressure

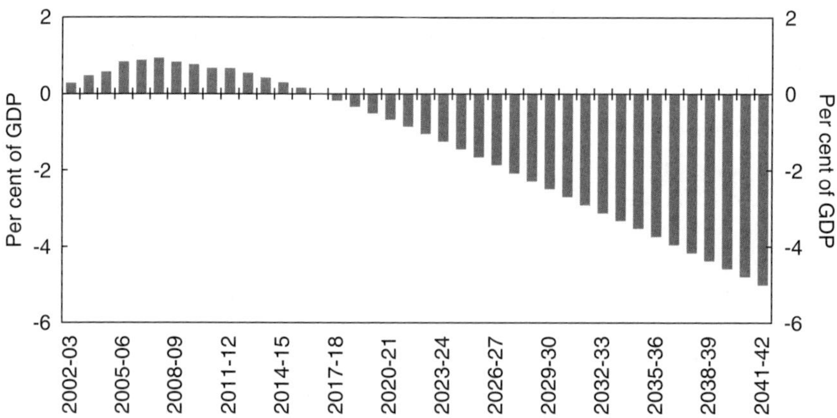

Source: Treasury projections (previously published as Figure 4 in the IGR)

2. Australia's Health System

Australians' life expectancies are among the highest in the world. In relative terms, Australia's health outcomes are achieved at a moderate cost, with total health spending around 8.5 per cent of GDP, which is about average for OECD countries.

Health and aged care services are funded and provided by both the public and private sectors. The Commonwealth is responsible for almost half of the total health spending for Australia, and is the major public funder, although State, Territory, and Local governments also fund health services.

2.1 Health

The Commonwealth spent around 4 per cent of GDP on health in 2001–2002. Less than 20 per cent of this was funded through the Medicare levy (on personal income). The Commonwealth funds the Medical Benefits Scheme (MBS) to provide patient subsidies for medical practitioner services, optometry, diagnostic imaging, and pathology. The MBS forms the core of Medicare — the Commonwealth's universal health programme. Under the Pharmaceutical Benefits Scheme (PBS), the Commonwealth subsidises a select list of pharmaceuticals to provide patients with timely, reliable and affordable access to necessary and cost–effective medicines. New procedures, tests and pharmaceuticals are added to the list of those subsidised under the MBS and PBS following Government approval of the recommendations of the relevant advisory bodies.

In addition to the MBS and PBS, the Commonwealth:

- makes a major contribution to the funding of public hospital services provided by State governments;
- provides a 30 per cent rebate to subsidise the cost of private health insurance; and
- provides financial support in other areas, including medical research, public health, indigenous health services, health information management and access, health safety and quality, and medical workforce development and infrastructure.

2.2 Aged Care

The Commonwealth provides funding for residential aged care and a range of community care services equivalent to 0.7 per cent of GDP in 2001–2002. For residential aged care, the majority of funding is provided directly to non-government organisations. The Commonwealth also contributes

Figure 2: Historical Commonwealth Health Spending

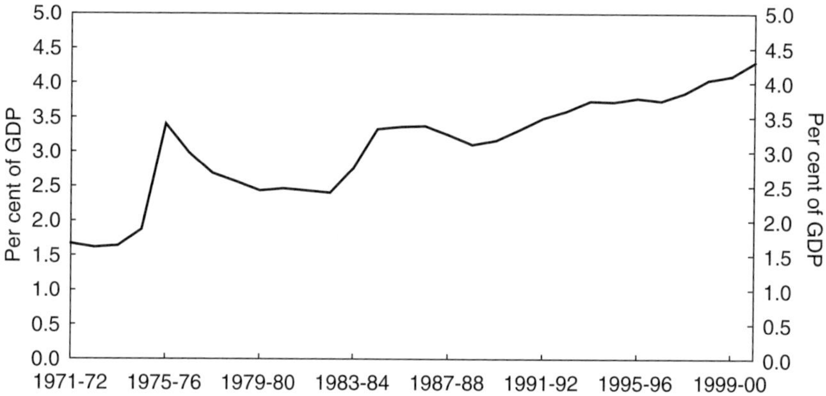

Source: Australian Institute of Health and Welfare health spending data base, Australian Institute of Health and Welfare 2000, ABS AusStats Cat. No. 5204.0 and Treasury. Data may differ from the functional data in the Budget Papers (previously published as Figure 20 in the IGR)
Note: The sharp increase in 1975–1976 reflects the introduction of Medibank and the increase in 1983–1984 reflects the introduction of Medicare.

significant funding towards community care services that are delivered by the States and Territories.

3. Key Trends and Assumptions

Over the 30 years up to 2000–2001, Commonwealth spending on health and nursing homes increased from 1.7 per cent of GDP to 4.3 per cent of GDP (Figure 2). While Commonwealth health spending fluctuated markedly during the 1970s, reflecting various policy changes (including the introduction and subsequent abolition of Medibank), growth steadied in the 1980s and 1990s following the introduction of Medicare.

In addition to this health spending, Commonwealth spending on hostels and community care in 2000–2001 was around 0.4 per cent of GDP. However, due to the recent shift in focus in aged care from residential care to community care, it is not yet possible to identify the underlying trend.

Non-demographic growth,[1] rather than population growth or changes in the age structure of the population, has been the key driver of real health

[1] Non-demographic growth refers to real per person age-adjusted compound growth.

Table 1: Real Growth Rates for Commonwealth Health Spending (per cent)

	1984–1984 to 2000–2001	1989–1990 to 2000–2001
Non-demographic (population and age structure removed)	2.1	3.2
Population	1.2	1.2
Age structure	0.5	0.5
Total	3.8	4.9

Source: Australian Institute of Health and Welfare and Treasury estimates. (previously published as Table 7 in the IGR)
Note: Growth trends of health spending are very sensitive to the start and end dates chosen and the inclusion or exclusion of policy changes. Both growth rates exclude the introduction of Medicare, the largest policy change over the last two decades, and the introduction of the Private Health Insurance Rebate (introduced on 1 January 1999). The start date of 1989–1990 excludes several years following the introduction of Medicare, allowing a more stable trend to appear.

spending over the past decade (Table 1). Non-demographic factors (such as listing new medications on the PBS and greater use of diagnostic procedures) are also likely to generate the greatest cost pressure in the future.

Technological change accounts for a significant proportion of non-demographic growth in health spending per person. As the Commonwealth exercises significant controls over whether to adopt new technology in the health system, past increases in spending partly reflect the Commonwealth's choice to fund new technologies.

This growth has occurred even though policies have been introduced to constrain costs whilst improving the quality of health care and introducing new treatments or services. For example, in 1998, the Government introduced the Therapeutic Group Premium policy to constrain spending on the PBS. Under the arrangements, the Government subsidises up to the price of the lowest priced product in the therapeutic group. Consumers make up the difference where the price charged is greater than the PBS subsidy.

Over the past decade, Commonwealth spending on health has grown at a faster rate than total national health spending. This indicates Commonwealth health spending increased faster than State government or private sector spending.[2] The Commonwealth's share in financing the nation's health spending grew from 43 per cent in 1991–1992 to 46 per cent in 2001–2002. Over the same period the States' share fell from 25 to 22 per cent

[2] The number of people with private health insurance has increased significantly since the introduction of Lifetime Health Cover in July 2000, (Private Health Insurance Industry Association Council, 2005) so the contribution of the private sector is likely to have increased since then.

and the private sector's share fell from 33 to 32 per cent (Australian Institute of Health and Welfare, 2003).

Different components of the health system have grown at different rates (see Table 2). Over the past decade, real non-demographic growth in Commonwealth spending on public hospitals has been 1.6 per cent per year. Real non-demographic growth for MBS subsidies has also been about 1.6 per cent per year since the introduction of Medicare in 1984.

By contrast, spending growth on the PBS has been very rapid. Real non-demographic growth for the PBS has averaged 6.1 per cent per year over the last 20 years. When the impact of the budget changes through to the end of the forward estimates period (2005–2006) is included, the growth rate is 5.6 per cent. The increased availability and use of newer and more expensive drugs, leading to increases in the total volume of prescriptions and the government cost per prescription, drive this rapid growth.

The 2002–2003 Commonwealth Budget included several initiatives to address the rapid growth in the PBS and reduce spending on the PBS by $1.9 billion over the following four years. These initiatives included increases in patient co-payments and safety net thresholds under the PBS, a review of controls on the prescription of certain drugs, better information for doctors on the restrictions that apply to PBS drugs and measures to facilitate the use

Table 2: Historical Health Spending Growth Rates in Components

	Non-demographic growth (real, per person, age adjusted where appropriate) (per cent)	Period
Historical expenditure growth rates in components		
Hospital	1.64	1989–1990 to 2000–2001
PBS subsidy	5.64	1983–1984 to 2005–2006
MBS subsidy (years)		
0–4	0.52	1984–1985 to 2000–2001
5–9	−0.12	
10–14	0.33	
15–19	0.94	
20–24	−0.11	
25–34	0.31	
35–44	1.45	
45–54	1.74	
55–64	2.43	
65–74	3.78	
75 and over	2.30	
Aged care	1.71	

Source: Commonwealth of Australia Budget Paper No.1 (various) and Department of Health and Ageing data. (previously published as Table C3 in the IGR)

of less expensive generic drugs. A number of these initiatives have not been approved by the Senate.

Spending on older people is growing faster than for the total population. For the MBS, the highest growth rates have been for those aged 55 and over (Table 2).

4. Health and Aged Care Projection Methodology

These models use historical trends of spending per person of given age and gender as the basis for projecting future spending per person of given characteristics. The projections combine these trends with projected population and projected economic factors. These trends in costs reflect the demand for and supply of services, the quality of services, government policies and contractual arrangements, and, importantly, technological change, as well as factors such as growth in wages of service providers.

The primary model for health spending allows for spending by age to grow at different rates in different programs. The areas modelled, the approach taken, and the relevant growth rates are in Tables 2 and 3. A more detailed description of the projection method is given in Appendix A using the PBS as the example. Appendix A also considers a range of modelling issues and the reasons for the decisions taken. A secondary model was also developed to project aggregate Commonwealth health spending and examine the sensitivity of health spending to variation of the growth rate.

Aged care spending was projected for the three components of nursing homes, hostels and Home and Community Care (HACC).

5. Projection Results

Commonwealth spending on health is projected to increase to 4.3 per cent of GDP by 2011–2012 and to 8.1 per cent of GDP by 2041–2042 (Table 4). This is roughly equivalent to a real non-demographic growth rate for all of Commonwealth health spending of about 2.6 per cent per year over the four decades.

Of all the components of Commonwealth health expenditure, spending on PBS subsidies is projected to grow the fastest, even after the budget changes. As a proportion of GDP, the PBS is projected to grow more than five-fold, from 0.6 per cent of GDP currently to 3.4 per cent of GDP in 2041–2042. Spending on MBS subsidies as a proportion of GDP is expected to grow by 60 per cent, with hospital and health services spending growing by 40 per cent (Figure 3).

Most of the projected growth in health spending reflects the increasing cost and availability of new high technology procedures and medicines, and

Table 3: Health Primary Model: Components and Modelling Approach

Component	Modelling approach	Non-demographic growth rates[a]
Pharmaceutical Benefit Scheme direct subsidies	Per person spending by sex and age group Same growth rate for all age groups	5.64 after allowing for 2002–2003 budget measures
Medical Benefits Scheme direct subsidies	Per person spending by sex and age group Separate growth rates for each age group	Age-specific rates vary from −0.12 to 3.78
Hospital and health services	Per person spending by sex and age group Same growth rate for all age groups	1.64
Other health spending[b]	Private health insurance was assumed to grow with the MBS, hospitals and nursing homes. The remainder of health spending was assumed to be a constant proportion of GDP	

[a] *Per capita real age-adjusted.*
[b] *Other health expenditures includes the Private Health Insurance Rebate, other PBS and MBS spending, community and public health, administration, aids and appliances and research. (Previously published as Table C2 in the IGR).*

Table 4: Projected Commonwealth Health and Aged Care Spending, by Components (per cent of GDP)

	2001–2002	2006–2007	2011–2012	2021–2022	2031–2032	2041–2042
MBS subsidy	1.09	1.10	1.15	1.33	1.56	1.78
PBS subsidy	0.60	0.63	0.79	1.31	2.15	3.35
Hospital and health services	1.16	1.16	1.20	1.34	1.51	1.63
Other	1.12	1.14	1.16	1.22	1.29	1.37
All health	3.96	4.02	4.30	5.20	6.51	8.13
Residential aged care	0.58	0.59	0.65	0.81	1.10	1.45
Community care	0.14	0.16	0.17	0.21	0.27	0.32
All aged care	0.72	0.75	0.82	0.01	1.37	1.77

Source: Treasury projections. (previously published as Table 8 in the IGR)

Figure 3: Projected Growth in Components of Commonwealth Health Spending

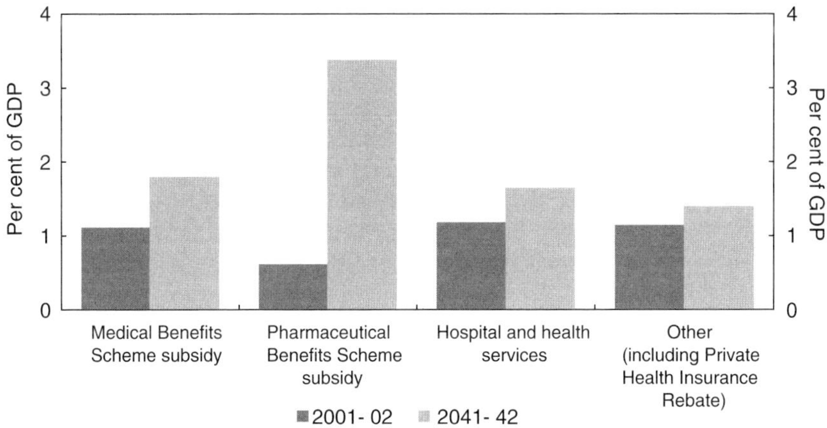

Source: Treasury projections (previously published as Figure 21 in the IGR)

an increase in the use and cost of existing services. Consumers have a high demand for more effective treatments, and expect these treatments will be provided to them soon after the technology first becomes available.

The ageing of the population also is projected to require increased health spending, as older people tend to have a greater need for health services. However, this is projected to have a much smaller effect on spending than the growing cost of new health care technology, increasing use of services and strong consumer demand and expectations.

Reflecting the ageing of the population, Commonwealth spending on aged care as a proportion of GDP is projected to more than double as a share of GDP, rising from 0.7 per cent of GDP in 2001–2002 to almost 1.8 per cent of GDP in 2041–2042 (Figure 4).

6. Sensitivity Analysis

6.1 Growth Assumptions

The projections for health spending are very sensitive to the non-demographic growth rate used. The growth rate, in turn, is quite sensitive to the starting point chosen and whether major policy changes are included or excluded.

A model of aggregate health spending was used to determine the sensitivity of health spending to varying the assumed non-demographic growth

Figure 4: Projected Growth in Commonwealth Aged Care Spending

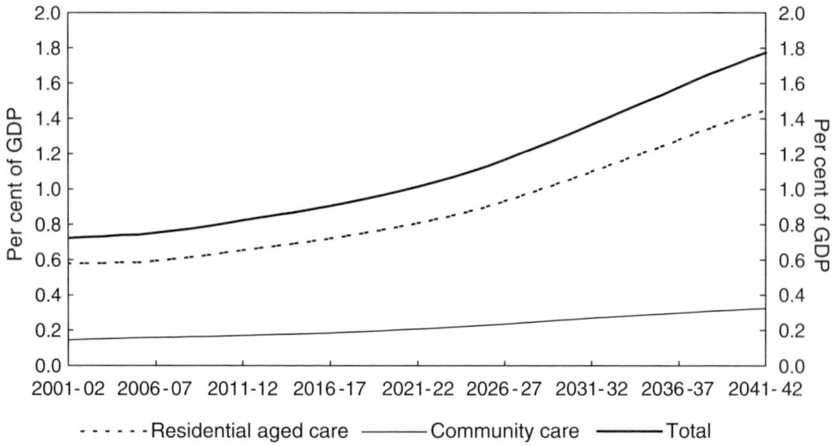

Source: Treasury projections (previously published as Figure 22 in the IGR)

Table 5: Projected Commonwealth Health Spending, Aggregate Model (per cent of GDP)

Underlying growth rate		2001–2002	2006–2007	2011–2012	2021–2022	2031–2032	2041–2042
Case A	3.0 per cent	3.96	4.26	4.84	5.99	7.69	9.65
Case B	2.5 per cent	3.96	4.14	4.55	5.36	6.49	7.67

Source: Treasury projections (previously published as Table 9 in the IGR)

rate. The main data for this model are the real growth rate in health spending (per person age-adjusted) and a distribution of Commonwealth health spending per person of a given age. Two cases were used to test the impact of varying the non-demographic rate.

For case A a non-demographic growth rate of 3.0 per cent was used, which is in line with growth experienced over the last 12 years if the impact of the Private Health Insurance Rebate on Commonwealth spending is excluded. In this case, health spending is projected to rise to 9.7 per cent of GDP (Table 5). This is higher than the result of the main model, largely because the growth rate does not account for the changes to the PBS in the 2002–2003 Budget. It was estimated that 82 per cent of projected growth, after compounding, is due to non-demographic factors, 9 per cent to population ageing and 9 per cent to population growth.

Case B used an average real per person age–adjusted growth rate of 2.5 per cent. This is an average of growth rates to 2000–2001, from starting points in each year from 1984–1985 to 1989–1990, inclusive. These growth rates ranged from 2.1 to 3.2 per cent and their averaging produces a representative rate. The growth rates differ because the spike of expenditure when Medicare was introduced in 1984 was followed by five years of around zero real growth. Case B is consistent with no further major upwards policy changes to Commonwealth health spending (such as occurred with Medicare or the Private Health Insurance Rebate) over the next four decades.

This case projects Commonwealth total health spending as a proportion of GDP to almost double by 2041–2042 compared with spending in 2001–2002. The relative impact of population growth and ageing is slightly greater than in case A.

Changing the real non-demographic growth by 0.5 percentage points (from 2.5 to 3.0) changes the projected value of Commonwealth health spending in 2041–2042 by 2.0 percentage points of GDP (Table 5). Further sensitivity testing (below) confirms that plausible changes in the assumed level of real non-demographic growth in health spending affect the projections far more than plausible changes in the demographic assumptions.

These projections of health spending cannot be directly compared with those for Australia published recently by the OECD (Dang et al., 2001), because of different coverage, use of more recent data and some revisions of methodology. The OECD placed Australia in the high health spending growth group (along with Canada, the Netherlands, New Zealand and the United States). However, the OECD study noted that the projection methodologies for health vary considerably by country, including the extent to which they take into account non-demographic growth factors.

6.2 Sensitivity Analysis: Demographic Assumptions

Significant uncertainty necessarily surrounds the assumptions underlying the IGRs health projections and their impact on government finances. Accordingly, the results represent a plausible central case and should not be viewed as specific forecasts. Nonetheless, as shown below, exploration of the impact of varying some key assumptions suggests that the projected size of the budget pressures is reasonably robust to changes in the underlying assumptions.

The demographic assumptions probably are the least uncertain, as they are based on relatively stable long-term trends. Greater uncertainty surrounds the assumptions -about productivity and spending and non-demographic growth.

Plausible variations in the assumptions were developed to illustrate the impact on GDP, and where effects were significant, on Commonwealth spending (Table 6).

Table 6: Assumptions Underlying Sensitivity Analysis

	Base case	Lower	Higher
Mortality			
Male life expectancy (years) in 2042	82.5	—	83.9
Female life expectancy (years) in 2042	87.5	—	88.5
Fertility (total fertility rate)[a]	1.6	1.5	—
Net migration (number of people per year)	90,000	80,000	135,000
Full-time labour force participation of older male workers	64.9% in 2011–2012	—	68.1% by 2011–2012
Labour productivity growth	1.75%	1.2%	2.0%
Unemployment rate	5%	4%	6%
Non-demographic health costs growth[b]	—	2.5%	

[a] *Represents the number of children a woman would bear during her lifetime if she experienced the current age-specific fertility rates at each age of her reproductive life.*
[b] *The annual real rate of growth per person age–adjusted. The health base case uses the component rather than the aggregate model. (Previously published as Table 14 in the IGR).*

In the lower mortality scenario more people live to older ages. However, it takes around 30 years to affect significantly the numbers of people in the older age groups.

Scenarios that involve a higher proportion of people in older age groups, a lower proportion of people employed relative to the population, lower productivity growth, and higher growth in the cost of programmes increase future pressures on government spending (Table 7).

In Table 7 the impact of changing the assumed non-demographic growth rate was examined by decreasing the average annual non-demographic growth rate for all health spending to 2.5 per cent. This can be interpreted as a drop of 0.1 percentage points of growth from the central scenario, which broadly corresponds to a non-demographic growth rate of 2.6 per cent. The lower growth rate decreases projected health costs by 0.5 per cent of GDP by 2041–2042.

Similarly, the potential impact of higher non-demographic growth was assessed. The higher growth (3.0 per cent) case is in line with growth experienced over the last 12 years, if the impact of the Private Health Insurance Rebate is excluded. This increases health costs, in comparison to the central scenario, by 1.5 per cent of GDP by 2041–2042.

The crucial implication of this analysis is that non-demographic growth arising from new technology and increased use and costs of services impacts

Table 7: Impact of Alternative Scenarios in 2041–2042 (Percentage Points)

Factors that increase budget pressure	**Lower mortality**	**Lower labour productivity**	**Higher health cost growth**
Spending impact (percentage points of GDP)			
Health	0.17	**	1.52
Aged care	0.12	**	0
Other	0.19	0.25	0
Total	0.48	0.25	1.52

Factors that decrease budget pressure	**Higher labour force participation (older workers)**	**Higher migration**	**Higher labour productivity**	**Lowest health cost growth**
Spending impact (percentage points of GDP)				
Health	−0.10	−0.25	**	−0.46
Aged care	−0.02	−0.13	**	0
Other	−0.13	−0.29	−0.05	0
Total	−0.25	−0.67	−0.05	−0.46

Source: Treasury projections (based on Table 15 of IGR)
Note: In the productivity scenarios health and aged care spending is assumed to increase to the same extent as the productivity-based wage increase. The potential impact of productivity growth on the cost of health care is difficult to quantify and has not been included here.

the projections much more than plausible changes in the demographic and economic assumptions, such as decreased mortality and increased labour force participation of older workers. The Productivity Commission recently produced a report on the impacts of advances in medical technology in Australia and noted that there are a number of new technologies on the horizon which may place upward pressure on health expenditure (Productivity Commission, 2005). For example, new vaccines, gene and stem cell therapies and artificial organs and joints. However, it is unclear whether introduction of such new technologies will increase non-demographic growth beyond its current levels over the long term partly because their costs may be mitigated by replacing current treatments or "downstream healthcare savings" (Productivity Commission, 2005). The Productivity Commission noted that the impact on expenditure of new technologies is particularly uncertain because it is dependant upon factors such as exactly when technologies will become available, who will access them, how the technologies will be used and funded, to what extent the technologies will be more effective than those currently available and whether the technologies will expand the range of conditions that are treatable (Productivity Commission, 2005). Similarly, the level of private health insurance coverage will also impact expenditure (coverage increased from about 30 per cent in the late 1990s to over 40 per cent in 2000 with the introduction of new private health insurance policies) (Private Health Insurance Industry Association Council, 2005).

7. Conclusions

The Commonwealth is the primary funder of health and aged care services in Australia. It funds Medicare, which incorporates the Medical Benefits Scheme, the PBS, which subsidises selected pharmaceuticals, and the Private Health Insurance Rebate. It also contributes to State funding of public hospital services and provides funding to non–government organisations for services such as residential aged care, community care and indigenous health care.

Over the past three decades, Commonwealth health spending has more than doubled, to 4.0 per cent of GDP in 2001–2002. In recent years, spending on the PBS has been the fastest growing component. In the decade to 2000–2001 PBS spending as a percentage of GDP more than doubled.

Although population growth and ageing affect health spending, these factors account for only around one–third of the recent growth. Much of the growth has come from the demand for new technology and treatments. Australians now expect to access more expensive diagnostic procedures and new (and more expensive) medications listed on the PBS. Unless addressed by policies even more effective in restraining costs than past policies and/or faster economic growth, these trends are likely to continue to drive health spending over the next four decades, pushing up Commonwealth health spending to 8.1 per cent of GDP in 2041–2042.

All areas of health spending are projected to increase, with PBS spending projected to rise from around 0.6 per cent of GDP in 2001–2002 to 3.4 per cent by 2041–2042 (Table 4), about a five-fold increase in its share of the economy. The reforms to the PBS implemented in the 2002–2003 Budget have helped reduce the overall cost of the scheme. Ongoing sound management of the PBS will be required to keep long–term growth in the scheme sustainable, to allow governments to continue providing access to affordable medicines for all Australians.

As the number of very old people increases, spending on aged care is also projected to increase from 0.7 per cent of GDP in 2001–2002 to 1.8 per cent of GDP in 2041–2042. Aged care is the most demographically sensitive area of government spending and the number of very old people is expected to increase significantly.

References

Australian Bureau of Statistics (1999). *Australian Social Trends*. Catalogue no. 4102.0, Australian Bureau of Statistics, Canberra.

Australian Institute of Health and Welfare (2003). *Health Expenditure 2001–2002*. Australian Institute of Health and Welfare, Canberra.

Dang, T., Antolin, P. and Oxley, H. (2001). *Fiscal Implications of Ageing: Projections of Age-Related Spending*. OECD Economics Department Working Papers, no. 305, Organisation for Economic Co-operation and Development, Paris.

Department of Health and Aged Care (1999). '*World Class Care*', *National Strategy for an Ageing Australia*. Discussion paper *(Draft)*. Department of Health and Aged Care, Canberra.

Eckerman, S. (1992). *Projected Health Expenditure and Ageing: Revised Methodologies*. Australian Institute of Health and Welfare, Canberra.

Goss, J., Eckerman, S., Pinyopusarerk, M. and Wen, X. (1996). *The Impact of Population Ageing on Health Expenditures in Australia in the 21st Century*. Australian Institute of Health and Welfare, Canberra.

Goss, J., Mathers, C., Pinyopusarerk, M., Wen, X. and Gillett, S. (1994). *Economic Perspective on the Health Impact of the Ageing of the Australian Population in the 21st Century*. Australian Institute of Health and Welfare, Canberra.

Lee, R. and Skinner, J. (1996). Assessing Forecasts of Mortality, Health Status, and Health Costs During Baby Boomer's Retirement, in Hanusheck, M.E. and Marritato, N. (eds), *Assessing Knowledge of Retirement Behaviour*, National Academy Press, Washington, DC.

Mathers, C. (1999). *International Trends in Health Expectancies: Do They Provide Evidence for Expansion or Compression of Morbidity*. Compression of Morbidity Workshop Paper, Occasional Papers Series no. 4, Department of Health and Aged Care, Canberra.

McCallum, J. and Geiselhart, K. (1996). *Australia's New Aged*. Allen and Unwin, Sydney.

Private Health Insurance Industry Association Council. (2005). Membership Statistics. Accessed 9 December 2005 http://www.phiac.gov.au/statistics/membership-coverage/hosquar.htm.

Productivity Commission (2005). *Impacts of Advances in Medical Technology in Australia*. Research Report, Productivity Commission, Canberra.

The Department of The Treasury (2002). *Intergenerational Report 2002–2003*. Budget Paper no. 5, The Department of The Treasury, Canberra.

Appendix A: Modelling Approaches Used to Project Health and Aged Care and Associated Issues

Health and aged care spending is projected using trends in cost per head of population by age and gender. This is then combined with the projected population changes. The primary model used in this report separately projects the main components of health spending to allow for different growth rates for hospitals, Medicare and the PBS.

The PBS is used to illustrate the methods used in the primary model.

Firstly, the distribution of the cost to the Commonwealth of the PBS per person of a given age range and gender was determined. The annual cost varies from about $40 per person to about $700 per person (aged over 80), with spending on women greater than that for men.

Secondly, historical information on the nominal total cost of the PBS each year was compiled and 1983–1984 chosen as the start year for the analysis. This start date includes 20 years of readily available data covering a number of policy changes, but none of a fundamental nature.

The factors influencing the raw growth rate were extracted to determine the real per person age-adjusted growth rate for the PBS. This growth rate separates the impact of population growth and population ageing (captured in the demographic projections) from the non-demographic growth.

Incorporating the 2002–2003 Budget measures, growth was calculated to the end of the forward estimates period (2005–2006) as follows:

- the nominal compound growth from 1983–1984 to 2005–2006 is 11.57 per cent;
- the real compound growth is 7.56 per cent;
- the real compound growth per person is 6.25 per cent; and
- the real compound growth per person, corrected for the changing age composition over the analysis period is 5.64 per cent.

The real per person age–adjusted growth rate of 5.64 per cent was used in the projection. This growth figure is assumed to apply for each age group and for all years of the projection.

Commonwealth PBS spending projections were then generated using the age by sex distribution of PBS spending, the real per person age-adjusted growth rate and population and CPI projections.

For the medical benefits component of health the greater availability of data allows a differential growth rate (per person in a given age range) to be calculated for different age ranges, with the calculated rates of growth being higher for older groups.

Health — Secondary Model

An aggregate model for health was used to project total health spending using a single growth rate and to test the sensitivity of Commonwealth health spending to variations in the growth rate.

The main data for this model are the real growth rate in health spending (per person age-adjusted) and a fine scale distribution of Commonwealth health spending per person of a given age.

The choice of starting date and inclusion or exclusion of major policy changes results in different growth rates, and the underlying growth rates and projected health spending are very sensitive to those assumptions. Sensitivity analysis was conducted to demonstrate the impact of a non-demographic growth rate of 3.0 per cent and a lower growth rate of 2.5 per cent. The component model results lie between these two projections.

Aged Care Projections

The aged care sector comprises nursing homes, hostels and community care (HACC and other programmes funded by the Department of Health and Ageing and the Department of Veterans' Affairs). The age structure for the Home and Community Care programme was used for all Commonwealth community care. There is no stable trend in these areas because of recent major policy changes which have shifted the expenditure balance towards community care. Therefore, because wages are a significant component of spending in these areas, the real per person age adjusted growth rate going forward was assumed to be strongly influenced by real wages growth, and taken to be 1.75 per cent beyond 2007–2008, reflecting the base productivity growth assumption. The same per capita growth rate was applied across all areas of aged care spending.

Some Modelling Issues

1. A number of authors have argued that as life expectancy increases, all additional life years are relatively healthy life years, with expensive medical care being shifted out to the end of the life course (Eckerman, 1992; Goss et al., 1994; Goss et al. , 1996; Lee and Skinner, 1996; Department of Health and Aged Care, 1999). It is argued that the years of expensive health care would not increase, thereby producing a compression of morbidity. No explicit adjustment was made for compression of morbidity, as the available evidence for Australia is insufficient and inconclusive. Recent evidence indicates that disability rates amongst the aged are rising (Australian Bureau of Statistics, 1999) and some authors argue that such trends may continue (Mathers, 1999). Further, to the extent that compression of morbidity occurs, it would have been captured implicitly as a factor constraining growth.
2. Trends were established during periods of structural stability and then continued without modification or softening. There was consideration as to whether a very fast growing trend such as PBS expenditure could continue for a very long period without weakening. It was decided not to

place an artificial limit on this growth for two reasons:

- the historical fit to an exponential growth by the PBS was extremely good over a 20 year period during which there was considerable concern about the rapid growth; and
- any constraint would be a matter of arbitrary specification and not based on data.

3. As noted above, an alternative aggregate (whole of health) model has been used as a secondary model for consistency and sensitivity analysis. An aggregate model has some intrinsic value in implicitly allowing some movement of resources between components and, to a degree, in effect providing some automatic stabilisation of a rapidly growing component such as the PBS. For a 5-year period ending June 2002, the aggregate model projections provided a good fit to actual data.
4. The issue also arises whether other factors such as increase in real income per person correlate strongly enough with growth of component expenditure to warrant inclusion in the projection equations alongside population and ageing. However, analysis of the Australian data does not give a strong case for such factors to be included. Note that in some common OECD methodologies such additional factors (reflecting affordability) are included but importantly, without the historical non-demographic growths being included.

Appendix B: GDP Projections

The IGR presents its projections as a percentage of Gross Domestic Product (GDP) so they are considered relative to the size of the economy. Growth in real GDP in the longer term reflects the net impact of productivity growth, employment growth and changes in hours worked. The results of the IGR analysis and projections are shown in Table B1.

Table B1: Growth in Real GDP and Real GDP Per Person[a]

Decade	Labour productivity growth	Employment growth	Real GDP growth[b]	Real GDP per person growth
1980s	1.2	2.4	3.4	1.8
1990s	2.0	1.3	3.4	2.2
2000s	1.7	1.5	3.1	2.1

(Continued)

Table B1: *Continued*

Decade	Labour productivity growth	Employment growth	Real GDP growth[b]	Real GDP per person growth
2001s	1.75	0.6	2.3	1.5
2002s	1.75	0.2	2.0	1.4
2030s	1.75	0.1	1.9	1.5

Source: ABS Cat. No. 5206.0 and 6203.0 and Treasury (previously published as Table 4 in IGR)
[a]*Average annual growth rates (per cent).*
[b]*1999–2000 dollars.*

Table B2: Projected Real and Nominal GDP ($million)

	Per cent of GDP	2001–2002	2011–2012	2021–2022	2031–2032	2041–2042
Nominal	1.0	7,100	12,179	19,467	30,236	46,559
	0.1	710	1,218	1,947	3,024	4,656
Real (2001–2002 dollars)	1.0	7,100	9,583	11,966	14,519	17,465
	0.1	710	958	1,197	1,452	1,747

Source: Treasury projections (previously published as Table 1 in IGR)

Small changes in proportions of GDP, even 0.1 per cent, are equivalent to significant amounts in dollar terms when prices are assumed unchanged (real terms). The amounts are even more significant in dollar terms when the effect of likely price changes over time is taken into account (Table B2).

Appendix C: Demographic spending projections

The central IGR projections of Commonwealth demographically-driven spending are summarised in Table C1.

Table C1: Projections of Commonwealth Demographic Spending(per cent of GDP)

	2001–2002	2006–2007	2011–2012	2021–2022	2031–2032	2041–2042
Medical Benefits Scheme	1.1	1.1	1.2	1.3	1.6	1.8
Pharmaceutical Benefits Scheme	0.6	0.6	0.8	1.3	2.1	3.4
Hospital and health services	1.2	1.2	1.2	1.3	1.5	1.6
Other (including Private Health Insurance Rebate)	1.1	1.1	1.2	1.2	1.3	1.4
Total health	*4.0*	*4.0*	*4.3*	*5.2*	*6.5*	*8.1*
Residential care	0.6	0.6	0.7	0.8	1.1	1.4
Community care	0.1	0.2	0.2	0.2	0.3	0.3
Total aged care	*0.7*	*0.8*	*0.8*	*1.0*	*1.4*	1.8
Total health aged care	**4.7**	**4.8**	**5.1**	**6.2**	**7.9**	**9.9**
Age and Service Pension	2.9	2.8	2.9	3.6	4.3	4.6
Disability Support Pension	0.9	0.7	0.8	0.8	0.9	0.9
Parenting Payment (Single)	0.6	0.6	0.6	0.6	0.6	0.6
Unemployment allowances	0.8	0.8	0.7	0.6	0.5	0.4
Family Tax Benefit (Parts A and B)	1.6	1.3	1.2	1.1	1.0	0.9
Total Payments of individuals	**6.8**	**6.3**	**6.2**	**6.8**	**7.2**	**7.4**
Schools	0.8	0.8	0.8	0.7	0.7	0.7
Higher education	0.7	0.6	0.6	0.6	0.6	0.6
Vocational education and training	0.2	0.2	0.2	0.2	0.2	0.2
Administration and other	0.1	0.1	0.1	0.1	0.1	0.1
Total education	**1.8**	**1.8**	**1.7**	**1.6**	**1.6**	**1.6**
Unfunded Government superannuation	**0.6**	**0.5**	**0.5**	**0.5**	**0.4**	**0.3**
Total Commonwealth demographically driven spending	**13.9**	**13.3**	**13.6**	**15.1**	**17.1**	**19.2**

Source: Treasury projections (previously published as Table A1 in IGR)

Chapter 8

The Australian Pharmaceuticals Benefit Scheme and Older Australians: Changes in Government Outlays and Consumer Costs from the 2002–03 Federal Budget Measures

Laurie Brown, Annie Abello, Ben Phillips and Ann Harding

NATSEM, University of Canberra, Australia

Abstract

Government outlays on the Australian Pharmaceutical Benefits Scheme have increased rapidly over the past 10 years. Finding ways of curbing government expenditure on the PBS, while maintaining social equity and access to 'essential' medicines is at the centre of ongoing public debate. The PBS is highly progressive, with 80 per cent of total PBS government outlays being directed at concessional patients, the majority of whom are elderly. Older Australians receive far greater PBS benefits than any other user group. An estimated 16 per cent of total PBS government outlays are directed towards persons aged 75 years and over. In the 2002–2003 federal budget, the Government aimed to introduce an increase of close to 28 per cent in PBS copayments and safety net thresholds. This paper, using PharmaSim, a microsimulation model of the PBS, examines the impact on the costs to government and patients of PBS listed medicines and estimates the distributional effects of this policy change, particularly for older Australians.

1. Introduction

In 2001, Australians aged 65 or more years accounted for 12.5 per cent (2.37 million) of the total population (18.77 million). Australia's current age structure already reflects the impact of population ageing. The trend of ageing of the population will continue as 'the inevitable result of sustained low fertility combined with increasing life expectancy at birth' (ABS, 2003).

International Symposia in Economic Theory and Econometrics, Vol. 16

ISSN: 1571-0386 DOI: 10.1016/S1571-0386(06)16008-1

Additionally, the first of the post-World War II baby-boomers will start reaching retirement age in the next decade or so. The proportion of the population aged 65 years and over is estimated to increase to 14.7 per cent in 2011, to 19.0 per cent in 2021 to 27.1 per cent in 2051 (ABS, 2003, Series B). The 'very old', i.e., those aged 85 years and over, who typically have very high demand for health and aged care services including prescribed medicines, currently make up 1.4 per cent of the total population. This group is projected to double in size by 2021.

Progressive population ageing has become a major driver of public policy formulation in Australia, especially in the social, welfare and health fields. The Australian Commonwealth Government's Pharmaceutical Benefits Scheme (PBS) was designed originally in 1948 to provide access for all Australians to a 'free-list' of life-saving medicines. In 2003, it aims to provide Australians with timely, reliable and affordable access to necessary and cost-effective prescription medicines.[1] However, the PBS is now under financial pressure with greater than expected growth in PBS expenditures in the last few years. Much of the current concern stems from the perceived unaffordability of prescribed medicines, and government and consumers' ability and willingness to pay for these drugs.

Federal government expenditure on the PBS has been one of the fastest growing areas of government outlays over the past decade, with significant increases in recent years. Since the early 1990s, PBS expenditures have grown at over 10 per cent a year (Figure 1), a rate well above growth in GDP (4 per cent) or in the total health budget (6 per cent). In 2001–2002, government expenditure on the PBS increased by 20.0 per cent (Figure 1). Although this was an anomaly and the increases have returned since to historical levels, this spike fuelled an ongoing and often emotionally charged public debate over the long-term fiscal sustainability of the PBS.

Three key factors are contributing to the increasing costs of the PBS: (a) increases in drug prices. Australia has had a long history of having been able to negotiate below world prices for PBS listed drugs. As on 30 June 2000, manufacturer prices for the top 150 pharmaceuticals — accounting for over 80 per cent of total PBS expenditures — were much lower in Australia than in the US, Canada, UK and Sweden (e.g., Productivity Commission, 2001). However, while the Australian Government has continued to secure low drug prices by international standards, the cost of pharmaceuticals, in general, have risen in excess of 1 per cent per annum over the last few years[2] and

[1] www.health.gov.au/pbs/general/aboutus.htm

[2] Although annual changes in CPI for pharmaceuticals have varied markedly over the last 5–10 years. Consumer Price Index, Australia, various years, ABS Cat No. 6401.0.

Figure 1: Government, patient and total costs of the PBS, 1992–2002

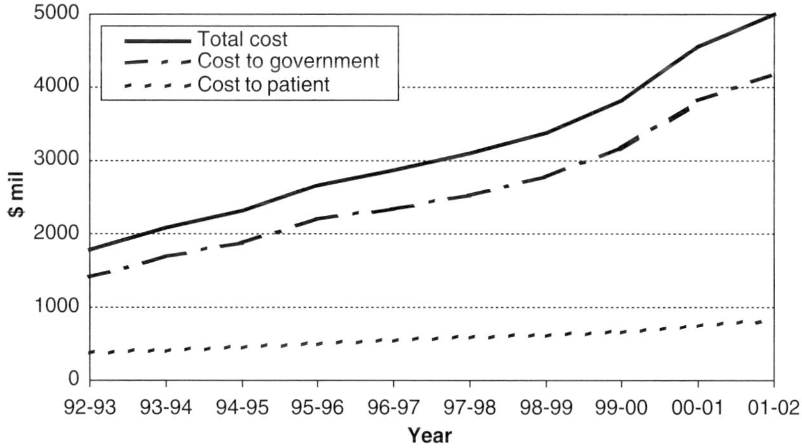

Data Source: DHA.

covered under the PBS by as much as 7.5 per cent[3]; (b) entry, and imminent entry, into the pharmaceutical market of new biotechnological drugs and other innovative targeted therapies. These new drugs have the potential to deliver significant health benefits, often to those with previously unmanageable conditions, but these new 'era' drugs are more expensive relative to the existing small molecule compounds that up to now have been listed on the PBS (Lofgren, 2001; Brown et al., 2002). These 'high-tech high cost' drugs are presenting new challenges to the PBS listing process, especially since doctors are prescribing larger volumes of newer, more expensive medications compared to older, cheaper drugs and Australian prices for these new drugs are much closer to prices in other developed countries. Growth in the costs of the PBS in real terms from non-demographic factors (such as price inflation and the listing of new medications) has averaged 6.1 per cent over the last 20 years (Department of Treasury, 2002); and (c) population ageing, including the growth in the numbers of people eligible for concession cards, increased patient demand for prescribed medicines, and increasing rates of diagnosis and treatment of chronic illness particularly asthma, diabetes, heart disease and mental illness (Donovan, 2002; Harvey, 2002; Rickard, 2002).

It is the older age groups who are the main consumers of prescribed medicines, largely reflecting their poorer health status and increased number of health problems compared with younger age groups, and to a lesser

[3] From HIC data on script volumes and costs.

degree their tendency to visit their 'family' doctor more. In Australia, the number of GP consultations is the most powerful predictor of the number of prescriptions written (Pritchard, 1999) and the number of per capita doctor visits per year has been increasing since the late 1970s (Walker and Abello, 2000).

The BEACH study of general practice activity in Australia, 2001–2002, showed the prescription rate per 100 GP encounters to be 117 scripts per 100 encounters for males aged 65–74 years and 122 for females, and 111 scripts per 100 encounters for males aged 75 or more years and 117 for females in this age group. These rates were approximately 80 per cent higher than for children and teenagers, 70 per cent for younger adults and 25 per cent for those aged 45–64 years (Britt et al., 2002).

The PBS is highly progressive, with 80 per cent of total PBS government outlays being directed at 'concessional' patients (basically individuals and families with low incomes and who receive social security benefits), the majority of whom are elderly. As will be shown in this paper, older Australians receive far greater PBS benefits than any other user group. Data from Western Australia shows that over 80 per cent of elderly residents (aged 70 or more years) use the PBS at least once during a year and on average they consume between 40 and 45 PBS items each year (Cooper and Hagan, 1999). This compares with an average of five PBS items per person per year for those aged less than 20 years.

The PBS is an uncapped scheme. It has been estimated that if current trends and rules governing the PBS remain unchanged then the cost of the Scheme to the Commonwealth Government could increase four–five fold by 2020 (Walker et al., 2000; Department of Treasury, 2002). The Federal Government's Intergenerational Report (Department of Treasury, 2002) predicts the PBS to be the fastest growing area of Commonwealth Government spending to 2040, with PBS Government outlays estimated to rise from around 0.6 per cent of GDP in 2001–2002 to 1.31 per cent in 2021–2022 and to 3.4 per cent in 2041–2042. While much of the projected increased cost of the PBS is due to non-demographic factors – particularly PBS listing of newer and more expensive pharmaceutical technologies – it also reflects the impacts of population ageing and consumers' ongoing demand for more effective medications, especially by older Australians. Over the coming decades, there will be significantly more senior pensioners who, under current policy settings, will be entitled to access PBS listed medicines at the much higher government benefit, i.e., concessional rates.Thus, the sustainability of the PBS, and in particular, the continued funding of what appears to be ever-increasing government outlays on subsidised prescribed medicines, is being keenly questioned within federal health and financial public policy circles. The Federal Government is seeking ways of curbing government expenditure on the PBS while maintaining social equity and access to 'essential' medicines. In the 2002–2003 federal budget, the Government announced a budget measure that aimed to introduce a near-28 per cent increase in the PBS policy settings, i.e., in patient copayments and safety net thresholds. Although these budget measures have been blocked in Senate, in releasing the 2003–2004 Budget, the Federal Treasurer re-iterated the need for such measures to be introduced.

The aim of this paper is to simulate, using PharmaSim, a microsimulation model of the PBS, the impact of this proposed budget measure in terms of changes in government outlays and consumer contributions, particularly focussing on the distributional effects on older Australians — the main users and beneficiaries of the PBS. The structure of the paper is as follows: a brief overview of the PBS is given as background; the proposed budget measures in changing the settings of the PBS are described; some methodological details of PharmaSim and the modelling of the budget scenario are provided; the results of the modelling are presented comparing the outcomes of the scenario to the base case, i.e., to no change; and finally a few concluding remarks are given.

2. Overview of the PBS

While a number of aspects of the PBS are of concern to the pharmaceutical industry and other key stakeholders, in general, the PBS is seen internationally as one of the best in the world (Brown et al., 2002). A comprehensive range of medicines is included on the PBS, with the majority of prescribed drug sales being covered by the scheme (Department of Health and Ageing, 2003). Medicines must be approved for use in Australia in terms of their efficacy and safety, and then be assessed as being 'cost effective' in order to be PBS listed. The aim of this cost effectiveness criteria is to ensure that new drugs listed on the scheme represent "value for money" to the Australian community and provide equity across disease groups. However, it is also seen as a cost containment measure and an additional barrier to market entry at subsidised prices (Cookson, 2000; Hill et al., 2000; Birkett et al., 2001; Dalton, 2001; Sansom, 2001; Brown et al., 2002).

About 2,500 medicines are currently listed on the PBS. As at 1 May 2002, the scheme covered 593 drug substances (generic drugs), available in 1,461 forms and strengths (items) and marketed as 2,506 different drug products (brands). However, many drug items have restrictions placed on their use in terms of their eligibility for government subsidy under the PBS — some 785 items are restricted to specific indications, patient groups or clinical settings that achieve the optimal clinical benefit and cost effectiveness (restricted listing); with 286 of these restricted items further requiring the prescribing doctor to obtain prior approval from the Health Insurance Commission

(HIC) to prescribe under subsidy to the individual patient ("Authority required" items).

The scheme covers Australian residents and eligible foreign visitors. Consumers are required to make a user-pays contribution to the cost of PBS benefit medicines via patient copayments. As stated in the introduction, low-income individuals and families eligible for certain Commonwealth Government (Centrelink) pensions and allowances are able, however, to access PBS medicines at concessional rates. Centrelink now issues three types of cards that confer concessional status. These are the Health Care Card, the Pensioner Concession Card, and the Commonwealth Seniors Health Card.

The PBS also has 'Safety Net' arrangements to protect individuals and families from large overall annual expenses for PBS listed medicines. Once a family that does not have concessional status records spending beyond the general patient safety net threshold (SNT) in a calendar year, they are required to pay only the concessional copayment for each further PBS medicine within the same year. For concessional patients, there is no cost once their families have a record of spending beyond the concessional safety net limit in a calendar year. In this case, the government pays the full price of all further PBS medicines prescribed within the year. Each year, on 1 January, the safety net for each family is reset to zero for administrative purposes. Levels of patient copayments and the PBS safety net arrangements are referred to as the 'PBS policy settings'. Patient copayments and safety net thresholds are normally indexed to movements in the Consumer Price Index from 1 January each year.

Patients may be required, however, to pay more than the copayment where a PBS item is priced above the benchmark price for different brands of the same drug, or the benchmark price for a particular therapeutic group of drugs. The Government pays the additional cost of drugs exceeding patient copayments up to the benchmark price only. Brand or therapeutic group premiums are met by the consumer and do not count towards safety nets.

On average, the government subsidises patients to the extent of 84 per cent of PBS drug costs with nearly 80 per cent of total government PBS subsidies accruing to concessional patients.

3. The 2002–2003 PBS Budget Measures

Despite the marked growth in government outlays on the PBS in recent years, the PBS settings, in general, have increased only in line with inflation. Apart from annual indexation, patient copayments have not risen since 1996–1997 (Department of Health and Ageing, 2003a). In his 2002–2003 budget speech, the Treasurer, the Honourable Peter Costello, outlined the

Government's approach to making the PBS more sustainable — defined as 'delivering access to medicines at affordable prices over the longer term'. A key measure, introduced alongside several changes aimed at ensuring PBS medicines are used more appropriately, was that from 1 August 2002, co-payments for concession cardholders such as pensioners and Seniors Health cardholders would rise by \$1–\$4.60 and copayments for others by \$6.20–\$28.60 per prescription, representing a near 28 per cent increase. Safety net arrangements would continue to protect people who need a large number of medicines. Consistent with the current arrangements, once concession cardholders have paid for 52 PBS prescriptions in the year, they will receive further PBS medicines free for the rest of the year. Non-concession cardholders who pay \$874.90 in a year for their PBS medicines will be eligible for further PBS medicines at the concessional rate for the rest of the year (Department of Treasury, 2002a).

The Treasurer argued that the proposed measures would ensure that consumers, industry, doctors and pharmacists all contribute to containing the rate of increase in the PBS, and that by making the PBS more sustainable, the Government could continue to fund the listing of new, highly effective, but expensive medicines. Notwithstanding the cost of the prescription, patients, especially concessional cardholders, were still expected to pay only a small part of the cost of many PBS medicines.

In May 2002, when the new PBS policy settings were announced, the proposed changes were estimated to result in about \$1,056 million in net savings to government over the following four years[4] (Commonwealth Treasury, 2002), i.e., the 28 per cent increase in patient copayments and SNTs was expected to generate between four and six per cent savings in government expenditure on the PBS per annum over the period 2002–2003 to 2005–2006.

These changes in the PBS policy settings were not passed by the Senate. However, the Treasurer remains committed to these measures — the forward estimates outlined in the 2003–2004 budget for the Pharmaceuticals Benefits Sub-function included the impact of the proposed increases in patient copayments as announced in the previous budget (Department of Treasury, 2003). It is also interesting to note that, in the 2003–2004 budget, the Government announced an initiative to enhance the capacity of the HIC to validate online the eligibility of Centrelink concessional cardholders to receive benefits under the PBS at reduced rates. The aim is to improve the

[4] These are the savings to the Department of Health and Ageing portfolio from changes in the PBS settings. Further savings of \$59.7 million accrue to the Department of Veterans' Affairs through savings from the Repatriation Pharmaceutical Benefits Scheme.

monitoring of PBS entitlements, a move expected to generate government savings of $30.7 millions over four years (DHA, 2003).

4. PharmaSim — Modelling the PBS

The cost and distributional impacts of the proposed budget measures were modelled using PharmaSim, a microsimulation model of the PBS. Harding (1996) and Gupta and Kapur (2000) provide an overview of microsimulation modelling — the basic concepts of this modelling approach, the various types of models available, some of the technical characteristics and considerations, and examples of model applications. Microsimulation models are distinctive in that they are based on microdata, i.e., "low-level" population data, typically the unit records of individuals from a national sample survey conducted by a national Bureau of Statistics, or administrative records of individual clients or consumers. One of the most important advantages of large-scale microsimulation models is, that being based on unit records, it is possible to examine the effects of policy changes for narrowly defined ranges of individuals or demographic groups (Creedy, 2001). They can mirror the heterogeneity in the population, replicate the complexity of the policy structures, transfers and settings, and be used to forecast in detail the outcomes of policy changes and 'what if' scenarios, i.e., the results can describe what may happen to particular individuals and groups under specified conditions (Brown and Harding, 2002).

PharmaSim improves earlier modelling work on the PBS by Schofield (1998, 1999), and Walker (Walker et al., 1998; Walker et al., 2000; Walker, 2000). PharmaSim incorporates variation in the number of drugs used by age, gender and PBS beneficiary (concessional cardholder) category; includes far more detailed imputation of drug prices within each of 19 drug groups and 157 drug subgroups; includes a forecasting capacity and has the capability to incorporate responses to changes in drug prices or PBS policy settings.

The conceptual and methodological constructs and technical features of PharmaSim are described in Abello et al. (2003) and Brown et al. (2004). In summary, the model is made up of two modules — an econometric Medicine Module and a forecasting microsimulation Patient Module. The Medicine Module is basically a deterministic time series model that projects total scripts and average costs per script for 19 drug classes. Trends in these data then serve as inputs to the forecasting version of the Patient Module.

The Patient Module is composed of two parts — an input dataset and a forecasting component. The main input dataset is at the person-level (i.e. each record pertains to an individual with a family identifier to link family members) with individual characteristics and data on drug usage across the

19 drug classes by sex, age and concessional cardholder status. The unit of analysis can be the individual, the family, or aggregate levels (e.g. groupings by demographic or income ranges) (Abello et al., 2003; Brown et al., 2004).

Individual-level data on demographic, socio-economic and drug usage patterns and costs are combined to construct the model's base dataset using four data sources. First, PharmaSim is based upon the unit record file of the 2001A version of NATSEM's STINMOD,[5] which is derived from the ABS 1998–1999 Household Expenditure Survey (HES). The HES microdata provide a rich source of information about the demographic and economic characteristics of a representative sample of Australian families. STINMOD/01A updates the incomes and housing costs of those captured in the original HES, reweighting the dataset to allow for demographic and labour market change between 1998–1999 and 2001, and imputing the receipt of a wide range of social security payments and the payment of income tax liabilities. Importantly, this latter step also means that the receipt of the variety of pharmaceutical concession cards was imputed for each family within the dataset (Harding et al., 2004).

The HES data do not, however, contain any information about the usage of prescribed pharmaceuticals — only about the spending of each household on prescription medicines. Accordingly, a second ABS unit record file, the 1995 National Health Survey (NHS), was used to derive information on the usage of prescribed pharmaceuticals across 19 drug classes, by age, gender and concessional (i.e. 'card') status. From this, the estimated number and type of prescribed pharmaceuticals used by age, gender and card status was imputed for each person within the HES. Ultimately, each person in the PharmaSim model selected to use prescribed pharmaceuticals had one or more of the 19 drug types allocated to them, so that within each card, age and gender cell, the drug usage pattern in the model matched the usage pattern in the NHS.

A third dataset on the costs of the pharmaceuticals consumed was then prepared, using a distribution of prices (average per script costs) at the ATC level observed administratively for each of the 19 drug classes in that year. The price distribution at the ATC level ranged from 1 to a maximum of 10 prices for each drug group, with a total of 157 prices being used. These cost data were then merged onto the patient-based dataset, allowing estimation of the costs of the drugs used by each individual in the Patient Module. By aggregating individual-level costs, the model is able to estimate total patient and government expenditures on PBS prescribed drugs over the base and forecast years.

[5] STINMOD is NATSEM's static microsimulation model that models the impact of the personal income tax and social security systems on Australian families.

Finally, the initial results generated from PharmaSim are aligned with HIC data on actual scripts, i.e., the model is aligned so that the results match actual administrative data on PBS scripts for the base year 2001–2002. In aligning the model to administrative data in this way, the pool of prescribed medicine scripts is separated into the three prescribed medicine groups: Group 1 scripts comprise the drugs that attract a government subsidy under the PBS, i.e., the PBS benefit drugs; Group 2 scripts comprise PBS listed medicines that do not attract a government subsidy, i.e., scripts with a total cost (or price) below the PBS copayment level — the below copayment drugs; and Group 3 scripts comprise private medicines, i.e., prescribed medicines not listed on the PBS. The focus of the model simulation is the segment of the population that uses Group 1 scripts, i.e., PBS benefit drugs.

In forecasting mode, the script data in the person-level dataset are revised each year to be consistent with the aggregate level of scripts estimated in the Medicine Module. The module can then project PBS scripts, government outlays and patient expenditure over a five-year forecasting period. The PBS is modelled by applying the rules of the scheme to each individual and family in the dataset over an 18-month period on a two-weekly basis starting on 1 January (that is when each family's SNT is reset to zero). The safety net operates on a calendar year basis and therefore needs to be modelled over this period. To reconcile this with the need to generate statistics on a financial year basis, statistics are produced on scripts and costs for both the first and last 12 months of the 18 months simulation period (Abello et al., 2003; Brown et al., 2004).

The model's population database is the non-institutionalised population that spends on prescribed drugs, i.e., the dataset contains only spenders on prescribed medicines within the two-week survey period of the HES. Given the two-week window within which data on prescriptions were collected, it is recognised that spenders are more likely to include high users of prescription drugs or those with chronic illnesses that use prescription drugs regularly, whereas a smaller proportion of those with acute or short-term conditions would be captured. If the survey period were lengthened then the number of spenders would increase proportionately with the less frequent users of prescribed drugs also being included in the population of prescription users. This is a deficiency of the model arising from the fact that the only data available on expenditure or usage of prescriptions covers only a fortnightly period. In recognition of this, the model is not used to examine the results of simulation at the level of the individual, but only at the aggregate or at reasonably large subgroup levels (whether by drug class, age and sex or concessional card status), and when the results are presented at the family level, the results are only for a fortnightly window (Brown et al., 2004). Further, since the model's input dataset is not based on persons living in institutionalised care, for example, hospitals or nursing homes, the results presented in the paper on prescribed drug usage by those aged above 75 years are likely to be under-estimated.

Another important and related limitation to the current version of PharmaSim is that, due to the reliance on the two-week survey data, difficulties are encountered in fully modelling the effects of the safety net (about 20 per cent of all scripts in a year are above safety net scripts). This is because the safety net rule applies to the total spending on PBS medicines by a family in a calendar year. However, data on the drugs used during the course of a year by a particular family are not available. Instead, all that is available is the two-week sample of drug use provided by the NHS. To derive annual estimates, a standard practice is to multiply the two-week figures by 26. For most purposes this provides fairly reliable estimates, but it is not adequate for modelling the PBS safety net. For chronic conditions (when drugs are used regularly throughout the year), multiplying the NHS two-weekly figures by 26[6] might give a fair estimate of annual drug consumption. For non-chronic conditions, multiplying by 26 would give correct aggregate estimates within the age-sex-card cells but would over-estimate drug consumption for particular individuals and families. Thus, families consuming drugs for non-chronic conditions may incorrectly be shown to reach the safety net when, in actuality, the consumption of such drugs should have been spread out over several families, none of whom may have reached the safety net. To roughly proxy the impact of the safety net, the current version of PharmaSim ensures that the proportion of scripts that reach the safety net limits is the same as that shown in administrative data (Harding et al., 2004).

Given these uncertainties, the results presented in this paper focus on the distributional impact of the PBS in the first fortnight of 2004 — when the safety net thresholds have just been reset to zero and before any families become eligible for the safety net. In future enhancements to the model, the population base will be extended to all prescribed drug users in the population and patterns of drug use across a full calendar year simulated. This will then allow the impact of the safety net to be assessed with greater precision.

Overall, microsimulation techniques bring a range of methodological advantages in assessing the impact of the type of policy changes evident in the 2002–2003 budget measures for example. Since microsimulation modelling is based on unit record files, the variance in the number and types of drugs

[6] Based on preliminary analysis of annual patterns of drug usage, 13 seems to be the more realistic factor as the majority of scripts cover a 30 day supply of the prescribed drug.

used by the population can be examined directly. A greater variety of parameters can be changed independently, and more accurate and detailed estimates of PBS services and benefits and the associated distributional effects of policy changes, generated. PharmaSim is able to simulate the effect of changes in the drugs listed on the PBS, in their prices, in the rules (policy settings) of the PBS, in government versus consumer outlays, and in the distributional impacts.

Results of scenarios simulated using PharmaSim are compared to the outcomes of the 'base case', i.e., the situation when no policy changes occur except CPI indexed increases in the PBS settings. Each scenario is based on 'static', i.e., non-behavioural modelling, in that it is assumed there is no patient response (behavioural change) to any changes proposed in copayment rates or prices. This type of modelling is commonly referred to as measuring the effects of policy changes on the 'morning after' the change, assessing what each individual would, counterfactually, spend on PBS benefit drugs under the new system or set of policy rules. This is a standard practice in microsimulation modelling. However, it is acknowledged that there are potentially important price responses by consumers and providers (Brown and Harding, 2002; Brown et al., 2004).

The PBS policy settings used in the modelling of the Budget Scenario are given in Table 1. For the purposes of the scenario, the proposed budget measures (28 per cent increase in copayments and SNTs) are introduced on 1 January 2003. The base case uses actual PBS settings for 2003 and then assumes a CPI increase of 2.5 per cent for 2004. The proposed PBS settings are used in the scenario for 2003, which are then up-rated by 2.5 per cent

Table 1: PBS Policy Settings for Budget Scenario

	Base case			Scenario	
	1/1/ 2002[a] ($)	1/1/ 2003[a] ($)	1/1/ 2004[p] ($)	1/1/ 2003[p] ($)	1/1/ 2004[p] ($)
Copayment — Concessional					
Below safety net	3.60	3.70	3.79	4.60	4.72
Above safety net	0	0	0	0	0
Copayment — General					
Below safety net	22.40	23.10	23.68	28.60	29.32
Above safety net	3.60	3.70	3.79	4.60	4.72
Safety net — Concessional	187.20	192.40	197.21	239.20	245.18
Safety net — General	686.40	708.40	726.11	874.90	896.77

Note: a = actual; p = projected.

from 1 January 2004. Aggregate results are generated for 2003–2004, the first financial year for which the effects of the scenario are felt over a full financial year. Distributional impacts are described for the fortnight window 1–14 January 2004.

PharmaSim has been validated previously by comparing the aggregate results produced by the model with the projected forward estimates documented in the budget papers. PharmaSim estimates of total PBS government expenditures for the period 2001–2002 were virtually identical to the Budget estimate and for the period 2002–2006 closely approximated government estimates (within 5.5 per cent). Differences in assumptions are likely to explain these small discrepancies (Abello et al., 2003).

5. Results

PharmaSim estimates that the PBS, with no changes to the policy settings aside from normal indexation, will subsidise 161.8 million scripts at a total cost of $5,758 million in 2003–2004. As is the current situation, government outlays will account for 84 per cent of the total costs, the remaining 16 per cent being met from patient copayments (Table 2). Introduction of the

Table 2: Scripts and Government, Patient and Total Costs, Base Case and Scenario, 2003–2004

	Base case	Scenario	Change from base	
			Actual	Percentage
Scripts	('000)	('000)	('000)	(%)
Concessional	135,814	135,814	0	0
General	25,964	22,522	−3,441	−13
All patients	161,778	158,337	−3,441	−2
Costs	($ mil)	($ mil)	($ mil)	(%)
Cost to patients				
Concessional	400	500	100	25
General	506	544	38	7
All patients	906	1,044	138	15
Cost to government				
Concessional	3,851	3,751	−100	−3
General	1,001	868	−133	−13
All patients	4,852	4,620	−233	−5
Total costs				
Concessional	4,251	4,251	0	0
General	1,507	1,412	−95	−6
All patients	5,758	5,663	−95	−2

budget measures, however, would result in total savings to government of \$233 million, a 5 per cent reduction in expected government expenditure. Concessional patients would pay an additional \$100 million in copayments, representing 43 per cent of the cost shifting, or a net increase in their expenditure of 25 per cent (recall the base case incorporates the standard CPI increase of 2.5 per cent in patient contributions). For general patients, however, some 13 per cent of scripts 'drop-out' of the subsidy scheme as their average price falls below the higher copayment rate of \$28.60, i.e., these benefit medicines become 'below copayment drugs'. As below copayment drugs, the cost (\$95 million) has to be borne in full by general patients, and they are eliminated from the modelling which only includes Group 1 drugs, i.e., PBS benefit medicines. Hence, in Table 2, government is shown to reduce its outlay to general patients by \$133 million, but general patients are shown to pay only \$38 million more — the gap of \$95 million representing the cost of the scripts that become below copayment drugs and are no longer eligible for government subsidy.

Older Australians, i.e., those aged 65 or more years are the main beneficiaries of the PBS. Under the scenario for 2003–2004, older Australians consume 45.5 per cent of total scripts – individuals aged 65–74 years using 24.9 per cent and those aged 75 or more years 20.6 per cent. An estimated 13 per cent of total PBS scripts are prescribed for women aged 75 years and over (Figure 2). The large majority of these Australians are concessional patients (92 per cent), and most of them (82 per cent) have a pensioner concession card but a significant number are self-funded retirees who do not qualify for the Age Pension but are accessing PBS medicines at concessional rates through the Commonwealth Seniors Health Card (CSHC).

The distributions of government and consumer costs, by age group and cardholder status, for the scenario, are given in Table 3. The results are

Figure 2: Distribution of Scripts by Age and Gender, 2003–2004 (Scenario)

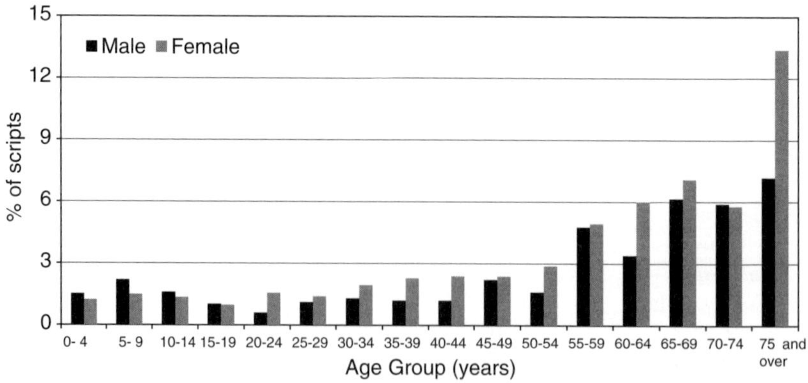

Table 3: Fortnightly Costs by Age Group — Scenario and Change from Base, January 1–14 2004

Age group	Concessional patients				General patients			
	Scenario	Share of total	Difference from base		Scenario	Share of total	Difference from base	
	($ 000)	(%)	($ 000)	(%)	($ 000)	(%)	($ 000)	(%)
Distribution of government costs								
0–14 years	11,174	8	–417	–4	4,311	13	–630	–13
15–24 years	4,862	4	–180	–4	2,592	8	–351	–12
25–44 years	16,882	12	–533	–3	8,094	23	–1,325	–14
45–64 years	37,994	27	–1,230	–3	16,568	48	–2,520	–13
65–74 years	40,276	29	–1,359	–3	1,441	4	–324	–18
75 years or over	27,692	20	–1,101	–4	1,474	4	–349	–19
All	138,880	100	–4,819	–3	34,479	100	–5,499	–14
Distribution of patients costs								
0–14 years	2,130	9	417	24	3,431	14	459	15
15–24 years	918	4	180	24	1,680	7	149	10
25–44 years	2,724	11	533	24	5,847	24	474	9
45–64 years	6,285	26	1,230	24	11,077	45	112	1
65–74 years	6,944	28	1,359	24	1,166	5	–126	–10
75 years or over	5,629	23	1,101	24	1,606	6	95	6
All	24,629	100	4,819	24	24,807	100	1,162	5

presented for the two-week window 1–14 January 2004. As expected, the budget measures impact evenly across the age groups for concessional patients, with a 3–4 per cent reduction in government costs for all age groups. Because different age groups use different types and number of drugs, there is more variability across the age groups for general patients due to differences in the type and numbers of drugs 'dropping out' of the scheme through the higher general patient copayment rate. However, these discrepancies did not significantly alter the relative share of government outlays to general patients or the consumer contributions made by each age group.

Nearly half of government outlays to concessional patients go to those aged 65 or more years, compared to only 8 per cent for general patients (Table 3). Elderly concessional patients did, however, contribute to 51 per cent of total patient contributions from concessional patients.

Figures 3 and 4 show the relative share of total government outlays and consumer contributions by age and cardholder status. Again the results are presented for the two-week window 1–14 January 2004, and compare the base case and scenario. The dominance of the older age groups as the main beneficiaries of government expenditure on the PBS is clearly evident in Figure 3 — almost 17 per cent of total government outlays went to individuals aged 75 or more years, i.e., of every six dollars spent by Government on the PBS, one dollar was received by a person aged 75 years or more. While this age group received almost 17 per cent of total PBS government outlays, they represented only 5.8 per cent of Australians. This group also

Figure 3: Share of Government Outlays, Base Case and Scenario, January 1–14 2004

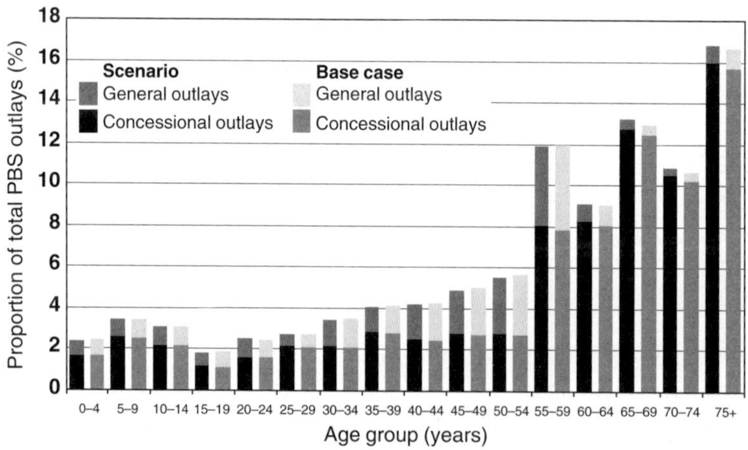

Figure 4: Share of Consumer Contributions, Base Case and Scenario, January 1–14 2004

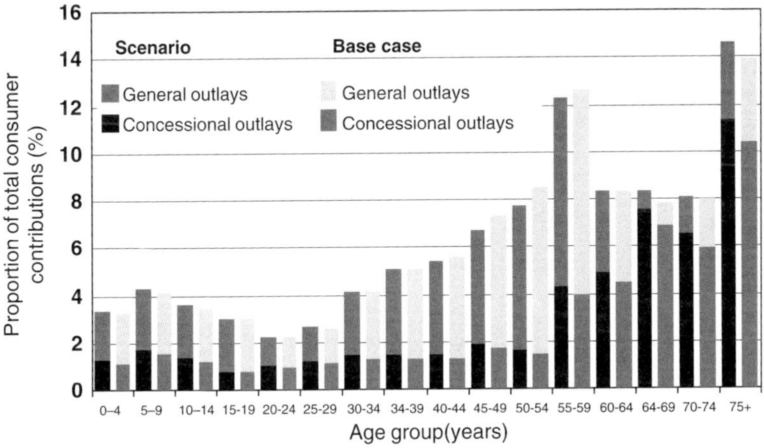

contributed the greatest share of consumer copayments (Figure 4). In contrast, Australians aged 15–19 years received the lowest share of total PBS government outlays at 1.9 per cent but represented 6.9 per cent of the Australian population.

Figures 3 and 4 also show individuals aged 55–59 years are an important group of PBS users receiving approximately 12 per cent of government outlays and contributing just over 12 per cent of consumer copayments — the major difference being that many of these individuals are general patients.

Figures 5 and 6 show government and consumer expenditure over the two-week window standardising for the number of concession cardholders in the Australian population in each age group, or the number of general patients in each group. Results are presented for the scenario only — these differ little from the base case. Older Australians who are concession cardholders receive on average just over \$40 per person per fortnight, with an additional \$5 of government expenditure per person for elderly general patients. On a per capita basis, the 55–59 year age group are also major recipients of government PBS subsidies, averaging \$42 per concessional cardholder and \$10 for general patients in the population. On a per capita basis, it is the very elderly concessional patients who have the highest out-of-pocket expenses — with the introduction of the budget measures concessional cardholders aged 75 or more years would pay on average \$8 per person per fortnight towards their PBS medicines and general patients in this age group would contribute \$6 per person.

Figure 5: Per Capita Expenditure By Government, Scenario, Jan 1–14 2004

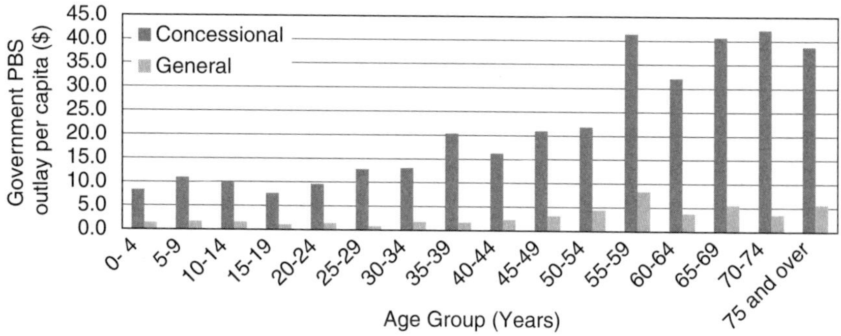

Figure 6: Per Capita Weekly Consumer Expenditure, Scenario, Jan 1–14 2004

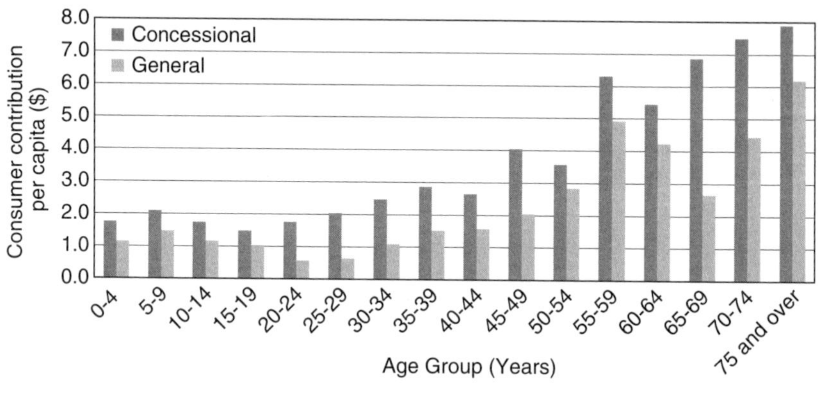

As stated earlier in the paper, one of the advantages of microsimulation is to examine distributional impacts by a range of demographic and household groups. Figure 7 and Table 4 present the distribution of government outlays on the PBS for various family types for the base case and scenario for the two-week reporting period 1–14 January 2004. Under the base case and scenario, the 'couple families without dependent children' and those who are concession cardholders are the main beneficiaries of government expenditure on PBS drugs, and in particular, the 'retired' concessional cardholder couples. This elderly family type received nearly 30 per cent of total government outlays — under the scenario settings, the Government subsidy on PBS drugs for this family type was in the order of \$47.00 per week per family, a level of benefit representing about nine per cent of weekly

Figure 7: Share of Total Government Outlays by Family Type, Jan 1–14 2004

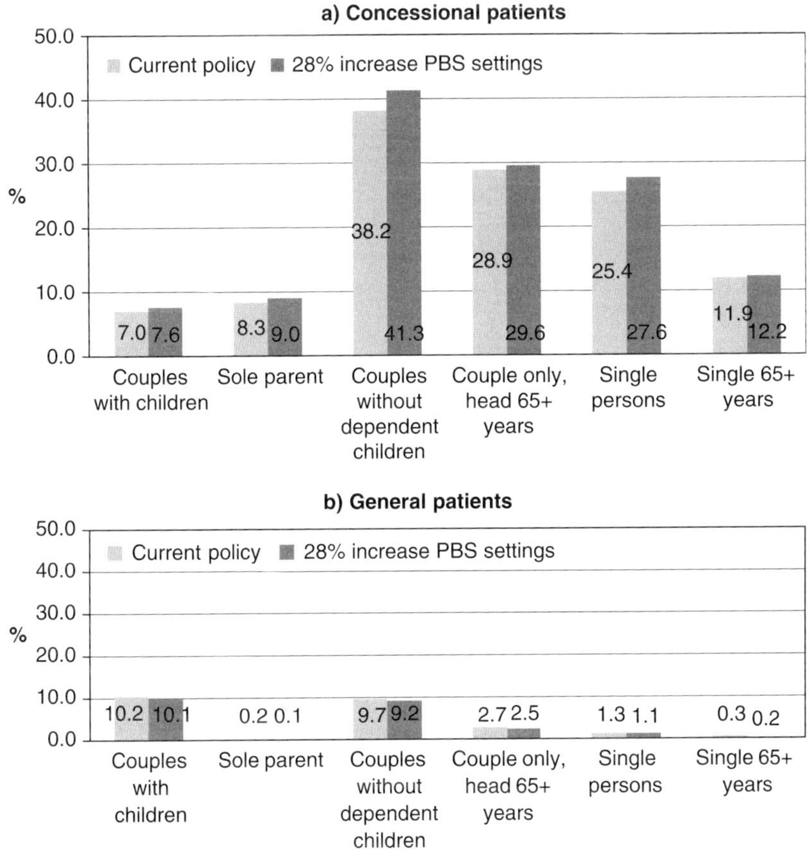

disposable income. This compares to an average government benefit per week of $20.75 for all concessional families or 5.73 per cent of average family weekly disposable income.

A further 12 per cent of government expenditure on PBS medicines went to elderly concession cardholders living by themselves. For these individuals, the Government subsidy on PBS drugs was around $14.20 per week per sole person family, representing about 5.3 per cent of weekly disposable income for this family type (these figures are not significantly different from the base case). Overall, the share of PBS outlays received by families without dependent children eclipses the slice of PBS outlays directed towards Australian families with children.

Table 4: Estimated Impact of The PBS by Family Type (1–14 January 2004)

	Unit	All couples with children	All sole parents	Couples without dependent children	Couple only, head aged 65 + years	Single Persons	Single aged 65 + years	All families
Concessional patients								
Base case								
Government subsidy per week on PBS drugs	$	23.95	16.95	41.85	48.55	12.9	14.75	21.50
Government subsidy as proportion of income	%	4.11	3.37	8.76	9.74	5.33	5.53	5.94
% of all PBS government subsidy received by this group	%	7.00	8.32	38.17	28.86	25.41	11.94	78.97
Scenario								
Government subsidy per week on PBS drugs	$	23.10	16.30	40.45	46.95	12.5	14.20	20.75
Government subsidy as proportion of income	%	3.96	3.24	8.47	9.42	5.17	5.33	5.73
% of all PBS government subsidy received by this group	%	7.56	8.96	41.33	29.57	27.59	12.18	85.38
Per cent difference (base vs scenario) *Government subsidy per week*	%	−3.55	−3.83	−3.35	−3.30	−3.1	−3.73	−3.49

General patients								
Base case								
Government subsidy per week on PBS drugs	$	5.15	1.25	5.25	11.05	0.4	1.05	2.87
Government subsidy as proportion of income	%	0.42	0.16	0.51	1.73	0.07	0.29	0.34
% of all PBS government subsidy received by this group	%	10.22	0.15	9.66	2.69	1.26	26.93	21.23
Scenario								
Government subsidy per week on PBS drugs	$	4.55	0.95	4.48	9.65	0.3	0.80	2.48
Government subsidy as proportion of income	%	0.37	0.12	0.44	1.51	0.06	0.22	0.30
% of all PBS government subsidy received by this group	%	10.11	0.13	9.23	2.49	1.14	21.74	20.59
Per cent difference (base vs scenario) Government subsidy per week	%	−11.65	−24.00	−14.68	−12.67	−19.2	-23.81	-13.44

6. Conclusions

The PBS is extremely important in reducing the financial pressures that Australian families, and particularly older Australians, would otherwise face in paying for prescribed pharmaceuticals. On the part of government, the key concern is rising public expenditure on the PBS and one solution was the proposal in the 2002–2003 budget to raise the PBS policy settings. The modelling indicates, in keeping with Treasury estimates, that by increasing patient copayments and SNTs by nearly 28 per cent, the Government would save in the order of 5 per cent of its annual expenditure on the scheme. As a flat rate increase, the proposed budget measures impact relatively evenly across the population. This is most evident for concessional patients and to a lesser degree for general patients for whom an estimated 13 of every 100 scripts would no longer be subsidised as their price drops below the higher general patient copayment rate. General patients would have to meet the cost of these scripts in full.

It must be noted that the PharmaSim's current base data contains little information about whether or not the health conditions suffered by families are chronic and, accordingly, it is not possible with this version to comprehensively model the safety net. As a result, the results presented in the paper were predominantly for the first two weeks of January 2004, before any families become eligible for the safety net. The annual distributional impact of the PBS will differ from the fortnightly impact shown here to the extent that the likelihood of reaching the safety net differs between the population groups examined.

While the Government's aim is to achieve fiscal sustainability of the PBS, there are a number of current 'structural' impediments to this, especially within the context of an ageing population. First, the Government remains the major funder of PBS medicines — even with the implementation of the proposed budget measures, consumer out-of-pocket contributions still represent only 18.4 per cent of the total costs of PBS benefit medicines. Donovan (2002) indicates that the approach of simply raising copayments does not address the reasons why the PBS cost is growing, and it is likely to produce negative consequences for those who use medicines the most — namely the elderly and those with chronic illnesses. While the intention of increased copayments is to send a price signal to consumers in order to reduce their use of unnecessary medicines, such a measure would restrict access to affordable medicines and could result in some patients not filling their scripts. This could have unintended consequences such as lost productivity of people with chronic conditions, and increased pressure on hospital and emergency services if health conditions deteriorate when medicines are not taken to treat or prevent the onset of medical conditions, all of which could ultimately increase rather than lower total government expenditure on health (Donovan, 2002).

Second, as the results show, the PBS is highly progressive with most of government outlays being targeted to concessional patients. As concessional patients are largely social security and family payment recipients on relatively low incomes, this immediately illustrates one of the key policy dilemmas facing government: reducing or restraining outlays on the PBS in any substantial way necessarily involves affecting low-income Australians, given that they are overwhelmingly the beneficiaries of the current scheme. It is these very groups of individuals that the PBS is designed to help access 'essential' medicines at affordable prices.

Third, the major user group is older Australians, nearly all of them access PBS medicines at the concessional rate. While partly related to income, age is a fundamental driver of the receipt of PBS benefits. Growth in numbers of age pensioners, ceteris paribus, will be reflected in increased script volumes and costs, and unless the eligibility criteria for concession cardholder status are changed, most of the rise in costs will be borne by government. In addition, in recent years, PBS concessional status has been granted to many self-funded retirees. The federal government raised the income thresholds for self-funded retirees' eligibility to the CSHC from 1 January 1999 and again from 1 July 2001. These two policy changes have increased the number of CSHC holders from around 46,000 pre-1999 to over 282,500 as at June 2003,[7] i.e., these two policy changes have increased the number of self-funded retirees accessing PBS medicines at the concessional rate by sixfold.

Raising copayments and SNTs is a mechanism for cost-shifting, but it does not by itself address the key drivers of the increases in PBS expenditures as discussed in the introduction. PBS costs are the outcome of an array of influences — the strategic negotiation between government and the pharmaceutical industry over the listing, pricing and indications for particular drugs, doctor-prescribing behaviour, and consumer need and demand, for example. The Government needs to address population ageing alongside the non-demographic drivers of growth in PBS costs. However, as Rickard (Rickard, 2002, p. ii) states 'PBS sustainability is just as much a matter of public and political decision as it is a matter of finance and expenditure. It is a decision about how the three PBS objectives [*universal access, comprehensiveness in the medicines available and responsible costs to the community*] are to be weighted against each other, and what sort of balance between them seems best for Australia, in the circumstances of its limited health care resources'. This is particularly relevant to ensuring the ongoing well-being of older Australians. As Harvey (Harvey, 2002) comments, reducing the use of essential medicines ultimately costs the community much more money than it saves.

[7] From Commonwealth Department of Family and Community Services Annual Reports 1998–1999 and 2002–2003.

7. Postscript

A number of changes have transpired since this paper was first written. The proposed budget measure to increase PBS copayments and safety nets was finally put into effect starting 1 January 2005, instead of mid-2002 as set-out in the paper. Due to the delay in getting the policy implemented, the magnitude of increase in copayments and safety nets relative to the previous year was lower at 21 per cent instead of 28 per cent, although 21 per cent is still a sizeable increase. Another measure that came into force in 2005 was the price of all drugs in a reference-pricing group, or medicines that produce similar health effects, were required to drop 12.5 per cent once one of them came off patent and the first generic version became available. Further, starting 2006, the safety net thresholds were legislated to increase by two scripts per year for both concessional and general PBS beneficiaries.

A new version of the model was completed in 2004. The new model, MediSim, has improved capability to model the safety net, and information on drug usage was imputed for the whole year. Given these enhancements, among others, distributional results can now be presented for the whole year instead of just for a fortnight.

Given all the above changes, in calendar year 2005, the volume of total PBS prescriptions decreased by 0.9 per cent relative to the previous year (Table 5). This is the first time since 1990–1991 (coinciding with another significant copayment increase) that PBS scripts showed any decline. The decline in scripts was a substantial 6.8 per cent for general patients, while a marginal 0.3 per cent increase was registered for concessional patients. Clearly, the 21 per cent increase in patient copayments had a significant effect on the number of prescriptions filled that year.

The aggregate impact of the scenario for the financial year 2003–2004 is summarised in Table 2. The 28 per cent increase in patient copayments was expected to translate into a 3.4 million decline in prescriptions filled by

Table 5: Volume of PBS Scripts, Calendar Year 2002–2005

	2002	2003	2004	2005
Scripts (million)	25.0	26.6	29.1	27.1
General	131.9	133.5	139.9	140.4
Concessional	156.9	160.1	169.0	167.5
Subtotal				
Annual per cent change		2002–2003	2003–2004	2004–2005
General		6.4	9.4	−6.8
Concessional		1.1	4.9	0.3
Subtotal		2.0	5.6	−0.9

general patients, and result in $233 million savings to government, representing a 5 per cent reduction in government expenditure.

What actually happened? In the 2005–2006 budget, the forecast expenditure on the PBS was $6.6 billion, but the 2006–2007 budget papers showed actual spending for 2005–2006 was only $6.2 billion, a savings of $337 million — equivalent to a 5 per cent reduction in government expenditure. While the magnitudes are not the same, given the time difference between the scenario and actual implementation of the copayment increase, the estimated impact in terms of government saving is remarkably close. As well, the simulation results show that general patients will be more affected by the copayment increase, and this is confirmed by the decline in scripts for this group of PBS beneficiaries.

Acknowledgements

The construction of the current version of the PharmaSim microsimulation model was funded by Medicines Australia. The authors wish to thank staff of Medicines Australia for their helpful advice and assistance with the project over the last two years. The preparation of this paper and future developments to the model are supported by an Australian Research Council linkage grant (no. LP0219571).

References

Abello, A., Brown, L., Walker, A. and Thurecht, T. (2003). *An Economic Forecasting Microsimulation Model of the Australian Pharmaceutical Benefits Scheme.* NATSEM Technical Paper no. 30, University of Canberra.

Australian Bureau of Statistics. (ABS). (2003). *Population Projections, Australia.* ABS Catalogue No. 3222.0, Canberra.

Birkett, D.J., Mitchell, A.S. and McManus, P. (2001). A Cost-Effectiveness Approach to Drug Subsidy and Pricing in Australia. *Health Affairs*, 20(3), 104–114.

Britt, H., Miller, G., Knox, S., Charles, J., Valenti, L., Henderson, J., Pan, Y., Sutton, C. and Harrison, C. (2002). *BEACH Bettering the Evaluation and Care of Health. General Practice Activity in Australia 2001-02.* AIHW Catalogue No. GEP 10, Canberra.

Brown, L., Abello, A., Phillips, B. and Harding, A. (2004). Moving Towards an Improved Micro-Simulation Model of the Australian Pharmaceutical Benefits Scheme. *Australian Economic Review*, 37(1), 41–61.

Brown, L.J. and Harding, A. (2002). Social Modelling and Public Policy: Application of Microsimulation Modelling in Australia. *Journal of Artificial Societies and Social Simulation*, 5(4), http://jasss.soc.surrey.ac.uk/5/4/6.html

Brown, L.J., Walker, A., Waters, A., Harding, A. and Thurecht, L. (2002). *Funding of High Cost Biotechnology and other Innovative Targeted Therapies under the*

Pharmaceutical Benefits Scheme. Refereed Position Paper, NATSEM, University of Canberra, p. 90.

Commonwealth Treasury. (2002). Budget Papers 2002, Budget Paper no. 1, Part 3 Revenue, Expenses and Budget Funding, Statement 6: Expenses and Net Capital Investment. Treasury, Commonwealth of Australia, Canberra, August.

Cookson, R. (2000), *ASTEC Non-EU Case Study on Australia*, The London School of Economics and Political Science, London, www.lse.ac.uk/Depts/lsehsc/healthresourceslinks/other.htm

Cooper, C. and Hagan, P. (1999). *The Ageing Australian Population and Future Health Costs: 1996 – 2051.* Department of Health and Aged Care Occasional Papers, New Series No 7, Department of Health and Aged Care, Commonwealth of Australia, Canberra.

Creedy, J. (2001). Tax Modelling. *Economic Record*, 77(237), 189–202.

Dalton, A. (2001). Australia's Pharmaceutical Benefits System: Flawed but Improving, and Better than Anywhere else. *Australian Health Review*, 24(2), 7–14.

Department of Health and Ageing. (2003a). 2003-04 Portfolio Budget Statements, PART C-Section 2: Information on Planned Outcomes and Outputs Outcome 2: Access to Medicare. Commonwealth of Australia, Canberra.

Department of Treasury. (2002a). *Intergenerational Report 2002-03, Budget Paper No. 5.* Treasury, Commonwealth of Australia, May.

Department of Treasury. (2003). Budget Paper No. 1, Part 3 Revenue, Expenses and Budget Funding, Statement 6: Expenses and Net Capital Investment. Commonwealth of Australia, Canberra.

Donovan, J. (2002). The Benefits of the PBS to the Australian Community and the Impact of Increased Copayments. *Health Issues*, 71, 1–8.

Gupta, A. and Kapur, V. (eds). (2000). Microsimulation in Government Policy and Forecasting, Contributions to Economic Analysis Series, North-Holland, Amsterdam.

Harding, A. (ed). (1996). *Microsimulation and Public Policy, Contributions to Economic Analysis Series* North-Holland, Amsterdam.Harvey, K. (2002). Securing the Future of the Pharmaceutical Benefits Scheme? *The Drawing Board: An Australian Review of Public Affairs*, Symposium: The 2002–03 Federal Budget, June 2003.

Harding, A., Abello, A., Brown, L. and Phillips, B. (2004). The Distributional Impact of Government Outlays on the Australian Pharmaceutical Benefits Scheme in 2001–02. *Economic Record*, 80(special issue), 583–596.

Hill, S.R., Mitchell, A.S. and Henry, D.A. (2000). Problems with the Interpretation of Pharmacoeconomic Analyses: A Review of Submissions to the Australian Pharmaceutical Benefits Scheme. *JAMA*, 283, 2116–2121.

Lofgren, H. (2001). Pharmaceutical Benefits in Australia and Welfare Policy and the Cost of Prescription Drugs. *Australian Journal of Social Issues*, 36(3), 207–220.

Pritchard, D. (1999). Severity of Illness in General Practice as Predictor of Prescribing in *GP Infonet*, Newsletter of the General Practice Evaluation Program, Vol 4, Issue 2, p. 6.

Productivity Commission. (2001). *International Pharmaceutical Price Differences:* Research Report, Canberra, AusInfo.

Rickard, M. (2002). *The Pharmaceutical Benefits Scheme: Options for Cost Control, Current Issues*, Brief no. 12 2001-02, Department of the Parliamentary Library, Common wealth of Australia, Canberra.

Sansom, L. (2001). The PBS — Its Future. *The Australian Journal of Hospital Pharmacy*, 31(4), 257.

Schofield, D. (1998). *Re-Examining the Distribution of Health Benefits in Australia: Who Benefits from the Pharmaceutical Benefits Scheme?* Discussion Paper no. 36, National Centre for Social and Economic Modelling, University of Canberra.

Schofield, D. (1999). Modelling Health Care Expenditure: A New Microsimulation Approach to Simulating the Distributional Impact of the Pharmaceutical Benefits Scheme, PhD in Information Sciences and Engineering, University of Canberra.

Walker, A. (2000). Distributional Impact of Higher Patient Contributions to Australia's Pharmaceutical Benefits Scheme. *Australian Health Review*, 23(2), 32–46.

Walker, A. and Abello, A. (2000). *Changes in the Health Status of low Income Groups in Australia: 1977–78 to 1995*, Discussion Paper No. 52, National Centre for Social and Economic Modelling, University of Canberra.

Walker, A., Percival, P. and Fischer, S. (1998). *A Microsimulation Model of Australia's Pharmaceutical Benefits Scheme*, Technical Paper No 15, National Centre for Social and Economic Modelling, University of Canberra.

Walker, A., Percival, P. and Harding, A. (2000). The Impact of Demographic and other Changes on Expenditure on Pharmaceutical Benefits in 2020 in Australia, in Mitton, L., Sutherland, H. and Weeks, M. (eds), *Microsimulation Modelling for Policy Analysis: Challenges and Innovations*, Cambridge University Press, UK.

Chapter 9

Modelling Medicare and Pharmaceutical Benefits Scheme (PBS) Utilisation and Costs

Chris Raymond and Brett Parsons

Health Insurance Commission (now Medicare Australia as of 1 October 2005)

Abstract

The Health Insurance Commission (HIC) administers many Australian government health programs. This paper discusses the modelling of the two largest programs, Medicare and the Pharmaceutical Benefits Scheme (PBS). The dynamic multilevel model and data exploration tool are designed to

- *enable visualisation and analysis of the historical time series data at any level of the classification variables. The classification variables for both Medicare and PBS are "type of service or drug", patient state, age and gender;*
- *forecast service or drug utilisation, total cost, government cost and cost to patient at the finest level of granularity. The exploration tool allows the forecasts to be viewed at the finest level or interactively aggregated to the users' specification;*
- *identify areas of Medicare and PBS that have unusual levels of growth; and*
- *take into account the changing age/gender distribution of the population at the state level as the population ages (i.e. the "dynamic" aspect of the model).*

1. Introduction

Medicare and the Pharmaceutical Benefits Scheme (PBS) outlays are a significant part of Commonwealth Government health expenditure. In the 2002–2003 financial year Medicare and PBS (including Repatriation PBS (RPBS)) expenditures were \$8.12 and \$5.06 billion, respectively. Table 1 below shows the size of this expenditure relative to total health expenditure (Australian Institute of Health and Welfare, 2003) and gross domestic product (GDP) (Australian Bureau of Statistics, 2003a). Data for 2001–2002

International Symposia in Economic Theory and Econometrics, Vol. 16

ISSN: 1571-0386 DOI: 10.1016/S1571-0386(06)16009-3

Table 1: Comparison of Medicare and PBS Expenditure to Total Health Expenditure and GDP (Current Prices)

Year	Total health expenditure (THE)	GDP	Medicare			PBS (including RPBS)			Medicare and PBS (including RPBS) combined		
	$bn	$bn	$bn	% of THE	% of GDP	$bn	% of THE	% of GDP	$bn	% of THE	% of GDP
2001–2002	66.6	714.4	7.83	11.8	1.10	4.60	6.9	0.64	12.43	18.7	1.74
2002–2003	na.	753.3	8.12	na.	1.08	5.06	na.	0.67	13.18	na.	1.75

are also included as total health expenditure but are not available for 2002–2003.

The data visualisation and modelling tool described here is designed to identify areas of interest (e.g. high growth) within this expenditure.

Government expenditure (i.e. benefit paid by HIC) is modelled using the following equation:

$$\begin{aligned}\text{Benefit} = {} & \text{Services per Capita} \times \text{Population} \\ & \times \text{Benefit per Service}\end{aligned} \tag{1}$$

Population is estimated and forecast by the Australian Bureau of Statistics (2003b). The model calculates and forecasts the other two quantities on the right-hand side of equation (1), i.e. Services per Capita (SPC) and Benefit per Service (BPS).

The modelling is multilevel. That is, the data are segregated by classification variables before equation (1) is applied. The classification variables are "type of service or drug", patient state, age and gender.

Charge (i.e. benefit plus patient contribution) is also modelled using an equation similar to equation (1), with BPS replaced by Charge per service. Patient contribution (Gap) is modelled simply as

$$\text{Gap} = \text{Charge} - \text{Benefit} \tag{2}$$

2. Data Description

The data are disaggregated to a level that makes it useful as a policy development and analysis tool. Further disaggregation of the data is possible if it is considered necessary in the future.

At the finest level of disaggregation, equation (1) becomes:

$$\begin{aligned}\text{Benefit}_{s,a,g,st} = {} & \text{Services Per Capita}_{s,a,g,st} \times \text{Population}_{s,a,g} \\ & \times \text{Benefit Per Service}_{s,a,g,st}\end{aligned} \tag{3}$$

where, s is the state/territory (8 levels); a the patient age range (10 levels); g the patient gender (2 levels); and st the service type (Medicare: broad type of service (9 levels), PBS: anatomical therapeutic chemical classification level 1 (ATC1, 15 levels)) and so the variable $\text{Benefit}_{s,a,g,st}$ denotes the benefit paid for Medicare/PBS services of service type st for population in state s, age cohort a and gender g.

Each data segment is a time series, thus Medicare consists of $8 \times 10 \times 2 \times 9 = 1{,}440$ separate time series that can be examined and forecast using time series techniques. For PBS the number of separate time series is $8 \times 10 \times 2 \times 15 = 2{,}400$.

2.1 Population

Population projections data constitute an exogenous variable in the model and are sourced from the Australian Bureau of Statistics (2003b). The medium fertility and migration and low mortality scenario (Series B) was chosen for this study. Series B is the medium growth assumption. See Table 2 for details of the growth assumptions.

2.2 Medicare

The Medicare data are administrative data and does not include health status information. Thus changing health status in the population will be reflected indirectly through changes in service utilisation.

The data are based on date of service from March 1991 to June 2003. Since there is a lag between date of service and date of processing the most recent data are marginally incomplete. An estimate of outstanding claims is used to make the "3-month-lag" and "6-month-lag" data as complete as the "9-month-lag" data. That is, Medicare data for a given month of service are estimated to be approximately 97.96%, 99.71% and 99.99% complete after 3, 6 and 9 months of claims processing respectively. For the purposes of this model the "9-month-lag" data are regarded as complete and the "3- and 6- months-lag" data sets are boosted by the factors 99.99/97.96 and 99.99/99.71, respectively to make them "complete" and thus comparable with previous quarters.

The data are summarised at the quarter level in the time dimension. To remove seasonality, each quarterly value is the annualised value (i.e. rolling 12 months = 4 quarter moving sum = 4 quarterly moving average * 4). This means that each quarterly data point is deseasonalised and smoothed. The forecasts are done on the annualised values, however, the raw quarterly figures are also displayed to show the seasonality/variability of the data.

The classification variables are patient state/territory (8 levels), patient age range (10 levels), patient gender (2 levels) and service type = broad type of service (9 levels).

Patient age range values are 0–4, 5–14,15–24, 25–34, 35–44, 45–54, 55–64, 65–74, 75–84 and 85+ years.

Medicare broad type of service values are:

1. UNREF ATTEND (unreferred attendances)
2. SPEC.ATTEND (specialist attendances)
3. OBSTETRICS
4. PATHOLOGY
5. DIAG.IMAGING (diagnostic imaging)
6. AMB.SURGICAL (ambulatory surgical — all anaesthetics, operations and assistance at operations services not rendered in a hospital)

Table 2: Australian Bureau of Statistics (2003b, p. 1)

Main projection series, Australia	Assumptions				Population as at 30 June	
	Total fertility rate[a]	Net overseas migration[b]	Life expectancy at birth (years)[c]		2,051 million	2,101 million
	Babies per woman	Persons	Males	Females		
Series A	1.8	125,000	92.2	95.0	31.4	37.7
Series B	1.6	100,000	84.2	87.7	26.4	26.4
Series C	1.4	70,000	84.2	87.7	23.0	18.9

[a] *From 2011.*
[b] *From 2005–2006.*
[c] *From 2050–2051.*

7. OPTOMETRY
8. RNT & OTHER (radio and nuclear therapy)
9. HOSPITAL (all MBS services that have been rendered in a hospital).

2.3 Pharmaceutical Benefits Scheme

The PBS data are based on date of supply (i.e. the date the patient received the drug from the pharmacy) from January 1996 to June 2003 and include RPBS data. Since there is a lag between date of supply and date of processing the most recent data are marginally incomplete. An estimate of outstanding claims is used to make the "3-month-lag" data as complete as the "6-month-lag" data. That is, PBS data for a given month of supply are estimated to be approximately 99.82% and 99.96% complete after 3 and 6 months of claims processing respectively. For the purposes of this model the "6-month-lag" data are regarded as complete and the "3-month-lag" data set are boosted by the factor 99.96/99.82 to make it "complete" and thus comparable with previous quarters.

The lag period for PBS (6 months) is shorter than for MBS (9 months) because the average supply to processing lag for PBS is shorter than the average service to processing lag for MBS. Thus PBS data require a shorter period to achieve the same degree of completeness as the MBS data.

The classification variables are the same as for MBS except that service type = ATC1, 15 levels. These are:

1. Alimentary tract and metabolism
2. Blood and blood-forming organs
3. Cardiovascular system
4. Dermatologicals
5. Genito urinary system and sex hormones
6. Systemic hormonal preparations, excluding sex hormones
7. General anti-infectives for systemic use
8. Anti-neoplastic and immunomodulating
9. Musculo-skeletal system
10. Nervous system
11. Anti-parasitic products
12. Respiratory system
13. Sensory organs
14. Various +
15. Other + +.

This classification is defined by the World Health Organisation. See the website, http://www.whocc.no/atcddd/ for more details.

The State variable is the patient state, however, if the patient is not identified (e.g. General scripts prior to May 2002), then the pharmacy state is used.

Imputation of Patient Age and Gender for PBS

The introduction of the Improved Monitoring of Entitlements (IME) program made the presentation of a Medicare Card at the pharmacy compulsory from May 2002 in order for the patient to prove entitlement to PBS benefits. This meant that the patient demographic data (i.e. age and gender) associated with prescriptions were greatly enhanced from May 2002.

Prior to this date there are a large number of scripts where patient age and gender are unknown. In order to provide continuous time series at the lowest level of granularity, the pre-May 2002 scripts with missing patient age and gender were apportioned to state/age range/gender/type of service categories on the basis of the state/age range/gender/type of service/patient category distribution of scripts in the post-May 2002 data.

3. Forecasting Methodology

The forecasting is done using the PROC FORECAST procedure in SAS. The following is the pseudo-code:

```
proc forecast    data = datain
                 interval = qtr
                 outest = FitStatistics
                 method = Expo
                 trend = 2
                 weight = 0.3;
by State AgeRange Gender ServiceType;
id QuarterOfService;
var ServicesPerCapita BenefitPerService ChargePerService;
run;
```

3.1 Data = datain

The actuals for the 3 variables forecast (ServicesPerCapita, BenefitPerService and ChargePerService) are deseasonalised, smoothed and log transformed before forecasting.

The variables are deseasonalised and smoothed by performing a "rolling 4 quarter sum" (i.e. each quarter becomes the value for the current quarter plus the 3 preceding quarters) for the services, benefit and charge variables. The transformed variables are hereafter referred to as "annualised actuals".

The annualised actuals are used to create the forecast variables ServicesPerCapita, BenefitPerService and ChargePerService. These are log transformed before forecasting. The forecast is linear for the transformed forecast variables, but is exponential (i.e. compound growth) for the untransformed variables. This approach is taken because it is assumed these variables have compound growth over time.

3.2 Method = Expo

The following documentation is from SAS OnlineDoc Version 8 (1999).

Exponential smoothing is used when the METHOD = EXPO option is specified. The term exponential smoothing is derived from the computational scheme developed by Brown and others (Brown and Meyers, 1961; Brown, 1962). Estimates are computed with updating formulas that are developed across time series in a manner similar to smoothing.

The EXPO method fits a trend model such that the most recent data are weighted more heavily than data in the early part of the series. The weight of an observation is a geometric (exponential) function of the number of periods that the observation extends into the past relative to the current period. The weight function is

$$\omega_\tau = \omega(1-\omega)^{t-\tau}$$

where τ is the observation number of the past observation, t is the current observation number, and ω is the weighting constant specified with the WEIGHT = option.

This method was chosen so that recent trends in the data influence the forecast more than older trends.

3.3 Trend = 2

A linear forecast of the log-transformed variables is chosen, so that the untransformed forecast has compound growth. The following documentation is also from SAS OnlineDoc Version 8 (1999).

You specify the model with the TREND = option as follows:

- *TREND = 1 specifies single exponential smoothing (a constant model)*
- *TREND = 2 specifies double exponential smoothing (a linear trend model)*
- *TREND = 3 specifies triple exponential smoothing (a quadratic trend model)*

3.4 Weight = 0.3

In the pseudo-code Weight = 0.3. If higher (e.g. Weight = 0.5), then the forecast is more responsive to recent trends. The disadvantage of this is that the long-term forecast can vary significantly from quarter to quarter (i.e. too sensitive to noise). If lower (e.g. Weight = 0.1), then the forecast takes more historical data into account. Weight = 0.3 has been chosen as the best compromise between being responsive to recent trends while not ignoring older trends.

3.5 By State AgeRange Gender ServiceType

PROC FORECAST performs a separate analysis on observations in groups defined by the BY variables. As previously noted, there are 1,440 MBS groups and 2,400 PBS groups.

3.6 Outest = FitStatistics

Instead of outputting the values of the forecasts, the parameters are exported instead (i.e. intercept and slope). The advantages of this are that the parameters can be exported to Excel and Outlier Analysis performed on them. That is, the slope parameter is the estimated future growth rate, so this parameter can be analysed to identify areas of high growth; and minimising data volume. Each time series forecast only requires two data values (intercept and slope) to specify the forecast. If the quarterly forecast is exported then a data point is required for each quarter forecast.

4. Data Exploration Tool

A data exploration tool was developed in Microsoft Excel to enable the viewing of the time series at the lowest level of granularity and at any level of aggregation. Figure 1 shows an example output for all of PBS. It shows 6 time series graphs:

- Services
- Services per capita
- ABS population
- Benefit
- Benefit per service
- Components of growth % p.a. — benefit.

The last graph divides overall benefit growth into the components defined in equation (1), that is, population, SPC and BPS (i.e. price) growth.

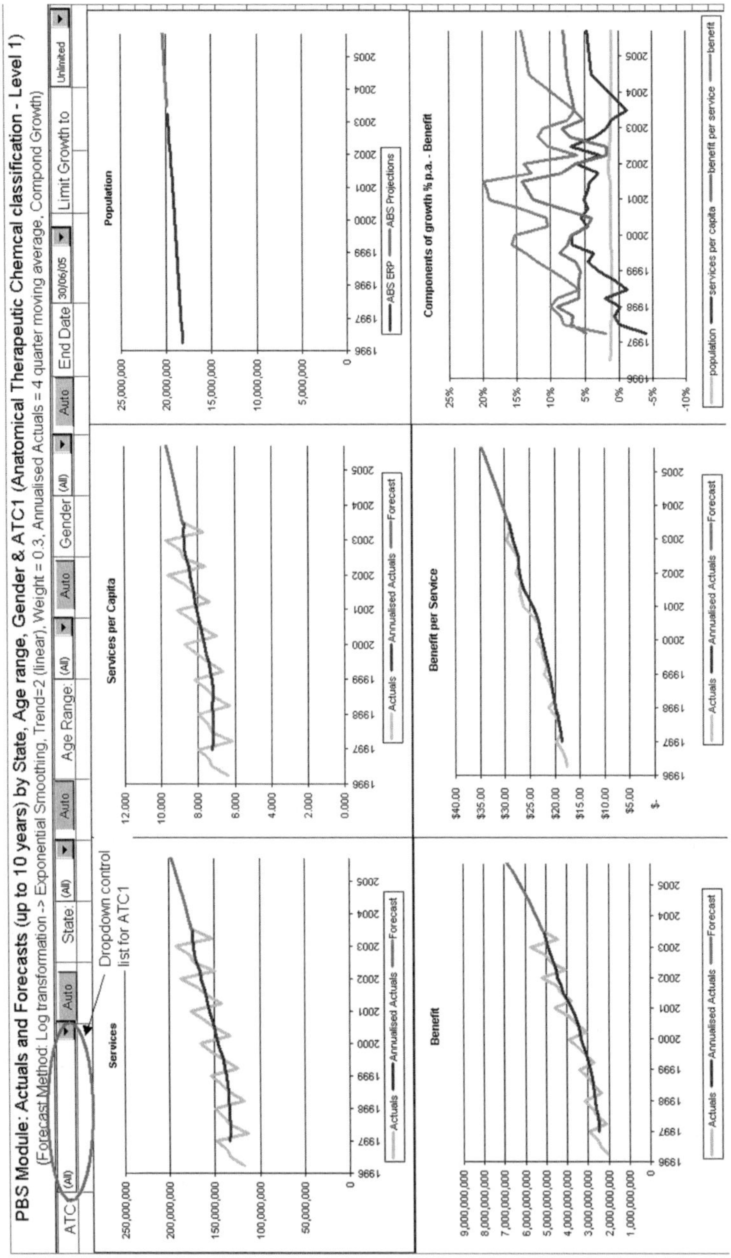

Figure 1: All PBS

Dropdown control lists appear above the graphs and enable the user to select particular values of

- Drug groups — ATC1
- Patient state
- Patent age range
- Patient gender.

Note that the actuals are seasonal. The forecasts (2 years in this example) are based on the annualised actuals (i.e. seasonal component removed).

Only 6 graphs are shown in the example, but the standard output contains a further 6 graphs which show

- Charge
- Charge per service
- Components of growth % p.a. — charge
- Gap (i.e. patient contribution)
- Gap per service
- Components of growth % p.a. — Gap.

4.1 Identification and Analysis of Outliers (i.e. Categories with High Growth)

Figure 2 shows the "Outlier Analysis" worksheet of the exploration tool. The "AutoFilter" feature of Excel can be used to identify areas of interest in the data. For example, Figure 2 shows the output when answering the question, "What are the current areas of rapid Service per Capita growth within the PBS where benefits paid are greater than $500,000 per annum"? The benefit column has been filtered to only show rows where benefit >$500,000.

To identify areas where the SPC growth is highest, the SPC% column has been filtered to give the rows with the top 100 values. It can be seen that the majority of the categories with high SPC growth have gender = female and ATC1 = musculo-skeletal system.

A similar procedure can be followed to identify areas of high BPS growth. That is, the BPS% column is filtered to show the top 100 values.

To explore the area identified in Figure 2, the standard time series graphs can be generated by selecting gender = female and ATC1 = musculo-skeletal system using the dropdown control lists (see Figure 3). It can be seen from Figure 3 that:

- rapid growth in SPC started in approximately June 2000; and
- initial growth in benefits was due more to BPS increase than SPC increase.

Figure 2: Identifying Areas of PBS with Benefit > $500,000 per Annum and High Service per Capita Growth

Outlier Analysis

Annualised growth in first forecast year

State	Age Range	Gender	ATC	ATC1 Description	population%	spc%	bps%	services	services %	benefit	benefit %
ACT	0-4	M	A	Alimentary Tract and Metabolism	-0.6%	30.2%	7.3%	29,109	29.4%	1,349,042	38.9%
ACT	0-4	M	C	Cardiovascular System	-0.6%	22.4%	1.0%	59,895	21.7%	1,235,779	22.9%
ACT	0-4	M	J	General Anti-Infectives for Systemic Use	-0.6%	20.3%	3.1%	16,054	19.6%	930,674	23.3%
ACT	0-4	M	L	Anti-Neoplastic and Immunomodulating	-0.6%	45.3%	38.1%	4,995	44.4%	2,542,516	99.5%
ACT	0-4	M	N	Nervous System	-0.6%	29.4%	-0.2%	45,230	28.6%	1,432,195	28.4%
ACT	0-4	M	R	Respiratory System	-0.6%	19.5%	14.2%	27,253	18.8%	770,288	35.6%
ACT	35-44	F	L	Anti-Neoplastic and Immunomodulating	0.1%	29.9%	12.2%	1,597	30.0%	633,067	45.8%
ACT	45-54	F	L	Anti-Neoplastic and Immunomodulating	0.6%	30.1%	12.4%	3,128	30.9%	1,104,876	47.1%
ACT	55-64	F	M	Musculo-Skeletal System	5.3%	29.6%	4.4%	25,802	36.5%	725,098	42.5%
ACT	65-74	F	M	Musculo-Skeletal System	3.5%	30.0%	9.2%	29,183	34.6%	1,031,578	47.0%
ACT	75-84	F	M	Musculo-Skeletal System	3.2%	30.6%	11.1%	26,233	34.7%	1,014,382	49.6%
NSW	45-54	F	M	Musculo-Skeletal System	1.6%	19.9%	-0.3%	332,447	21.8%	8,134,703	21.4%
NSW	45-54	M	B	Blood and Blood Forming Organs	1.4%	19.3%	20.1%	49,913	21.0%	2,094,776	45.3%
NSW	65-74	F	M	Musculo-Skeletal System	0.8%	21.1%	9.3%	839,919	22.0%	29,419,075	33.4%
NSW	75-84	F	M	Musculo-Skeletal System	2.2%	22.8%	10.6%	765,217	25.4%	28,850,268	38.8%
NSW	85+	F	M	Musculo-Skeletal System	2.9%	24.8%	11.3%	233,307	28.4%	8,896,170	43.0%
QLD	45-54	F	M	Musculo-Skeletal System	2.5%	20.7%	1.0%	191,297	23.7%	4,862,957	25.0%
QLD	65-74	F	M	Musculo-Skeletal System	2.7%	22.7%	9.0%	425,507	26.1%	15,336,034	37.4%
QLD	75-84	F	M	Musculo-Skeletal System	2.8%	24.6%	9.2%	372,487	28.1%	14,287,636	39.9%
QLD	85+	F	M	Musculo-Skeletal System	4.1%	26.5%	10.2%	113,118	31.7%	4,410,352	45.2%
SA	45-54	F	M	Musculo-Skeletal System	0.8%	21.1%	2.1%	74,465	22.2%	1,865,652	24.7%
SA	55-64	F	M	Musculo-Skeletal System	3.9%	18.6%	6.9%	138,528	23.3%	4,021,542	31.8%
SA	65-74	F	M	Musculo-Skeletal System	0.6%	21.7%	10.5%	179,777	22.5%	6,130,375	35.3%
SA	75-84	F	M	Musculo-Skeletal System	2.1%	23.1%	11.9%	175,473	25.7%	6,359,784	40.7%
SA	85+	F	M	Musculo-Skeletal System	2.5%	23.3%	13.0%	58,209	26.4%	2,121,948	42.8%
TAS	45-54	F	M	Musculo-Skeletal System	1.2%	21.0%	2.9%	28,871	22.5%	714,410	26.0%
TAS	65-74	F	M	Musculo-Skeletal System	1.3%	19.2%	10.0%	53,820	20.7%	1,710,305	32.8%
TAS	75-84	F	M	Musculo-Skeletal System	1.9%	19.4%	13.5%	48,974	21.7%	1,725,882	38.1%
TAS	85+	F	M	Musculo-Skeletal System	2.3%	20.9%	12.5%	15,484	23.7%	542,220	39.2%
VIC	45-54	F	M	Musculo-Skeletal System	1.6%	21.4%	1.1%	226,241	23.4%	5,564,486	24.7%
VIC	55-64	F	M	Musculo-Skeletal System	3.9%	18.7%	5.6%	396,856	23.3%	11,501,722	30.2%
VIC	65-74	F	M	Musculo-Skeletal System	1.1%	21.2%	9.9%	524,732	22.6%	17,856,586	34.8%
VIC	75-84	F	M	Musculo-Skeletal System	2.7%	22.4%	10.9%	488,876	25.6%	17,785,435	39.3%
VIC	85+	F	M	Musculo-Skeletal System	2.4%	23.5%	11.7%	158,808	26.5%	5,826,037	41.3%
WA	45-54	F	M	Musculo-Skeletal System	2.0%	21.0%	1.8%	94,192	23.3%	2,289,970	25.6%
WA	45-54	M	B	Blood and Blood Forming Organs	1.6%	21.5%	27.3%	13,907	23.5%	737,079	57.2%
WA	45-54	M	M	Musculo-Skeletal System	1.6%	18.8%	-1.7%	69,477	20.7%	1,440,071	18.6%
WA	75-84	F	M	Musculo-Skeletal System	3.3%	19.3%	11.6%	166,854	23.3%	6,035,672	37.6%
WA	85+	F	M	Musculo-Skeletal System	2.1%	23.5%	12.9%	58,515	26.2%	2,209,681	42.5%

Filtered for high values of SPC%

Filtered for benefits > $500,000 per annum

Figure 3: PBS where ATC1 = Musculo-Skeletal System and Gender = Female

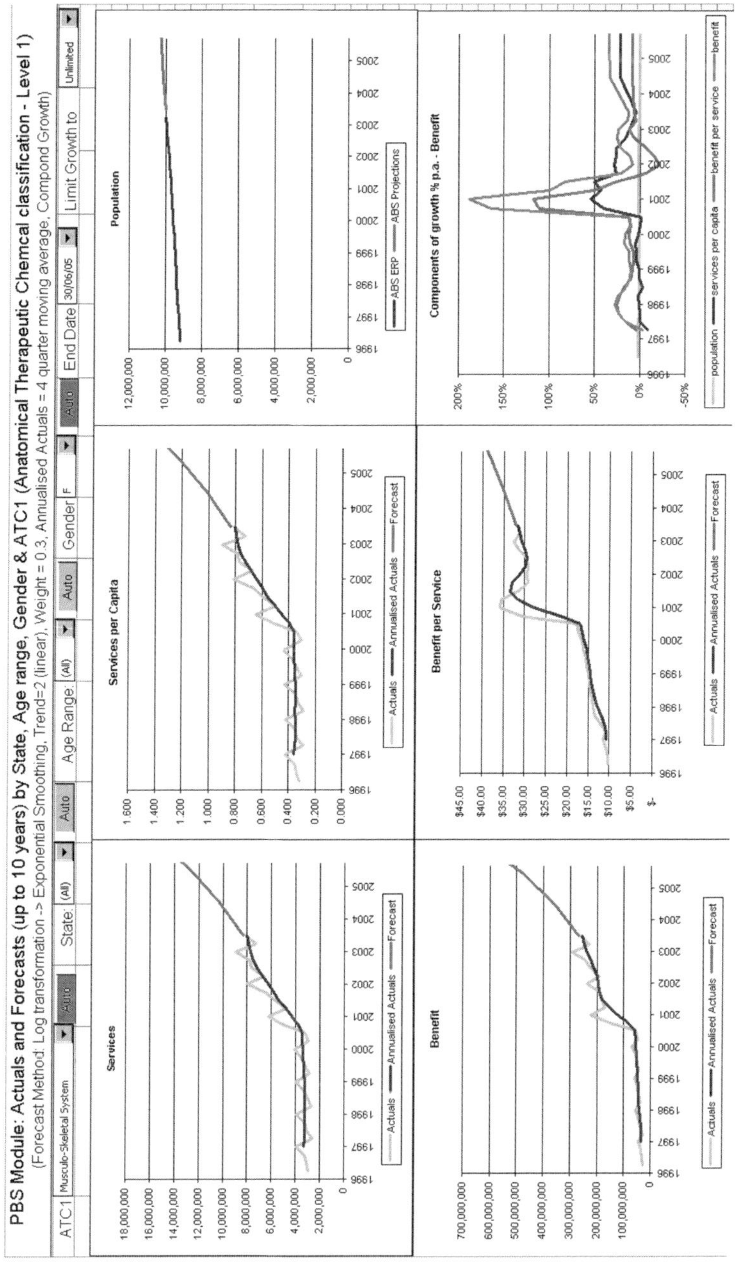

After June 2001 benefit growth slowed and was made up almost entirely of SPC growth.

Questions raised by this are:

- Why is the growth in SPC higher for females?
- Why did the BPS peak and then fall slightly?
- Which particular drugs are involved?

The answer to these questions requires the involvement of a PBS domain expert. In this example a PBS expert was able to attribute the observed behaviour to the introduction of a new class of anti-inflammatory drugs. This could have been ascertained, without the use of an expert, by enhancing the model to include drilldown to smaller drug groups and individual drugs.

4.2 Limiting Forecast Growth

Some areas within PBS may have very high growth rates (e.g. when a new drug is first listed). If this high growth rate is applied to a long-term forecast, then the services and benefit can increase unrealistically and even distort the global figures. To correct for this the exploration tool also has a "limit growth to" parameter (see dropdown control list on far right of Figure 3), which imposes an upper bound on the growth rate that can be used for SPC and BPS in any area.

5. Conclusions

The forecasting model and data exploration tool are being developed by the HIC to aid identification and understanding of service utilisation and cost trends within Medicare and PBS. It is currently being used by the Research and Analysis Section of the HIC for this purpose. The next development priority is to enable drilldown into the service groups to enable identification of smaller service groups or individual services (i.e. PBS or Medicare items) that are responsible for the behaviour of interest.

References

Australian Bureau of Statistics. (2003a). *5204.0 Australian System of National Accounts*. Dennis Trewin, Australian Statistician, Embargo, 11:30 Am (Canberra Time) 05/11/2003.

Australian Bureau of Statistics. (2003b). *3222.0 Population Projections, Australia, 2002 to 2101*. Dennis Trewin, Australian Statistician, Embargo, 11:30 Am (Canberra Time), Tuesday, 2 September 2003.

Australian Institute of Health and Welfare. (2003). *Health Expenditure Australia 2001–02*. Health and Welfare Expenditure Series no. 17, Canberra, AIHW.

SAS OnlineDoc® Version 8. (1999). SAS Institute Inc., Copyright ©1999, Support Web site at http://www.sas.com/ts.

Chapter 10

A Microsimulation Model for Pharmacare: Development, Analysis and Policy Applications

Vishnu Kapur and Anil Gupta

Applied Research and Analysis Directorate, Health Policy Branch, Health Canada, Canada

Abstract

Drugs are emerging as an increasingly important part of the health care system. In Canada, the fraction of health care expenditures devoted to drugs has been rising faster than other components. For example, drugs now constitute a greater share of total health expenditures than physicians. Two recent reports on Health Care in Canada — the Kirby report and the Romanow report — focus on relief to families for the rising cost of drugs. This paper presents our efforts in building a microsimulation model for drug-related programs including a pharmacare program. The paper also presents analysis based on the model. One big problem in putting together the model has been non-availability of a comprehensive data source to make cost and distributional impact analysis for such plans. The first part of the paper describes the methodology we have developed for creating such a database at the micro level. The database contains variables related to individual/ family drug coverage and drug expenses along with a diversity of socio-economic characteristics and health-related variables. The second part of the paper describes the microsimulation model. The third part presents results of simulations made on the model for a hypothetical drug benefits program. The paper presents the cost and distributional impacts of the simulation, analysing those impacts on a number of socio-economic and demographic variables.

1. Introduction

Drugs are emerging as an increasingly important part of the health care system. In Canada, the fraction of health care expenditures devoted to drugs has been rising faster than other components. The share of drugs in total health expenditures rose from 9.5 per cent in 1985 to 15.4 per cent in 2000

International Symposia in Economic Theory and Econometrics, Vol. 16

ISSN: 1571-0386 DOI: 10.1016/S1571-0386(06)16010-X

and is estimated to have risen to 15.9 per cent in 2002. Drugs now constitute the second largest component of health expenditures behind hospitals (Canadian Institute for Health Information, 2003). This trend is expected to continue in the coming years for a number of reasons, i.e. development of new drug therapies, possibility of developing genetically tailored drugs, substitution for other medical interventions (Canada, 2000a, 2000b).

While every Canadian has free access to physician and hospital services, not all citizens are covered for medically necessary use of prescription drugs. Canada has a fragmented system of drug coverage across the country (Gergoire et al., 2001). There is a mix of private and public coverage. Private sector drug plans are mostly sponsored by employers/unions as part of employment benefits. Public plans — federal, provincial or territorial plans — subsidize the cost of prescription drugs for their residents, particularly social assistance recipients and seniors. There is a considerable variation among these plans in terms of who is covered, for which drugs, and what kind of co-payments and deductibles. The federal government provides drug coverage for parts of the aboriginal population (Canada, 2000b). In summary, public plans cover approximately 44 per cent of prescription drug costs, private plans cover 34 per cent, while individual Canadians pay 22 per cent (Canadian Institute for Health Information, 2003). Despite the availability of both public and private plans, many Canadians have no coverage at all for prescription drugs. Moreover, among those with some coverage (either public or private), there is substantial variation in its nature and quality (Canada, 2000a). Financial hardship due to high drug expense is increasingly a real risk — indeed, it is a reality — for many individuals and families in Canada (Canada, 2000a). There is evidence that patients' health may be compromised if they do not have access to drug therapy (O'Brien, 1989; Soumerai et al., 1991; Martin and McMillan, 1996; Johnson et al., 1997). Further, several studies have shown that patients may reduce or abruptly terminate their use of prescription drugs in the absence of insurance or in the presence of high levels of deductibles/co-payment, if insured (Leibowitz et al., 1985; Soumerai et al., 1987; O'Brien, 1989; Martin and McMillan, 1996). A more recent study assessed the recent changes to the Quebec prescription drug plan and the effect of co-payment on drug consumption. It found that many beneficiaries of the plan — in particular social security recipients and Guaranteed Income Supplement seniors — significantly reduced their drug consumption with the introduction of co-payments in the Quebec plan (Tamblyn, 1999).

Given the expanding role of prescription drugs in Canada's health care system, a strong case can be made that prescription drugs are just as medically necessary as hospital or physician services (Canada Health Action, 1997). A recent report by the Commission on the Future of Health Care in Canada — the so called Romanow report — notes that, because the immediate integration of all prescribed drugs into the health care system has significant cost implications, the goal should be to move in a gradual way towards that integration (Canada, 2000b). Both the Romanow and the Senate Committee reports have advanced proposals for protecting Canadians against catastrophic prescription drug expenses (Canada, 2000a, 2000b).

In view of these developments, there is considerable pressure on provincial governments in Canada to provide relief to individuals and families facing high drug expenses. Proposals for setting up a general pharmacare program have been made over a number of years. In order to properly quantify such proposals, we require sophisticated tools that would provide fiscal as well as distributional impacts. Two major problems in developing proposals for public drug programs have been the lack of data and modelling capabilities.

In order to fill these and other such research gaps, Health Canada created Applied Research and Analysis Directorate in 1999 and Microsimulation Modeling and Data Analysis Division (MSDAD) as part of that Directorate. MSDAD supports the federal health agenda by developing tools that promote evidence-based decision-making at all levels of health care. As part of its mandate, the Division undertook the task of developing a database and a microsimulation model for pharmacare. This paper presents the methodology behind the development of the database and the model. The paper uses those tools to present fiscal and distributional analysis of a hypothetical scenario.

There is no single source of data which one could use to conduct pharmacare type modelling. So as to avoid the pitfalls of making a piecemeal type of modelling and analysis, the first task the authors undertook was to assemble the data from disparate sources into a cogent whole. These efforts resulted in putting together a comprehensive and cohesive micro database at the level of individuals/families that contains pertinent information on drug coverage and drug costs. In addition, the database contains a number of important demographic and socio-economic variables. Further, the database contains important tax-related variables, which are useful for determining the interaction between health- (including drug) related provisions of the income tax system and drug benefits plan. The paper describes in fair detail the methodology used in assembling the database. The paper also describes the modelling effort. Using the database and the model, the paper conducts a comprehensive analysis of a proposal for a hypothetical national drug plan.

The rest of the paper is divided into six sections. Section 2 is devoted to the processes of assembling the database. Section 3 describes the model. Section 4 presents summary results on the extent and depth of coverage based on the new database. Section 5 conducts an application of the model towards a hypothetical national drug plan. Section 6 concludes the paper.

2. Database Development

2.1 General

This section describes, in general, the methodology we employed for putting together the database behind the model.

There is no single source from which a comprehensive database required for such a complex model can be built. We, therefore, took recourse to assembling the database from diverse sources. Table 1 shows the variables each data source contributed towards synthesizing the database.

We provide further particulars of each of these data sources below:

1. The Survey of Consumer Finances (SCF) public-use micro-data file served as base data. It carries detail on incomes of individuals/families and other useful socio-economic and demographic information.
2. The Statistics Canada Survey of Household Spending (SHS) public-use micro-data file provided health-related expenditure variables, including out-of-pocket drug expenses and private health care insurance premiums — a limited and indirect measure of drug coverage.
3. Personal income tax data (aggregated) from Canada Revenue Agency served as parameters for imputation of tax-related income and deduction variables. We required these variables to simulate the personal income tax system and also to compute family net income as defined in certain existing and proposed drug benefit programs.

Table 1: Data Sources and the Variables Available in Each Data Source

Source data	Variables available			
	Socio-economic	**Drug coverage**	**Tax deductibles**	**Drug expenses**
Survey of Consumer Finances (SCF)	Detailed	No	No	No
Survey of Household Spending (SHS)	Summary	Partial	No	Out-of-pocket only
Personal income tax system	Some	No	Yes	No
National Population Health Survey (NPHS)	Summary	Yes	No	No
Private insurance claims data	Some	Not explicitly	No	Yes
Public claims data	Some	Not explicitly	No	Yes

4. The National Population Health Survey (NPHS) public-use micro-data carry explicit information on drug coverage in response to a direct question. We used these data to impute drug coverage.
5. To impute private drug costs, we obtained data from a private company collecting information on prescription drugs dispensed. The data were in the form of aggregate distributions of cost of drugs consumed by individuals participating in a number of representative private drug plans.
6. For imputation of public drug costs, we made use of the following data:

   a. A representative sample of prescription drugs dispensed under a public drug program in a large Canadian province. These data were in the form of a microdata file of individuals for prescriptions dispensed.
   b. Distributional data (aggregate) drawn from the administrative data file for public drug programs in another large Canadian province.

We employed the following processes to synthesize data from these sources:

1. Statistically merge SCF with SHS for health-related expenditure variables. The purpose of merging was to "impute" health-related variables to SCF (the main database). The merge used a hybrid between constrained and unconstrained methodology. The merge was conditioned on a number of important determinants of household health expenditures including household composition and size, age and gender of household head, ages of children in the household and household income (forming a set of common variables). The matching process maintained the correlations between the donated health-related variables as only one "donor" SHS observation contributed those variables to the matching recipient SCF case. The results showed that the frequencies, aggregate amounts and the distributions of each variable contributed to the SCF matched those observed in SHS. For details, consult Gupta and Kapur (2001).
2. Impute income tax-related variables (tax deductions and credits) to the SCF using aggregate distributional data obtained from Canada Revenue Agency. Again, see Gupta and Kapur (2001).
3. Impute drug-insurance coverage to resultant file using data from external sources (e.g. NPHS). Section 2.2 summarizes the imputation methodology. Basu and Kapur (2002) and Kapur and Basu (2003) provide details on the methodology.
4. Impute gross drug cost to individuals in our database using sources 5 and 6 listed above. Section 2.3 presents the imputation methodology in brief.

Figure 1 sketches these procedures.

Figure 1: Process of Assembling Database

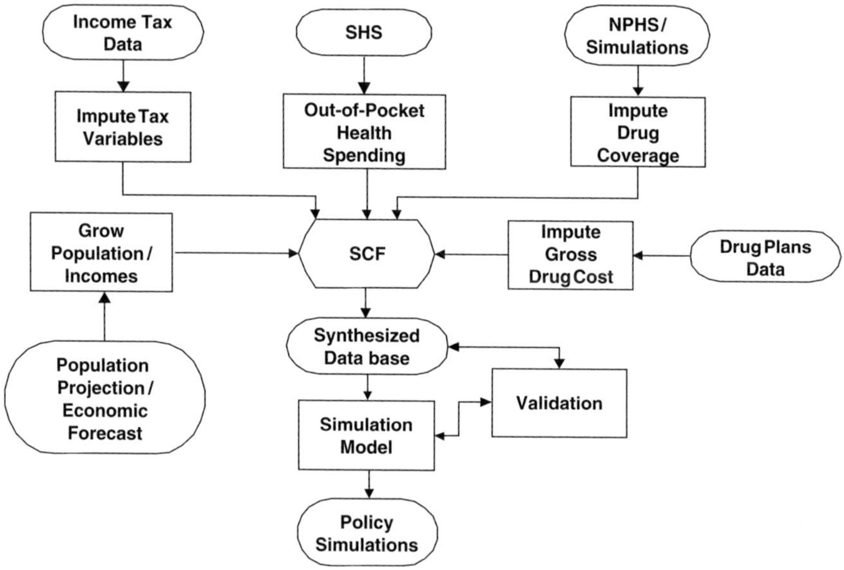

2.2 Database Development: Methodology for Imputation of Drug Coverage

We employed the following two-step procedure to impute drug coverage variable to the merged SCF-SHS-Tax (henceforth SCF-SHS) database assembled as per description in sub-section 2.1 above:

Step 1. Impute coverage for Premium Type Plans using NPHS data and

Step 2. Simulate coverage for Public Benefit Type Plans using variables present in the SCF-SHS database.

There is some overlap between the two steps. In other words, these steps do not generate mutually excusive sub-populations. Some persons, especially seniors, may be covered under both types of plans.

For the first step, we used data from the following two sources:

1. SCF-SHS: This database contains a variable showing the amount of household expenditure on premiums for private health-related insurance plans, including drug plans. However, many individuals covered by such plans do not pay premiums as part of benefit of employment. Thus, SCF-SHS database contains only partial information on drug insurance coverage.
2. NPHS: The coverage information in the NPHS, on the other hand, is based on response to the question: "*Do you have insurance that covers all or part of the cost of your prescription medications?*" Thus, NPHS contains full information on coverage.

Our quest is to impute full information to SCF-SHS.

The methodology imputes coverage in the following steps:

1. Determine probability, P_{1i}, of insurance coverage for drugs from NPHS using a logit model for all i.
2. Determine probability of paying premiums, P_{2i}, for such coverage from SCF-SHS database, again using a logit model.
3. From these probabilities, calculate the probability of coverage for the non-premium paying population, $P_i = (P_{1i} - P_{2i})/(1 - P_{2i})$ for all i. We then use this probability in a Monte Carlo model to impute presence of insurance coverage.

For a full treatment of the methodology behind this imputation and validation of the methodology, see Basu and Kapur (2002).

The above imputation process covered private premium type plans. We now turn to public plans.

For public benefit plans, we determined eligibility or otherwise by means of a simulation that emulates provincial drug plans. For this purpose, the simulation used socioeconomic variables in the SCF-SHS database. For example, all provinces cover social assistance recipients and low-income seniors. Some provinces (Ontario, Quebec, Alberta and British Columbia) provide universal coverage to all seniors. The simulation also determined coverage for other parts of the population, including that for public premium plans in Nova Scotia (seniors only) and Quebec. For details, see Kapur and Basu (2003).

2.3 Database Development: Imputation of Gross Drug Expenses

The database assembled in the above steps contains information on drug coverage and out-of-pocket drug expenses of individuals. However, for implementing a drug proposal, we still need a crucial variable, i.e. gross cost of drugs. In this section, we describe the methodology we used to impute that variable to our database.

As in the case of imputation of coverage described in the preceding section, we imputed gross drug expenses in two stages. In the first stage, we imputed drug expenses to those covered by private insurance plans. In the second stage, we imputed expenses to those on provincial drug benefit plans. In both the stages, imputations were made to individuals in the database with positive (non-zero) out-of-pocket drug expenses. In the case that an individual is not covered by any plan, the gross drug cost is the same as out-of-pocket drug expenses in the original SCF-SHS database.

Methodology

In both stages, the imputation process employed a set of distributions of gross drug expenses. Each such distribution took the form of upper limits of deciles of gross drug expenses. We employed a Monte Carlo procedure in the actual imputation. This procedure ensures that the imputed values capture the underlying distribution of drug expenses as observed in the source dataset.

The distributions were conditioned on a number of variables in order to capture as much variance as the data could provide. These variables are listed below:

1. Province of residence;
2. Age of individual;
3. Gender and
4. Amount of out-of-pocket drug expenses.

Imputation of Gross Drug Expenses — Private

As already stated, for imputing private drug expenses, we used data in the form of aggregate distributions of cost of drugs consumed by individuals participating in a number of representative private drug plans. We took account of the following two considerations in these imputations:

1. In case total gross drug expenses of a person are less than or equal to the deductible applicable to him or her, then out-of-pocket drug expenses are the same as the gross. We determined the size of the deductible from distributions obtained from external insurance data.
2. Drug insurance companies do not reimburse fully a higher cost brand name drug in the presence of a generic equivalent.

Table 2 shows the results of the imputation process described above. Note that we do not have firm estimates for targets. The ones used in the table are estimates derived from data published by the Canadian Institute of Health Information (2003) and tabulations made from SHS microdata. Therefore, we must use the target numbers in Table 2 with extreme caution.

Overall, the data and the process resulted in imputing \$5.1 billion compared to the target of \$4.9 billion, or about 4 per cent higher. Ontario and Quebec are right on target. The Atlantic provinces are reasonably close given small sample sizes and so is Manitoba. The results for the remaining three western provinces diverge from the respective target. This is attributable to (1) small sample sizes and (2) CIHI estimates being approximate at best.

Table 2: Amount of Private Drug Expenses: Imputed vs. Target

Province	Imputed ($M)	Target ($M)
Newfoundland	92.0	87.9
PEI	31.8	28.8
Nova Scotia	178.7	170.5
New Brunswick	149.0	143.9
Quebec	1221.3	1227.2
Ontario	2123.3	2103.4
Manitoba	203.0	186.7
Saskatchewan	207.2	161.2
Alberta	443.5	403.5
British Columbia	459.2	412.2
All provinces	5109.1	4925.3

Imputation of Gross Drug Expenses — Public

These imputations cover general drug benefit plans of various provinces, e.g. those for social assistance recipients and seniors. We used the following parametric data:

1. Ontario: Ontario Drug Benefit plan distributional data;
2. Quebec: Distributional data derived from 10 per cent sample of individuals using prescription drugs and
3. Other provinces: Distributional data derived by means of simulation of each drug benefit program made on Quebec micro-data. We assumed that the patterns of drug prescription, dispensation and use in these provinces are similar to those in Quebec.

We have had to make some adjustments on these data in order to achieve total target values.

Table 3 presents the results. Overall, the algorithm imputed over 93 per cent of target total dollars. For seven of the ten provinces, the total amount imputed is 5 per cent higher or lower. For Quebec and Ontario, the difference is larger because (1) the program data includes disease-specific and catastrophic programs and (2) the imputation process excludes very high-end drug users.

Figures 2 and 3 compare the observed and the imputed distributions for Quebec and Ontario, respectively. These charts show that the imputation process has been successful in capturing the underlying distributions.

Table 3: Provincial Drug Benefit Plans: Number of Beneficiaries and Total Expenditures — Simulated vs. Program

Province	Beneficiaries ('000s)		Expenditures ($M)	
	Simulated	Program	Simulated	Program
Newfoundland	101	110	49.4	52.4[b]
PEI	26	26	7.3	9.1[b]
Nova Scotia	153	166	112.3	117.1[c]
New Brunswick	114	111	55.3	53.8[b]
Quebec	2,215	2,203	763.8	823.0[a]
Ontario	1,878	2,009	1,213.4	1,344.0[a]
Manitoba	136	0	75.8	73.7[b]
Saskatchewan	112	126	54.1	54.8[a]
Alberta	382	0	234.6	244.7[d]
British Columbia	801	849	371.4	376.0[a]
All provinces	5,918[e]	5,600[e]	2,937.4	3,148.6

Source: 1998–1999/1999–2000 data from Brogan Guidebook
[a] *Program data.*
[b] *CIHI data.*
[c] *CIHI and program data.*
[d] *CIHI data, includes non-plan premium subsidy.*
[e] *Excluding Manitoba and Alberta.*

3. The Model

The micro database described in the previous section is composed of records of individuals with the ability to link all individuals in the same family and all families in the same household. This hierarchical nature of the database is very useful for simulating a number of public programs including drug programs.

Some of the important variables in the database at the individual level are the following:

- *Socio-demographic*: Province of residence, age and gender of individual, his/her marital status, characteristics of family the individual belongs to, type of household and number of persons in family.
- *Economic*: Individual annual income by component (e.g. employment, self-employment, investment and government transfers by type), level of education of the individual, whether at school (full-time or part-time) and a number of labour force variables.
- *Tax related*: A set of variables showing amount of annual tax deductions and credits.
- *Health expenditures*: A set of variables showing components of annual out-of-pocket expenses.

Figure 2: Distribution by Size of Public Drug Benefits, Quebec 1997: Observed vs. Imputed

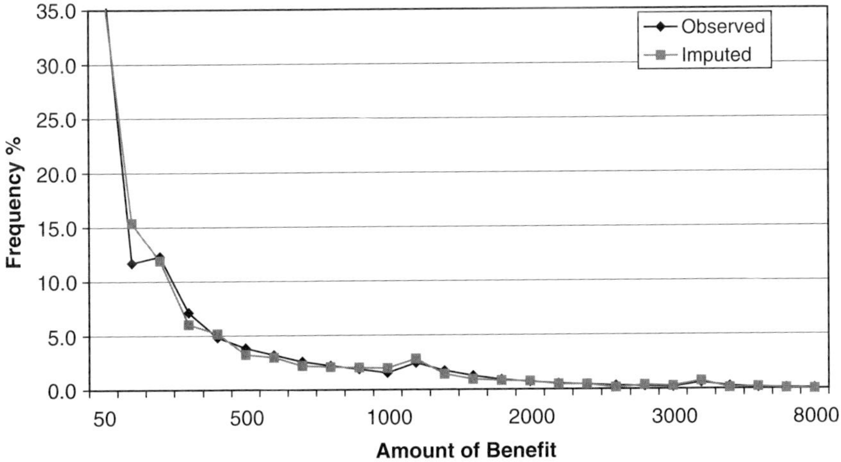

Figure 3: Distribution by Size of Total Drug Cost, Ontario 1997: Observed vs. Imputed

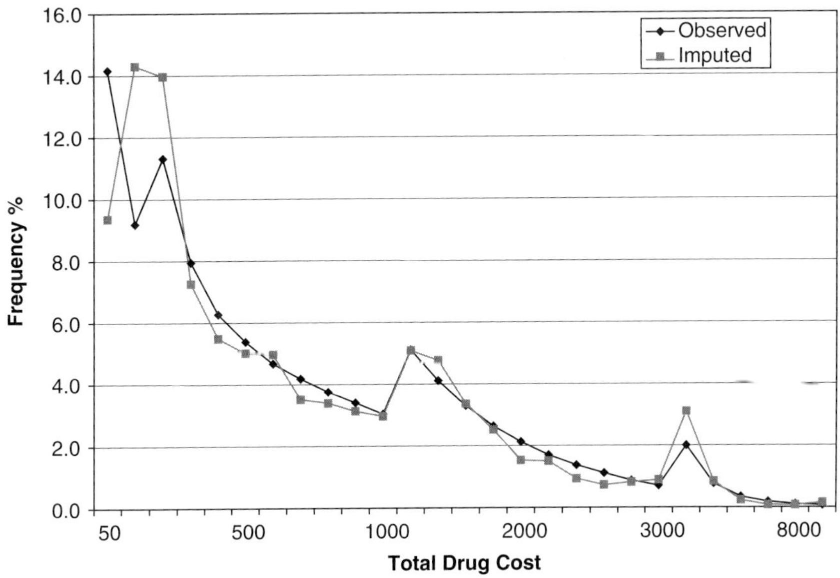

- *Prescription drugs*: Total annual cost of drugs consumed broken down by (1) portion paid by private insurers, (2) portion paid by public drug plans and (3) out-of-pocket drug expenses. The database also has drug coverage information, i.e. private insurance, public plan coverage and type of public plan. Further, it contains a variable showing the number of prescriptions dispensed during the year.

Using this set of comprehensive variables, the model simulates the following set of tax/transfer and drug benefit programs:

1. Federal and provincial personal income tax programs.
2. In particular, the model is capable of simulating the health-related exemptions allowable in the personal income tax system such as the disability credit and the medical expenses tax credit for out-of-pocket health expenses. A unique feature of the model is that it can make simulations involving individual components of the medical expenses tax credit, e.g. prescription drugs. (Under the provisions of the medical expenses tax credit, a taxpayer can claim a number of health-related expenses, e.g. physician care, hospital care, eye care, dental care, prescription drugs and home care).
3. Federal and provincial child benefit programs.
4. Federal Old Age Security and related programs for seniors.
5. Provincial drug benefit plans for select sub-populations and universal plans as well. The model is capable of these and all their features.
6. Alternative drug benefit plans with the existing plan parameters or the following features, individually or in combination:

   - Deductible: A flat amount or a proportion of income (adjusted for family size);
   - Co-pay: A proportion of drug cost; and
   - Maximum out-of-pocket drug expenses.

It should be noted that the model simulates the interactions between the various programs. For example, an increase in provincial drug benefits would lead to a decrease in out-of-pocket drug expenses and thus to a lower amount of tax exemption on account of the medical expenses tax credit allowable in the personal income tax system.

The model uses a detailed set of parameters of the above programs as inputs in making the simulations. The model makes two sets of simulations using the rich parameters set, (1) existing system and (2) option system involving changes to the existing programs and/or introduction of new programs. For each set, the model calculates the dollar impact of each program simulated at the individual or family level.

The output of the model shows, at the aggregate level, program dollar estimates for each program simulated for both the existing and the option systems with differences. The model also produces distributional impact on individuals/families by region of residence, by income, by age and gender, by family type, and by any other variable on the database. The control and shock feature of the model enables one to produce net impact of program changes and winner–loser analysis as well. The model outputs a micro-data file at the individual/family level for further statistical analysis of model results.

Figure 4 depicts the flow involved in a typical policy process employing a microsimulation or other quantitative model. The figure shows that the demands on the model could be challenging depending on the policy process. The model we have described above is fully capable of meeting those requirements in so far as they are consistent with the variables available on the database.

Figure 4: Sketch of Flow in a Typical Policy Development Process

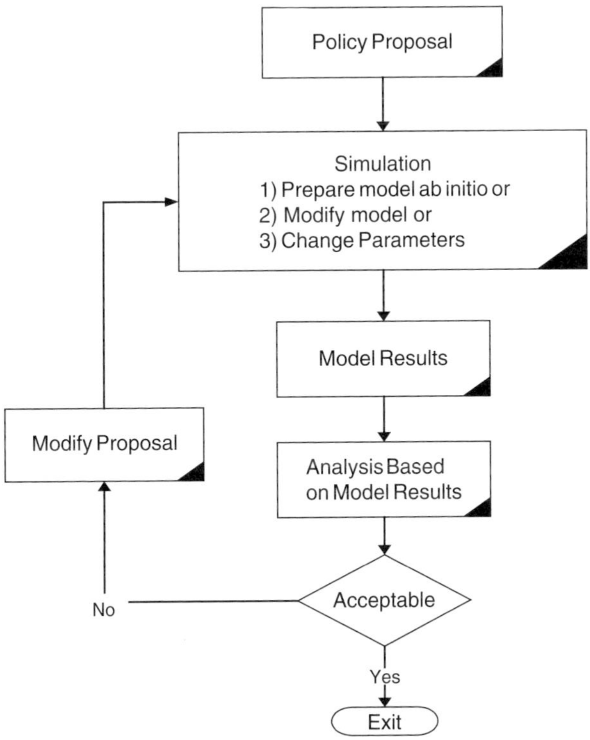

In summary, the model can simulate a varied array of the existing provincial drug benefit plans and any changes to those plans consistent with the variables available on the database behind the model. As the database contains a variable showing private plan benefits, the model can show the interaction between these two types of plans. Further, the model simulates the existing tax/transfer programs. Therefore, its results show interactions between those programs and the drug benefit plans simulated.

Major weaknesses of the model are data related, i.e. lack of data or weak data. We list some of the weaknesses in the following:

- The database behind the model has annual values on drug costs. However, many drug plans simulated in the model work on a sub-annual basis. For example, drug benefits for social assistance recipients are delivered month by month. We have attempted to overcome this weakness by making suitable assumptions and the results we get are very comparable to those shown in program data.
- For many individuals covered by both public and private plans, the interactions between plans depend upon who is the first payer. In many cases, these are hard to emulate given the nature of the database.
- As we saw in the preceding sections, construction of the database is quite complex. The model may not, therefore, be able to meet demands to produce robust estimates for relatively small population groups.
- Similarly, the model may fail to deliver demands for analysis involving interactions between a diversity of variables.

4. Results: Extent of Coverage

Overall, we estimate that a drug plan in one form or another covers 96 per cent of Canadians. However, there is a considerable provincial variation in coverage. Table 4 presents these results, comparing them with those in a recent study made by Canadian Life and Health Insurance Association Inc. (1999). Both the studies appear to lead to an almost identical set of coverage estimates.

Table 4 data includes both catastrophic and non-catastrophic types of plans. Catastrophic plans are public plans that provide protection to Canadian individuals/families with relatively high drug expenses. Table 5 compares coverage under non-catastrophic or conventional plans with that under both conventional and catastrophic plans. Using this definition, we find the coverage drops from 96 to 85 per cent, that is 15 per cent of Canadians, about 4.5 million, did not have appropriate coverage in 1997. Only Quebec has 100 per cent coverage. Western provinces are roughly in the same situation as their Atlantic counterparts.

Table 4: Proportion of Canadians with Drug Coverage 1997 CLHIA Study vs. this Study

Province	CLHIA (%)	Our study (%)
Newfoundland	65	68
Prince Edward Island	73	71
Nova Scotia	76	78
New Brunswick	67	75
Quebec	100	100
Ontario	100	100
Manitoba	100	100
Saskatchewan	100	100
Alberta	83	80
British Columbia	100	100
All provinces	97	96

CLHIA: Canadian Life & Health Insurance Association.

Table 5 also shows the split between public and private conventional plans. Because public plans are, generally, the first payers, we assume that those covered by both (mainly seniors) fall under public plans. Overall, about 60 per cent of Canadians are covered by private plans while about 25 per cent are covered by public conventional plans. There is a considerable variation by province in this pattern.

4.1 Who is not Covered?

We have conducted further analysis on coverage using a set of statistical models (logit and tobit). The results of these models show the following profile of persons lacking coverage under a conventional plan:

- These persons are more likely to reside in one of the Atlantic Provinces, Manitoba or Saskatchewan.
- They are prone to be young (less than age 25 or, to a lesser extent, age 25–34).
- They are more likely to have no post-secondary education.
- They are also more likely to be self-employed.
- They tend to work part year or part time.
- They are prone to be single persons living on their own.
- They are likely to live in a rural area.
- They are more likely to belong to households with lower middle income ($10,000–$30,000).

Table 5: Extent of Coverage in Canada

Province	Conventional and Catastrophic Plans (%)	Conventional Plans		
		Total (%)	Public (%)	Private (%)
Newfoundland	67.8	67.8	20.5	47.3
Prince Edward Island	71.5	71.5	24.4	47.1
Nova Scotia	78.1	78.1	19.7	58.4
New Brunswick	75.1	75.1	17.9	57.2
Quebec	100.0	100.0	43.3	56.7
Ontario	100.0	83.3	22.8	60.4
Manitoba	100.0	69.0	8.8	60.2
Saskatchewan	100.0	67.3	15.3	52.0
Alberta	80.1	80.1	16.5	63.7
British Columbia	100.0	76.8	21.6	55.2
All provinces	96.1	84.5	26.1	58.4

The above analysis answers a binary type question, i.e. who is covered and who is not. It does not throw light on the depth of coverage. We have chosen out-of-pocket drug expenses as an indirect indicator of depth or quality of coverage.

Table 6 shows how out-of-pocket drug expenses are distributed by level for each of the coverage categories. The data presented in the table shows that 80 per cent of households had expenses of \$350 or less on prescription drugs in 1997, 90 per cent had expenses of about \$600 or less, and 95 per cent of \$1,000 or less.

We have conducted further analysis on burden in terms of out-of-pocket drug expenses using a tobit model. Our analysis shows that persons living in Ontario have the lowest burden when compared to persons in other provinces; persons age 25–34 have a lower burden compared to other age groups; males have a slightly lower burden than females; urban households have a lower burden compared to their rural counterparts; persons with private coverage have a lower burden than those with public coverage; and persons without any coverage have a higher burden. Details on these and other results can be found in Kapur and Basu (2003).

5. Results: Application of the Model

As already stated, both the Kirby and the Romanow reports (Canada, 2000a, 2000b) made proposals for protecting Canadians against

Table 6: Distribution of Out-of-Pocket Drug Expenses by Level and by Type of Coverage, 1997

Level of Expenses ($)	Coverage			
	None	Private	Public	All
0	13.5	20.8	13.4	17.8
01–50	18.3	16.9	15.8	16.8
51–100	15.1	14.6	12.9	14.2
101–150	12.9	11.6	11.3	11.7
151–200	6.7	5.6	6.1	5.9
201–250	7.6	7.3	7.3	7.4
251–300	2.8	2.6	3.5	2.9
301–350	4.7	3.9	5.2	4.3
351–400	1.8	1.9	3.5	2.3
401–450	2.2	2.1	2.8	2.3
451–500	1.6	1.4	2.8	1.8
501–600	2.5	2.6	3.5	2.8
601–800	3.7	3.2	4.3	3.5
801–1000	1.7	1.4	2.0	1.6
1001–1500	2.6	2.2	2.9	2.5
1501–2000	0.9	0.8	1.3	0.9
2000 +	1.6	1.2	1.3	1.3
All	100.0	100.0	100.0	100.0

"catastrophic" drug expenses. While catastrophic drug expenses are not defined in the literature, they generally refer to the drug expenses that are beyond the means of a household. The proposals recommend that the federal government transfer funds to provinces/insurance plans so that they may be able to better protect Canadians for catastrophic drug expenses. The Kirby proposal calls for the federal government to take over responsibility of annual prescription drug expenses of an individual that exceed a certain limit that qualify them as catastrophic ($5,000). In order to qualify for federal assistance, provinces would have to put in place a program that would ensure that residents of the province would never pay more than 3 per cent of their family income for prescription drugs. Private drug insurance plans would have to guarantee that no member would be obliged to incur out-of-pocket expenses that exceed $1,500 per year in order to qualify for federal assistance. The Romanow report (Canada, 2000b) recommends that the federal government reimburse 50 per cent of the costs of provincial drug insurance plans above a threshold of $1,500 per person per year (i.e. the point at which drug expenses for an individual would be considered "catastrophic"). Note that the recommendations made in both the Kirby and the Romanow reports relate to federal transfer of funds to provinces.

Based on the design and the parameters used in the Kirby and Romanow reports, we have developed a hypothetical drug benefits plan to protect individuals/families from catastrophic drug expenses. The following defines this benefit plan:

- Benefit equals family *out-of-pocket drug expenses* in excess of a progressive deductible.
- The deductible is a function of family income starting from 1 per cent of family income for low income families and rising to 3 per cent of family income for high income families.
- The deductible is capped at $1,500. In other words, the maximum amount of the deductible for families at all income levels is $1,500.
- In summary, the deductible is the lesser of:
  - 1 per cent of family income up to $15,000 of annual income, 2 per cent of family income between $15,000 and $30,000 and 3 per cent for income above $30,000.
  - $1,500.

Our plan assumes status quo in terms of benefits available under existing public or private plans, i.e. we assume no other change in the existing system. The plan is specifically designed to cover families for catastrophic drug expenses.

We have simulated the plan on our microsimulation model. Note that there would be no losers in this plan because we have assumed that all existing plans would stay in place. Overall, the simulation results show that the new benefit would reduce out-of-pocket drug expenses of families by about a third. The number of families that would gain at least $1 from the plan is about 30 per cent of all families who use prescription drugs.

The distributional results of the simulation are depicted in Figure 5. The chart shows that benefits under the plan are progressive. As a proportion of existing out-of-pocket drug expenses, the total amount of benefits delivered would be about 65–80 per cent for families with low income (up to $20,000) dropping to about 10 per cent for high income families (incomes over $80,000). Similarly, the proportion of "winner" families (i.e. those gaining at least $1 from the new plan) would be almost 50–65 per cent for families with incomes under $20,000 falling to about 10 per cent at high levels (incomes over $80,000).

We have assumed a 100 per cent take up of the new program. Further, we have assumed no behavioural change on the part of individuals/families and on the part of the existing plans to which they belong. In other words, the new plan would be the last payer. However, our model is capable of implementing take up as a function of variables existing on our database, e.g.

Figure 5: Distribution of the Hypothetical Plan Benefits by Family Income

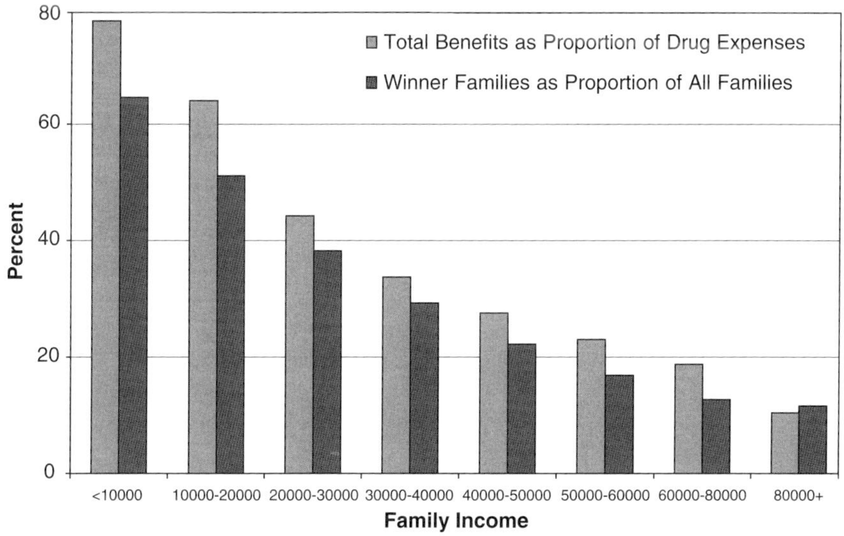

income and region of residence. Further, the model is capable of implementing any such behaviour under reasonable assumptions, again, using variables on the database. For example, the model is capable of assuming that the existing plan is the first payer instead of being the last, the assumption we made in our simulation above. Or, it could assume that the new plan replaces all or some parts of the existing public (provincial) plans. To that extent, therefore, the model is quite flexible.

There would be an interaction of the hypothetical plan we have simulated with the medical expenses tax credit provisions of the personal income tax system. As the model simulates both the new plan and the tax system, its results show that some of the families/individuals would experience an increase in their income taxes because their out-of-pocket drug expenses would drop by the amount of the new benefit.

We have also simulated on the model the proposals made in recent public reports (Canada, 2000a, 2000b) for catastrophic drug expenses. Our estimates are quite close to those published in these reports, which were made by other models or from other data sources.

6. Conclusions

Prescribed drugs are playing an increasingly important role in health care. However, while all Canadians have free access to physician and hospital services, not all are as generously covered for medically necessary use of prescription drugs. Many studies have shown that patients' health may be compromised due to lack of full and free access to drug therapy. Two recent public reports (Canada, 2000a, 2000b) have highlighted these problems and made proposals for protection of families against catastrophic drug expenses.

This paper describes the tools we have developed to enhance the knowledge base in the area of drug insurance benefits and to strengthen the evidence base for decision-making. Specifically, we have developed a comprehensive micro database from a number of different sources. We have conducted extensive analysis to validate the database. Further, we have developed a microsimulation model to simulate drug benefits proposals.

Using the database, we have conducted detailed analyses of drug coverage in Canada. The paper presents some of the results of these analyses. The paper also illustrates an application of the model for a hypothetical plan. We have also used the model to simulate recent public proposals for drug benefits reform. The results shown by our database and model are comparable to the estimates in the literature. In summary, our database and model are robust policy tools that enrich the evidence base for decision-making. This is, perhaps, the first model of its kind in Canada.

References

Basu, K. and Kapur, V. (2002). Imputing a Binary Variable from Donor to Recipient Dataset when Recipient Dataset holds Restricted Information on the Variable. *Health Outcome Research and Methodology*, 3(314), 279–288.

Canada. (2000a). *The Health of Canadians — The Federal Role*. Final Report on the State of Health Care System in Canada. Vol. 6: Recommendations for Reform, Ottawa, Standing Senate Committee on Social Affairs, Science and Technology.

Canada. (2000b). *Building on Values: The Future of Health Care in Canada.* Commission on the Future of Health Care in Canada.

Canada Health Action (1997). *Building on the Legacy: Vol II: Synthesis Reports and Issue Papers*, National Forum for Health. Ottawa, February.

Canadian Institute for Health Information Publication. (2003). *Drug Expenditures in Canada 1985–2002.*

Canadian Life and Health Insurance Association Inc. Publication. (1999). *Health Insurance Benefits in Canada — 1999.*

Gergoire, J.P., MacNeil, P. and Skilton, K. (2001). Inter-Provincial Variation in Government Drug Formularies. *Canadian Journal of Public Health*, 92(4), 3073–3112.

Gupta, A. and Kapur, V. (2001). *Closing the Data Gap*. Microsimulation Modelling and Data Analysis Division, Health Canada.

Johnson, R.F., Goodman, M.J. Hornbrook, M.C. (1997). The Impact of Increasing Patient Prescription Drug Cost Sharing on Therapeutic Classes of Drugs

Received and on the Health Status of Elderly HMO Members. *Health Services Research*, 32(1), 103–122.
Kapur, V. and Basu, K. (2003). *Drug Coverage in Canada: Who is at Risk?* Paper Presented at International Microsimulation Conference on Population Ageing and Health, Australia (December).
Leibowitz, A., Manning, W.G. and Newhouse, J.P. (1985). The Demand for Prescription Drugs as a Function of Cost-Sharing. *Social Science and Medicine*, 21(10), 1063–1109.
Martin, B.C. and McMillan, J.A. (1996). The Impact of Implementing a more Restrictive Prescription Limit on Medicaid Recipients. Effects on Cost, Therapy and Out-of-Pocket Expenditures. *Medical Care*, 34(7), 686–701.
O'Brien, B. (1989). The Effect of Patient Charges on the Utilization of Prescription Medicines. *Journal of Health Economics*, 8, 109–132.
Soumerai, S.B., Avorn, J. Ross-Degnan, D. (1987). Payment Restrictions for Prescription Drugs Under Medicaid: Effects on Therapy, Cost and Equity. *New England Journal of Medicine*, 317, 550–556.
Soumerai, S.B., Ross-Degnan, D. Avorn, J. (1991). Effects of Medicaid Drug-Payment Limits on Admission to Hospitals and Nursing Homes. *New England Journal of Medicine*, 325(15), 1072–1077.
Tamblyn, R. (1999). *Evaluation de L'Impact du Regime General D'Assurance Medicaments*. Canada, McGill University-University of Montreal-McMaster University (CHEPA).

Part III: Financing, Caring and Health Delivery

Chapter 11

Microsimulation Model of Medical Insurance Reform for Government Employees and Workers in China

Xiong Linping, Li Yiping, Ma Xiuqiang, Meng Hong and Lin Guohong

Second Military Medical University, Shanghai, Balance Center of Health Insurance, Zhenjiang, and Military Hospital, Zhenjiang, China

Abstract

The medical insurance system acts as an important part of the social security system in China. Since 1995, the medical insurance reform for government employees and workers has been extended to the whole country and has produced some significant achievements. This research discusses the modelling theory and programming of a medical insurance microsimulation model of medical expenses for urban employees in Zhenjiang, Jiangsu Province. Using the model, the medical insurance policy was simulated over the five-year forecast period 2002–2006.

1. Introduction

Medical insurance reform is a hot topic among the average Chinese population. Surveys indicate that the issue topped the list of most serious matters among urban residents (Gao et al., 2001; Akin et al., 2004). Established in the 1950s, China's decades-old medical insurance system for urban workers had many limitations — due in part to the planned economy — and was extremely wasteful. The State and enterprises bore almost all of the medical expenses of workers. In a bid to solve these problems, the country began to explore the establishment of a new and more efficient medical insurance system in the mid-1980s and has made outstanding achievements in medical insurance reform (China's State Council, 1998, 2004).

Given China's considerable size and diversity, further extension of pilot programmes and implementation to all cities and localities will still take a

International Symposia in Economic Theory and Econometrics, Vol. 16

ISSN: 1571-0386 DOI: 10.1016/S1571-0386(06)16011-1

long time. The reform still faces several problems, such as the optimization of medical insurance settings, ceiling and co-payment levels, and reasonable levels of deductibles from the unified medical funds (Ma, 2000; Wang and Zhong, 2001).

This paper describes a static microsimulation model that simulates the implementation course of the medical insurance policy for all insured urban employees in Zhenjiang. Zhenjiang is a medium-size city (with urban population of 1.01 million) on the south bank of the Yangzi River, 200 km northwest of Shanghai. The city was chosen as one of the two pilot programmes for medical insurance reform in early 1995. The implementation effect of the medical insurance policy is predicted on the basis of a microsimulation model. The simulation commences in 2002 and forecasts results over five years until 2006. The model simulates policy settings according to the current medical insurance scenarios for government employees and workers in Zhenjiang.

Through the model, the actions of unified medical funds and personal accounts are simulated in the process of payment, disbursement, and surplus. The aim of the simulation is to measure the possible change and difference in policies in the process of implementation of the medical insurance scenarios for government policy makers, and support them to further improve and perfect the policy settings and rules. In the remainder of this paper, we discuss the construction of the model for the medical insurance settings and present some findings.

2. State Variables of Microsimulation Units

The model took each insured employee as the base simulation unit (or microsimulation unit), and selected those items (from the insured employees' personal records datasets) that had direct or indirect relations with the medical insurance reform as state variables (Table 1). Moreover, the model

Table 1: State Variables of Microsimulation Units

Variables	Attribute
Personal number	Exclusive identification code of participants
Employer number	Identification code of employers
Sex	Gender of participants
Birthday	Year/month
Insured time	Year/month
Personal characteristics	Employee, retired or person with disability, etc.
Characteristics of employers	Enterprise, government unit, social organization, etc.
Total amount of wages	Income in the previous year

involves some derived variables and running variables, such as participants' personal accounts surplus in the previous year (which was obtained by analyzing the medical consumption records of insured employees in 2001).

3. Framework of the Model

Zhenjiang's model adopted static simulation methods (Harding, 1996; Brown et al., 2004), which simulate the medical insurance policy by basic datasets, produce exported datasets, and then aggregate the implementation effects of the policy. Figure 1 shows the overall framework.

Figure 1: Overall Framework of Zhenjiang Microsimulation Model

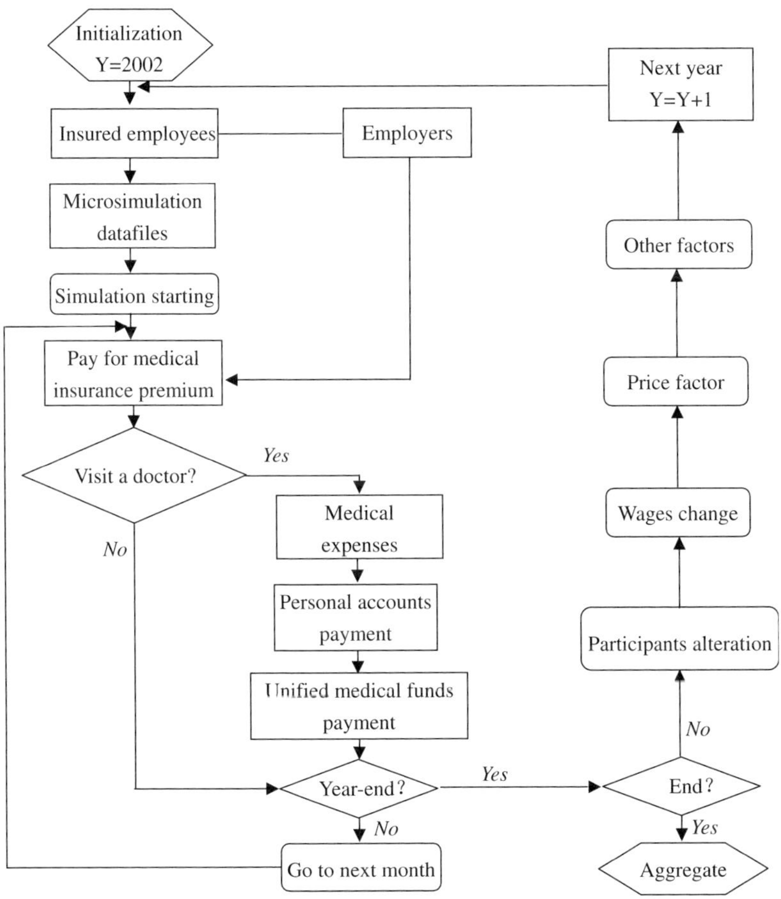

The process and the amount of charge and payment of basic medical insurance funds were influenced by various factors, such as participants' sex, age, personal group-type (characteristics), annual income, medical consumption level, and so on. The basic time unit that the model simulates is a month. The model firstly simulates participants' medical consumption behaviour, and the disbursement of medical insurance premium month by month until the end of the forecast year. The model then considers the change of participants' age structure, the increase or decrease of their wages, the increase of outpatient and inpatient medical expenses, and so on. The model proceeds into the next year until the end of the simulation period. Finally, the model aggregates the annual participants' outpatient and inpatient medical expenses, total consumption, and surplus of the unified medical funds and personal accounts for the full simulation period.

The parameters contained in the model are as follows: the payment proportion of employees and employers to the medical insurance premium respectively, the allotment proportion of unified medical funds and personal accounts, the distribution of outpatient and inpatient medical consumption, the standard ceiling and the disbursement proportion of various medical expenses, etc.

4. Construction of Micro Datafiles

The microsimulation input datafiles (Li and Gao, 1999) were constructed from a sample of original administrative individual data of Zhenjiang in 2001, and the medical consumption data of all participants from 1997 to 2001. This information was provided by the medical insurance management bureau of Zhenjiang. Building up the micro datafiles included the following steps: (1) sampled the original administrative data of participants in 2001; (2) took the sample as the principal part of microsimulation datafiles and then analysed the medical consumption data of participants from 1997 to 2001; and (3) created the derived variables that the simulation needed.

4.1 Data Sampling

In 2001, the number of medical insurance participants in Zhenjiang was 279,423, with males numbering 156,952 (56.17 per cent) and females 122,471 (43.8 per cent). Adopting the method of random sampling, more than 50,000 records from the participants' personal records datasets were obtained, giving a sampling ratio of 20 per cent.

Considering the influence of participants' sex, age, and group-type (employees, retired or person with disability, etc.) to their medical consumption behaviour, a stratified sampling method was used to acquire samples.

In addition, reflecting the structure of the current medical insurance policy, employees were classified into three age groups. For each stratum we used random sampling with a fixed sampling ratio of 20 per cent. In the process of sampling, each individual was given a random number within the interval [0 1]. If the random number was less than the sampling ratio, then this individual was selected. At the conclusion of this process, a total number of 55,720 individuals were selected, with an actual sampling ratio of 19.941 per cent.

4.2 Representativeness of the Sample

When undertaking random sampling, the representativeness of the sample should be checked. The sample datafiles, the participants' group-type, age, income, etc. were analysed and then the outcomes compared with the original full datafiles. Tables 2 and 3 present the representativeness of sex and average age in the sample data respectively.

The deviation of frequency distribution between the sample and the population in Table 2 is negligible (all under 0.5 per cent), showing the representativeness of the sample. From Table 3, one can see that the average age of the sample is in accordance with that of the population: the deviations are again very small, the largest discrepancy being for individuals with disabilities.

Table 2: Representativeness of Sex in the Sample

Items	Number of participants			Proportion (%)		
	Male	Female	Total	Male	Female	Total
Population	156,952	122,471	279,423	56.17	43.83	100.00
Sample	31,386	24,334	55,720	56.33	43.67	100.00

Table 3: Representativeness of Age in the Sample

Items	Employees (age)				Retirees	Senior retirees	Persons with disabilities	Total
	≤34	35–44	≥45	Subtotal				
Average age (year)								
Population	28.3	39.3	50.0	38.4	63.0	73.5	57.4	45.4
Sample	28.2	39.3	50.0	38.4	62.9	73.5	54.7	45.5
Standard deviation (year)								
Population	3.98	2.88	4.17	9.57	9.30	4.36	12.62	14.74
Sample	3.96	2.87	4.16	9.58	9.21	4.29	10.26	14.71

Results for income for the different groups of participants also suggest good representativeness of the sample. Because the medical expenses and unified medical funds payment rate of individuals with disabilities resembled those of the senior retirees (who joined the Chinese revolutionary party before 1949), in the following process of simulation, individuals with disabilities are united with senior retirees in order to decrease the sampling error for these individuals. These results show that the sampling method was very effective in achieving excellent representiveness of the population.

5. Function Modules and Model Parameters

The microsimulation state model includes three function modules: these are the participants module, the outpatient module, and the inpatient module, respectively. The following sections describe the structure of these modules and their model parameters.

5.1 Participants Module

The aim of this module is to simulate the changes in the group-type of participants (Figure 2). Through analyzing the alteration in participants' personal characteristics over the period 1997–2001, it was found that the proportion of individuals under the age of 34 years had a step-down trend year by year, while the proportions of the other two age groups of employees and the retirees showed an increasing trend year by year. Moreover, the number of senior retirees is also decreasing year by year (due to death). The proportion of employees under the age of 34 years decreased 2.10 per cent annually, while the rates of the other two age groups of employees and retirees increased by 0.19, 0.29, and 1.62 per cent, respectively, and senior retirees (including individuals with disabilities) decreased 1.73 per cent annually. For the five year forecast, the model assumed that the total number of participants had a trend like that over the period 1997–2001.

While forecasting the year 2002, the model took a sample of participants in 2001 as the base, firstly random sampling 2.10 per cent of employees under 34 years of age, changed their group-type to the 35–44-year-old group employees, then a certain proportion of individuals in the 35–44-year-old group went above to the 45-year-old group, and then to retirees. The number in the latter three groups increased by the rates of 0.19, 0.29, and 1.62 per cent, respectively. The annual wages of these group-changed individuals were adjusted correspondingly. At the same time, 1.73 per cent of senior retirees were dropped off due to death. And then we combined the remaining senior retirees with the other types of participants. After changing

Figure 2: Flow of Participants Module

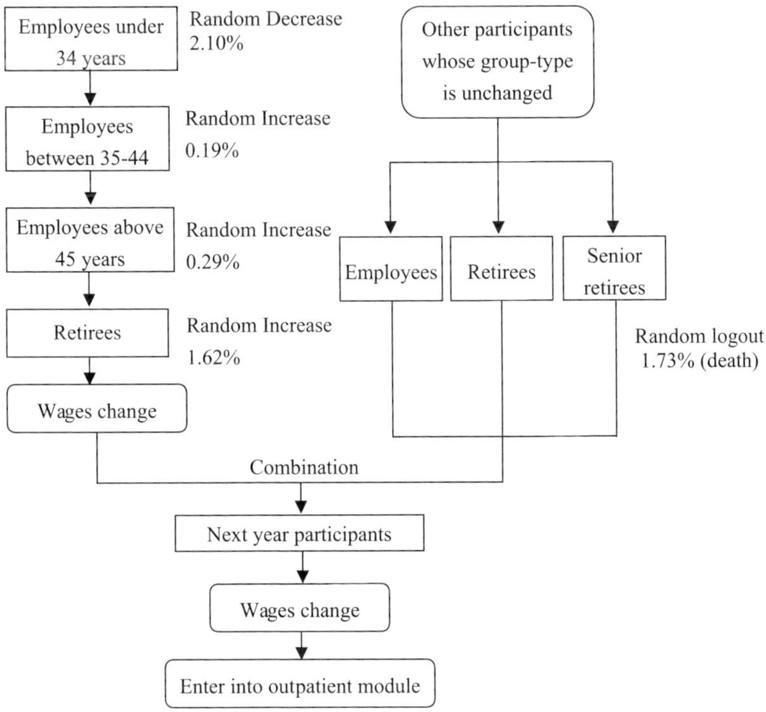

the participants' wage levels, the final datafiles of participants in 2002 were obtained.

In the same way, when forecasting the year 2003, the equal proportions of participants (as in the year 2002) were again changed to alter the group-type of participants. Their wage levels were then changed, and so on, until the end of simulation in 2006.

5.2 Outpatient Module (Clinic)

In China, employees receive outpatient care from clinics that are usually located in hospitals. If employees require inpatient care, they will be admitted to hospitals for more than one night.

Flow of Outpatients

The main mission in the outpatient module is to simulate the behaviour process in participants' consumption of clinics, using month as the time unit. Figure 3 presents the flow of this process. Before simulation, an important

Figure 3: Flow of Outpatient Module

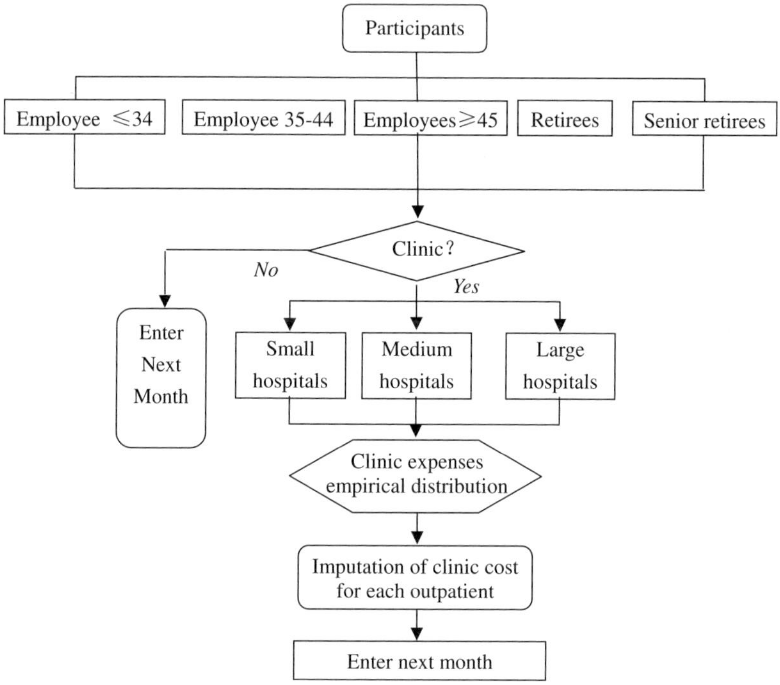

task was to calculate the clinic rates and the empirical distribution of clinic cost. The clinic rates determine whether an individual will attend clinic service. If he/she attends clinic, the cost will be determined by the empirical distribution of clinic cost.

Clinic Expense Parameters

The clinic rates and outpatient consumption levels of participants in 2001 were taken as the simulating parameters of the forecast year. In order to acquire the distributions of participants' behaviour in visiting doctors and clinic expenditure in 2001, certain classifications were made according to hospital levels in which the clinic was located, participants' sex, and type-group. Within each of these classifications, the participants' clinic expenses in 2001 were analysed, and then the clinic rates and clinic cost empirical distribution for each month in 2001 were calculated, which were necessary parameters for this module.

In analyzing the clinic expenses, 100 Chinese Yuan (US$1 is about 8.27 Chinese Yuan) was taken as the subsection interval, and we divided the outpatient medical expenses into 16 segments (namely "0–99", "100–199",

"200–299", , "1,500 and over"). The medical cost frequencies were analysed monthly, distinguishing individuals' sex, group-type, and hospitals which patients visited. The number of individuals whose monthly clinic expenses were above 1,500 Chinese Yuan is very few, and the variation of their expenses was quite large. (In 2001, individuals whose monthly clinic expenses were above 1,500 Chinese Yuan accounted for only 0.52 per cent of the total outpatients' expenses, but the largest cost reached 51,044 Chinese Yuan.) These individuals were classified into the "1,500 and over" segment. The amount of monthly clinic expenses in this segment was estimated as the actual monthly average clinic expenses.

Through the above analysis, the distribution of the participants' clinic expenses in small hospitals, medium hospitals, and large hospitals in 2001 had been obtained respectively. Table 4 illustrates this for large hospitals. During the imputation of clinic cost for each outpatient's step, for example, Table 4 shows us that about 69 per cent of all those male employees aged <35 years who visited a large hospital clinic in month 1 cost <100 Yuan to treat.

5.3 Inpatient Module (Hospital)

Hospitalization Rates and Medical Consumption Parameters

The main purpose of the inpatient module is to simulate the behaviour process in the hospitalization of participants, using a month as the basic time unit. Figure 4 shows the flow of this process. The important task is to calculate the hospitalization rates and the empirical distributions of inpatient expenses. The hospitalization rates determine whether an individual will be admitted to a hospital. If he/she is admitted to a hospital, imputation of hospitalization cost for each inpatient will be made by using the empirical distributions of inpatient expenses.

As in the Outpatient Module, the hospitalization rates and inpatient consumption levels of participants in 2001 were taken as the simulating parameters of the forecast year. In order to acquire the distributions of hospitalization expenses in 2001, certain classifications were made according to hospital level, individuals' sex, and group-type. The hospitalization expenses in 2001 were analysed by these classifications. And then the hospitalization rates and the empirical distributions of inpatients cost for each month in 2001 were obtained.

When analyzing the hospitalization expenses, 1,000 Chinese Yuan were taken as the subsection interval, and the inpatient medical consumptions were divided into 16 segments, namely "0–999", "1,000–1,999", "2,000–2,999", ... , "15,000 and over". Distinguishing by individuals' sex, group-type, and different level of hospitals, medical consumption

Table 4: Participants' Clinic Rates and Expenses Empirical Distribution in Large Hospitals in 2001

Month	Sex	Group	Utilization	0–99	100–199	200–299	…	1,400–14,99	1,500 +	Mean*
01	1	1	0.0705	0.6881	0.2120	0.0557	…	0.0000	0.0021	1,874
01	1	2	0.0764	0.6614	0.2095	0.0701	…	0.0004	0.0035	3,028
01	1	3	0.1047	0.6076	0.2368	0.0717	…	0.0002	0.0055	2,787
01	1	4	0.1101	0.5736	0.2343	0.0838	…	0.0003	0.0055	3,686
01	1	5	0.4151	0.2333	0.2570	0.1717	…	0.0032	0.0043	2,683
01	0	1	0.0951	0.6874	0.2088	0.0630	…	0.0000	0.0013	3,408
01	0	2	0.0931	0.6603	0.2206	0.0619	…	0.0000	0.0011	3,237
01	0	3	0.1402	0.6174	0.2302	0.0719	…	0.0000	0.0030	3,668
01	0	4	0.1270	0.5807	0.2310	0.0916	…	0.0002	0.0037	2,943
01	0	5	0.3992	0.3263	0.2526	0.1526	…	0.0000	0.0000	
…	…	…	…	…	…	…	…	…	…	…
12	0	4	0.1706	0.5461	0.2087	0.0877	…	0.0000	0.0223	2,217
12	0	5	0.4706	0.3170	0.2143	0.1429	…	0.0017	0.0093	2,848

The average cost of outpatients whose monthly clinic expenses were above 1,500 Chinese Yuan.

Figure 4: Flow of Inpatient Module

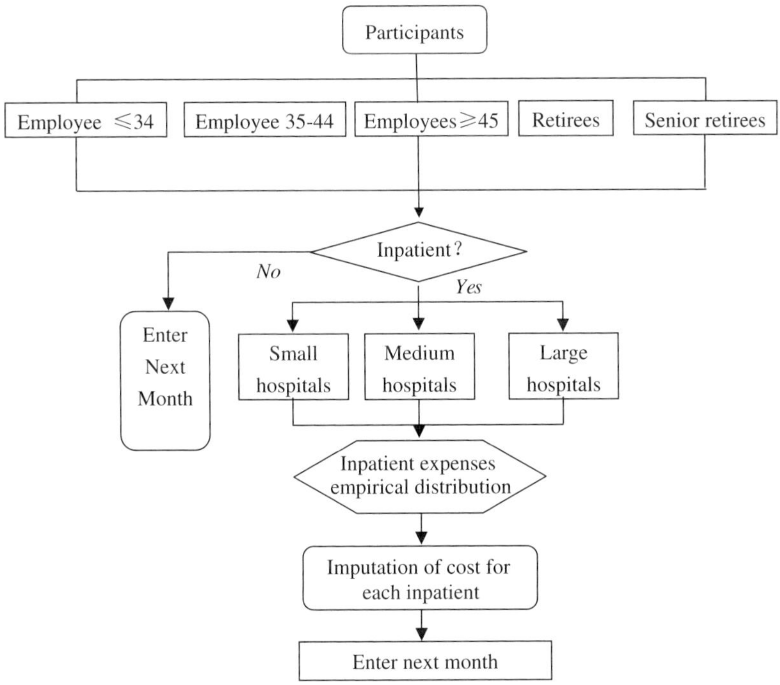

frequencies were analysed month by month. The proportion of individuals whose monthly hospitalization expenses were above 15,000 Yuan was very low, and the variation of their expenses was quite large. (In 2001, individuals whose monthly hospitalization expenses were above 15,000 Yuan were 2.71 per cent of the total participants, yet the largest expense reached 296,427 Yuan.) And so, these individuals were put into the "15,000 and over" segment. The amount of monthly hospitalization expenses in this segment was estimated as the actual monthly average inpatient expenses. Through the above calculations, the empirical distributions of the inpatients cost in three levels of hospitals in 2001 were obtained, respectively.

During simulation, if an individual's inpatient expense falls into one of the former 15 segments, same for outpatients, then his/her medical expense would be the mid-value of that segment. For example, if an individual's expense falls into the "1,000–1,999" segment, his/her medical treatment expense is estimated as 1,500 Yuan. If an individual's hospitalization expense falls into the 16th segment, namely "15,000 and over" segment, then his/her medical treatment expense is taken as the monthly average expense in that segment.

6. Moving Forward through Time

Those parameters, which have important effects on policy simulation — such as participants' age structure, annual income level, and outpatient or inpatient medical expenditure level, etc. — need to be adjusted annually. Those input variables, which are necessary in the process of simulation, such as participants' number, age structure, sex structure, and the changing level of inpatient or outpatient medical costs, were obtained from the participants' personal database and medical expense databases over the period 1997–2001.

The changing rate of participants' annual income is a very important parameter in the process of simulation, as it has a direct effect on the results of the policy simulation. We took the average changing rate of participants' annual wages from 1997 to 2001 as an estimate of this parameter (Table 5).

We also used the annual average increase in participants' outpatient and inpatient medical expenses from 1997 to 2001 as an estimate of the annual increase in expenses, with the annual increasing rates being 11.11 and 14.30 per cent, respectively.

7. Models of Medical Insurance Policy of Urban Employees

7.1 Regulations of the Basic Medical Insurance System

As one of the two earliest pilot cities selected for reform in China, Zhenjiang commenced the medical insurance reform for all employees in January 1995.

Table 5: Changing Level of Annual Wages of Different Types of Participants' from 1999 to 2000

Type of participants	Increasing wages (%)	Increasing rate (%)	Decreasing wages (%)	Decreasing rate (%)	Unchanged wages (%)
Employees (≤34)	75.08	16.50	11.82	8.00	13.10
Employees (35–44)	71.81	14.00	13.31	8.75	14.87
Employees (≥45)	70.11	12.75	15.69	10.25	14.21
Retirees	70.01	10.75	11.25	7.50	18.73
Senior retirees	81.62	16.25	9.95	6.50	8.43
Persons with disabilities	71.24	14.50	11.00	10.13	17.76
Total	73.31	14.13	12.17	8.52	14.52

Under the basic medical insurance system, there are two accounts systems, Personal Accounts (personal-saving system) and Unified Medical Fund (social insurance system). Each caters to a different kind of medical care need: ordinary and serious illness, respectively. During the implementation of the new medical insurance policy, Zhenjiang Government continually made adjustments and improvements to the laws and regulations of the medical insurance reform, according to economic level, employees' revenue, and medical security level. From January 1, 2002 onwards, Zhenjiang has implemented the basic medical insurance system as follows.

Basic Medical Insurance Premium

Employers pay 9 per cent of the total amount of their employees' annual wages, while participants in the social insurance scheme pay 2 per cent of their wages in the previous year as the basic insurance premium. Retirees and their work units do not need to pay for the medical insurance premium. For senior retirees, their units will pay 7,500 Yuan to the medical insurance fund for each person.

Rate Allocated to the Participants' Personal Accounts

(1) For employees under the age of 34 years, 3 per cent of the amount of employee's wages in the previous year will be allocated to their personal account.
(2) For employees between the age of 35 and 44 years, 4 per cent of the amount of the employee's wages in the previous year will be allocated to their personal account.
(3) For employees above the age of 45 years, 5 per cent of the amount of the employee's wages in the previous year will be allocated to their personal account.
(4) For retirees, 6 per cent of the amount of retiree's income (mainly pension) in the previous year will be allocated to their personal account.
(5) For senior retirees, 3,000 Yuan will be allocated to their personal account annually. This is a large amount compared with the annual average wages of about 14,000 Yuan in 2002 in Zhenjiang.

Ceiling for Reimbursement of Unified Medical Funds

(1) For employees, the ceiling for reimbursement is 10 per cent of their wages in the previous year.
(2) For retirees, the ceiling for reimbursement is 5 per cent of their income (pension) in the previous year.

Implementation Mode and Individual Disbursement Rate

(1) Clinic payments: There are two kinds of cases when the "personal account" (including savings in both the present year and previous years) has been exhausted. One case is that if the remaining expense is within the ceiling of reimbursement, then the individual should pay the bill out of their own pocket; the other case is that if the remaining expenses exceed the ceiling, then the amount of money exceeding the ceiling will be paid jointly by the individual and the unified medical fund. The rate of fund's payment varies with the level of hospitals as shown in Table 6.
(2) Hospitalization expenses: For incurred expenses of hospitalization, participants will first pay the bill by "personal account". Whenever the personal account has been exhausted, the individual pays the bill if the cost is within the ceiling; when the cost exceeds the ceiling, it will be covered by the individual and the unified medical fund jointly (Table 7; note that the rate of hospitalization expenses paid by retirees is half of that by employees).
(3) Reimbursement ceiling of social medical funds: For employees and retirees the ceiling will be 30,000 Yuan. This reimbursement includes the clinic expenses and hospitalization expenses paid by the funds, exclude the payment by personal account, within the ceilings and the special medical treatment.

Figure 5 shows the premium of the basic medical insurance and the allocation to personal accounts and unified medical funds.

Table 6: Reimbursement Rate by Individual and the Fund whenever Clinic Expenses Exceed the Ceiling

Hospital level	Rate by individual (%)	Rate by unified fund (%)
Large hospital	35	65
Medium hospital	30	70
Small hospital	25	75

Table 7: Reimbursement Rate by Individual and the Fund whenever the Hospitalization Expenses Exceed the Ceiling

Hospitalization expenses	Rate by individual (%)	Rate by the fund (%)
Within 5,000	20	80
From 5,001 to 10,000	10	90
From 10,001 to 30,000	5	95

Figure 5: Premium of Basic Medical Insurance and the Allocation

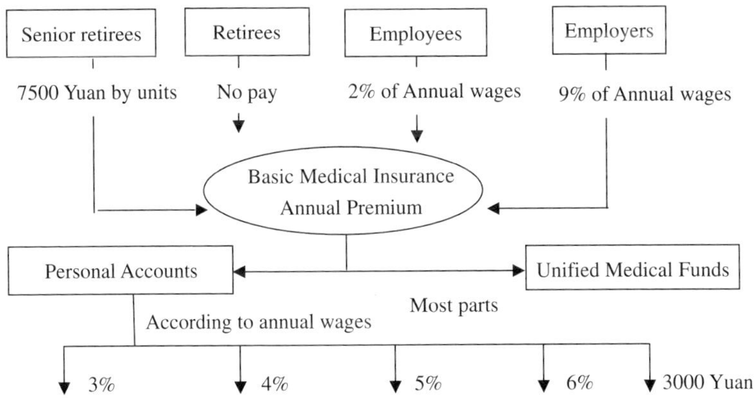

Large Sum Medical Expenses Fund

For those seriously ill patients whose medical cost are very high and cannot be covered by the ceiling 30,000 Yuan in basic medical social fund, there is a large sum medical expenses fund. Submit criterion: Employees, retirees submit 5 Yuan, 4 Yuan per capita each month, respectively. There are three cases of how the medical costs are to be covered by large sum fund according to the participants' annual medical expenses (Table 8). This research regards this large sum fund as a part of the basic medical funds.

Maximum Expenses Paid by the Individual

The maximum ceiling paid by participants, who joined in basic medical insurance system, is 3,500 Yuan out of pocket annually. This includes all the amount of money paid by individuals themselves within the limited ceiling of 30,000 Yuan.

7.2 Medical Insurance Policy Model for Urban Employees

Simulation Framework

The policy model had been structured according to Zhenjiang's medical insurance policy in 2002. Through simulating and analyzing the cases of revenue collection, disbursement of funds and the balancing of these two factors from 2002 to 2006, the implementation and function of selected medical insurance policies have been predicted. The framework of the policy model is shown in Figure 6.

Table 8: Reimbursement rate by Individual and Large Sum Fund for Seriously Ill Patients

Annual medical expenses	Rate by individual (%)	Rate by large sum fund (%)
Between 30,000 and 100,000		100
Between 100,000 and 200,000	5	95
Above 200,000	10	90

Figure 6: Policy Model's Framework for Urban Medical Insurance Reform

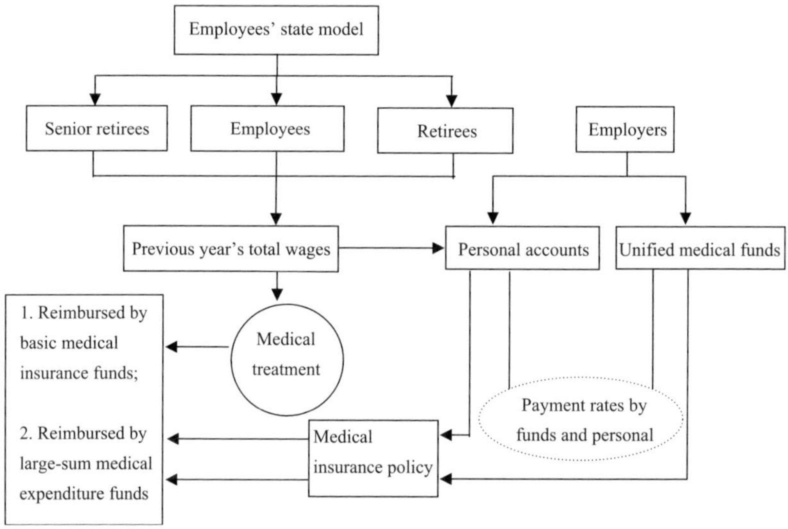

Analysis of Policy Items

Selection of policy parameters: Different combinations of policy parameters can be simulated. These policy parameters are as follows: Proportions allocated to personal accounts and unified medical funds when financing the basic medical insurance; and the ceiling of reimbursement.

Adjustments of policy parameters: The goal of policy simulation is to research under what condition the basic medical insurance funds can make ends meet, under the precondition of guaranteeing the employees' basic needs for medical treatment. Through adjusting the payment rates of employers and employees, and the expenditure proportion paid by unified medical funds and individuals, we can see if the employers have the ability to meet the fund requirements and submit payments on time.

Structure of Policy Models

Design of running variables: For calculating the total amount of medical funds, additional data are put into the model besides the variables representing unified medical funds and the personal account. This database includes the following variables: total amount of money submitted by participants each year, total amount of personal account, total amount of unified medical funds, the remaining amount of the funds, total amount of money submitted by employers, and total amount of money for the seriously ill.

Design of running scheme: This includes simulation time, adjustment time of parameters and the time for output. The goal of the microsimulation model established in this research is to predict and analyse the implementation effect of the present medical insurance reform scheme. In addition, the model allows us to predict the result for different parameters — so the model will provide the theoretical evidence for optimizing the medical insurance schemes. The simulation period is 5 years, commencing in 2002. Adjustment for parameters and outputs is undertaken annually.

7.3 Validation and Adjustment of the Models

When the running programmes were completed, the model first predicted Zhenjiang medical insurance policy. The output results were then compared with actual data to estimate the precision of output. By analyzing the actual data, adjustment factors for clinic expense, hospitalization expense and reimbursement were obtained. Finally, on the basis of these adjustment factors, the model can be regulated accordingly.

8. Microsimulation Results

The model for Zhenjiang urban employees' medical insurance policy simulation has been established under the following conditions:

(1) Participants and their employers submit their medical insurance payments entirely and on schedule.
(2) Participants enter different levels of medical institutes by the clinic rates and hospitalization rates as in 2001.
(3) Employees' age and group-type vary with years following the trends as for 1997–2001.

8.1 Basic Analysis

Table 9 presents the participants' demographic distribution from 2002 to 2006. The total number of participants is estimated to decrease slightly year

Table 9: Projected Proportion of Different Groups of Participants (%), 2002–2006

Year	Employees (age)			Retirees	Senior retirees	Total
	≤34	35–44	≥45			
2002	25.81	24.06	21.18	28.02	0.94	100.00
2003	25.22	24.10	21.28	28.48	0.92	100.00
2004	24.66	24.13	21.38	28.92	0.91	100.00
2005	24.10	24.16	21.49	29.35	0.90	100.00
2006	23.55	24.20	21.59	29.78	0.88	100.00

by year, due to problems in ensuring that younger people enrol in the "compulsory" medical insurance scheme. The distribution of the different groups of participants also varies with time — that is, the proportion of employees under the age of 34 years is estimated to decrease over time. In addition, the proportion of senior retirees is reducing slightly. In the meantime, the proportions of the other groups of participants, especially for retirees, are estimated to increase. As predicted, the proportion of retirees will reach nearly 30 per cent in 2006.

From Table 10, the expenses for clinics and hospitals mount up each year, with the average annual rate of increase being 11.35 and 13.68 per cent, respectively. One can see that the proportion of total expenses due to clinic expenses from 2002 to 2006 has a slow downward trend, although clinic expenses still account for about 61 per cent of total expenses.

Table 10 shows the prediction results of the total medical expenses for both clinic and hospital use over the period 2002–2006.

Table 11 presents the proportions of medical expenses for the different groups of participants during the period 2002–2006. Overall, the amount of medical expenses for different groups of participants changes over the forecast period. The proportion of total medical expenses devoted to employees under the age of 34 years is estimated to decrease to 11.41 per cent by 2006. Conversely, the proportion of total expenses going to retirees is estimated to rise continuously until 47.72 per cent in 2006. The proportion spent on senior retirees is estimated to decrease slightly. The proportion for the other groups remains nearly unchanged.

Table 12 presents the simulation results of the average expenses for clinic and hospitalization respectively per participant. One can see that the medical expenses for all groups of participants will increase. It is estimated that fee-for-service for each senior retiree will reach 13,393 Yuan by the year 2006 (including clinic and hospitalization expenditure). Collectively, the average growth rate of clinic expenditure over the 5 years will be 11.36 per cent, while that for hospitalization will be 13.69 per cent.

Table 10: Projected Medical Expenses for Year 2002–2006

Year	Medical expenses (1,000 Yuan)			Proportion of clinic (%)
	Clinic	Hospitalization	Total	
2002	199,349	122,202	321,551	62.17
2003	221,887	139,343	361,230	61.94
2004	246,248	159,180	405,428	61.51
2005	274,746	180,895	455,641	61.35
2006	306,410	204,050	510,460	61.28

Table 11: Projected proportions (%) of Expenses for Different Groups of Participants over the Period 2002–2006

Year	Employees (ages)				Retirees	Senior retirees	Total
	≤34	35–44	≥45	Subtotal			
2002	12.96	14.54	19.96	47.46	45.59	6.95	100.00
2003	12.50	14.65	20.03	47.18	46.03	6.79	100.00
2004	12.25	14.49	20.13	46.87	46.45	6.69	100.00
2005	11.98	14.32	20.13	46.43	47.03	6.54	100.00
2006	11.41	14.30	20.10	45.81	47.72	6.47	100.00

Table 12: Estimated Average Expenses for Clinic and Hospitalization per Participant, 2002–2006

Item	Employees (age)			Subtotal	Retirees	Senior retirees	Total	Annual growth rate (%)
	≤34	35–44	≥45					
Clinic expenses (Yuan)								
2002	452	511	730	555	986	4,613	714	
2003	502	570	815	620	1,088	5,098	794	11.32
2004	557	629	901	687	1,207	5,571	882	10.99
2005	620	701	1,003	766	1,342	6,201	984	11.59
2006	686	780	1,113	852	1,495	6,982	1,097	11.54
Hospitalization expenses (Yuan)								
2002	126	185	355	214	887	3,902	437	
2003	139	216	402	244	1,003	4,404	499	14.04
2004	164	243	465	283	1,124	5,096	570	14.25
2005	191	266	525	320	1,272	5,717	648	13.66
2006	200	300	589	356	1,435	6,411	731	12.81

8.2 Microsimulation Analysis of Medical Insurance Policy

For the medical insurance policy put in practice in Zhenjiang from 2002 onwards, the predicted effects for the years 2002–2006 are outlined below.

Table 13 presents the payment distribution of incurred medical expenses. The proportion paid by personal accounts is expected to decrease over time. It is estimated that the rate in 2006 will be reduced by 4.07 percentage points compared with the year 2002. The proportion paid by the unified medical funds increases over time. It is estimated that the rate in 2006 will be 3.65 per cent higher than in 2002. The amount paid by the individuals increases slightly (0.39 per cent). The proportion shared by employers remains almost unchanged.

Table 14 predicts the distribution of the expenses paid by the unified medical funds for different groups of participants over the period 2002–2006. The table shows that the proportion paid by the unified funds for all groups increases slightly. It is estimated by the year 2006 that the proportion of retirees' medical expenses covered by the unified medical funds will reach nearly 62 per cent. In the meantime, the proportion paid by the funds for employees is about 36.71 per cent. By the year 2006, the total proportion of expenses covered by the funds will be 50.37 per cent.

Table 15 shows the trends in the total amount of unified medical funds and personal accounts. From 2002 to 2006, the average increase in the amount of medical insurance funds will be 9.59 per cent, and it is estimated that by 2006, the total amount of funds will be nearly 364.08 million Yuan. The amount of deposits in personal accounts grows substantially,

Table 13: Medical Expenditure and its Disbursement, 2002–2006

Items	Paid by personal account	Paid by the unified medical funds	Paid by individuals	Paid by employers	Total medical expenses
Disburse fee (1,000 Yuan)					
2002	116,755	150,222	50,278	4,296	321,551
2003	126,191	172,562	57,601	4,877	361,231
2004	137,129	197,759	65,037	5,502	405,427
2005	150,034	226,078	73,328	6,201	455,641
2006	164,558	257,126	81,828	6,948	510,460
Percentage (%)					
2002	36.31	46.72	15.64	1.34	100.00
2003	34.93	47.77	15.95	1.35	100.00
2004	33.82	48.78	16.04	1.36	100.00
2005	32.93	49.62	16.09	1.36	100.00
2006	32.24	50.37	16.03	1.36	100.00

Table 14: Proportion Paid by the Unified Funds for Different Groups of Participants (%), 2002–2006

Year	Employees (age)				Retirees	Senior retirees	Total
	≤34	35–44	≥45	Subtotal			
2002	30.75	33.38	37.19	34.27	58.72	53.05	46.72
2003	30.94	34.08	38.49	35.12	59.62	55.38	47.77
2004	31.79	34.36	39.58	35.93	60.42	57.95	48.78
2005	32.20	34.28	40.30	36.35	61.25	60.10	49.62
2006	31.68	34.55	41.10	36.71	61.86	62.35	50.37

Table 15: Total Amount of Unified Social Medical Funds and Personal Accounts, 2002–2006

Year	Total fund (1,000 Yuan)	Personal account (1,000 Yuan)	Unified medical fund (1,000 Yuan)	Accumulative add up of personal account (1,000 Yuan)
2002	252,380	227,643	144,988	110,888
2003	275,937	245,448	156,040	119,257
2004	302,177	267,790	168,390	130,661
2005	331,435	294,710	182,168	144,677
2006	364,084	325,975	197,599	161,417

with such accounts estimated to have about 161.42 million Yuan in them by 2006.

9. Conclusions

The basic simulation for participants shows that the number of employees under the age of 34 years is estimated to decrease over time. In the meantime, the number of the other groups of participants is estimated to increase, especially for retirees. The age structure of participants shows the ageing trends currently occurring within China's urban population.

The simulation result of medical expenses shows that both clinic and hospitalization expenditure of participants will continue to increase annually. The average annual rate of increase in clinic expenditure over the 5 years was estimated at 11.35 per cent, and 13.68 per cent for hospitalization. Among the different groups of participants, retirees will still be the main group accounting for most of the medical expenditure, with the proportion of medical expenditure for this group estimated to reach 47.72 per cent in 2006.

The results from the model show the age population of medical insurance participants. It is estimated that the proportion of retirees (including senior retirees) will reach more than 30 per cent by 2006. The ageing of the population puts more pressure on medical care expenditure. Under these circumstances, effective measurements need to be taken by government, for example, (1) further broaden the medical insurance coverage by encouraging people employed in a flexible manner and the young who are not covered by medical insurance to participate in the social medical insurance; (2) establish deposit accounts to accumulate funds for younger people for their old age, in order to reduce the risk of medical insurance funds and to release the burden of medical expenditure; (3) have retirees pay a small percentage of their pension to compensate the shortage of medical insurance funds; (4) increase contribution rates (either by employers or employees); and (5) change the percentage distribution of medical expenses between participants and unified medical funds for those with expenses above the ceiling.

This paper predicted the implementation effect of Zhenjiang's medical insurance policy on the basis of a static microsimulation model [9]. It shows that a microsimulation model is a powerful tool to represent the complexity of the medical insurance policy and forecast future cost impacts. Based on individual data, the model can both examine the effects of medical insurance policy changes for different groups of individuals and forecast in detail the outcomes of different policy settings. This paper established a base case using existing policy settings. Other counterpart research investigated what happens to key output variables if the policy settings are changed, for example, if contribution rates by employees are increased (see Xiong et al., 2005).

Acknowledgements

The authors are very grateful to the revisions and comments from Dr. Laurie Brown, National Centre for Social and Economic Modelling, University of Canberra, ACT, Australia.

This work was financially supported by the National Natural Science Foundation of China (No. 79970047).

References

Akin, J., Dow, W. and Lance, P. (2004). Did the Distribution of Health Insurance in China Continue to Grow Less Equitable in the Nineties? Results from a Longitudinal Survey. *Social Science and Medicine*, 58, 293–304.

Brown, L., Abello, A., Phillips, B. and Harding, A. (2004). Moving Towards an Improved Microsimulation Model of the Australian Pharmaceutical Benefits Scheme. *Australian Economic Review*, 37(1), 41–61.

China's State Council. (1998). The Decision on Establishing Basic Medical Insurance System in Urban Employees. December 14, Monograph.

China's State Council. (2004). *China's Social Security and Its Policy*. September, Beijing. http://english.people.com.cn/200409/07/eng20040907_156193.html.

Gao, J., Tang, S. Tolhurst, R. (2001). Changing Access to Health Services in Urban China: Implications for Equity. *Health Policy Plan*, 16(3), 302–312.

Harding, A. (Ed). (1996). *Microsimulation and Public Policy*, Contributions to Economic Analysis Series, North Holland, Amsterdam.

Li, S. and Gao, J. (1999). *Microsimulation Model and its Application*. Mechanical Industry Publisher, Beijing, China.

Ma, J. (2000). Reform of Government Employee and Labor Health Insurance in China. *Chinese Health Economics*, 2, 60–62.

Wang, B. and Zhong, J. (2001). Analysing the Payment System of Medical Insurance Scheme. *Chinese Health Economics*, 11, 8–10.

Xiong, L., Li, Y. and Ma, X. (2005). Model Medical Insurance Reform of Urban Employees in China. *The 27th Australian Conference of Health Economists*, Auckland, New Zealand, September.

Chapter 12

The View from the Middle: Taking Care of the Young and the Old

Chantal Hicks, Geoff Rowe and Steve Gribble

Statistics Canada, Ottawa, Ontario, Canada

Abstract

This paper looks at issues surrounding population ageing from a multi-generational perspective by focussing on people who are in a "sandwich generation" — people who have both children living at home and living parents who are aged 65 or older. Using LifePaths, a longitudinal microsimulation model developed at Statistics Canada, it compares outcomes for four cohorts: people born in Canada during the 1930s, 1950s, 1970s, and 1990s. It finds that the proportion of life spent in a "sandwich" situation does not vary significantly across the cohorts but that the characteristics of time spent in this situation will vary with the more recent cohorts having younger children, older parents, fewer siblings, and increased labour force participation.

1. Introduction

In recent times, Americans [and to some extent Canadians] are living longer, retiring earlier, and saving less (Wise, 1997), all of which ultimately may make them all the more reliant (in the long run) on their family networks. Family networks are likely the most important source of care for people in need, whether they are young children, elderly parents, or other people in need of temporary or permanent help. Parents are normally the main caregivers for their own young children. The situation is more complex when it comes to the elderly who need care. They get a mix of formal and informal care — the latter often provided by their adult children (see Keating et al., 1999; Cranswick, 2003; Cranswick and Thomas, 2005). That being said, most elderly in Canada do not need care and are healthy and independent. They are often caregivers themselves: 20 per cent of seniors provided help to their adult children and 23 per cent provided help to their own parents (Lindsay, 1999).

International Symposia in Economic Theory and Econometrics, Vol. 16

ISSN: 1571-0386 DOI: 10.1016/S1571-0386(06)16012-3

Declining fertility, marriage, and mortality rates mean that its quite possible that as seniors live longer, the size of their family networks may decrease. But the combined impacts of these interacting factors are far from certain. For example, Rowland (1984) argues that historical Australian data show: "Mortality decline has had a dual effect, augmenting the potential supply of relatives in later life, yet at the same time increasing the potential demand for such support. Fertility decline tended to reduce the stock of relatives, but its effects have been overshadowed by those of mortality decline and changes in marriage. Also other social changes accompanying the demographic transition have probably reduced the availability of family members to provide continuing support."

The identification of what might drive demand for social supports for the elderly (e.g., declining mortality) is one question, and what the trends are in the availability of such supports is quite another. In order to answer the latter question, we have to look at the problem from the perspective of the generation that provides the care. And, in particular, we have to consider what other competing demands there might be (e.g., childcare, work) and what secondary supports may exist (e.g., Is a spouse present? Are other siblings available?). Secondly, to understand the trends we may need to adopt a cohort perspective and examine the evolution of need for support and of capacity to provide support over individual and family life cycles.

Important though they are, analysis of these issues is problematical due to lack of data (particularly longitudinal data) on kin-networks. Post et al. (1997) discuss the only practical alternatives as being either a theoretical model (microsimulation is cited as the most popular current form of such models) or somewhat painstaking reconstruction of family lines from vital statistics and civil registers. Post and her colleagues are able to achieve intriguing results with Dutch genealogical data. However, their approach would inevitably be much less successful in Canada (except in Quebec) and in other countries that have less historical depth in their official statistics or more immigration (and therefore less well-defined historical populations) than the Netherlands.

Pennec (1997) constructed a microsimulation model designed to determine current and future probabilities of being in a four-generation family (for selected cohorts of women living in France). But here too, data limitations and concerns about complexity constrained the model that she built: she was unable to account for marital status and (even with that simplified model) was unable to obtain the data required to simulate circumstances applying to men.

Watkins et al. (1987) worked with American data (which suffers from some of the same limitations as does Canadian) to approximate (using hybrid multi-state, life-table methods) adult years lived with both children (<18) and living parents (≥ 65) for cohorts born in the years 1800, 1900,

1960, and 1980. They found growth in the number of adult years spent as part of a multi-generational family up to the 1960 cohort (from about 6 years for those born in 1800 to about 9 years for those born in 1960), but a decline thereafter (to about 7 years for those born in 1980). The greater part of the decline was related to reduced years spent as a parent (i.e., declining fertility rather than mortality). These authors concluded that "contemporary cohorts have chosen to spend a smaller proportion of their adult years as a spouse, as a parent, especially of a young child, or as a member of a conjugal family unit. ... although some of the obligations associated with family membership and with family status have been persistent, others have been redefined. ... we expect continued redefinition and blurring of family roles. Just as cohabitation smudges the distinction between married and unmarried, so also divorce blurs the distinction between single parents who are once married and those who have never married."

Microsimulation of family networks, while accounting for some aspects of co-residence, is a complex task: for example, fertility and marital (legal and consensual) unions need to be modelled. But these depend on individual educational, fertility, and employment histories, while in turn fertility and employment are strongly influenced by marital status. The investment involved in constructing a comprehensive microsimulation model that is capable of realistic views of the past is considerable. This has been accomplished with the LifePaths microsimulation model.

LifePaths has already been used to study the family networks of the Canadian elderly population. Carrière et al. (2003) found that the proportion of elderly women with no surviving children will increase in the upcoming decades, but that the proportion of elderly people with spouses would remain constant. Wolfson et al. (2003) found that the prevalence of disabled individuals who have neither a spouse nor adult children was unlikely to increase.

The present paper examines issues surrounding population ageing from a different multi-generational perspective. We have narrowed the focus from the entire family network to a specific subgroup within the network: the sandwich generation here defined as persons having children under the age of 25 at home and at least one living parent aged 65 or older. These people are a key part of the multi-generation family network and are of special interest. They are the people who are the primary providers for their own children and who are potential caregivers to their parents.[1] Williams (2004) found that 27 per cent of them performed some form of eldercare. These people may also be at most risk of adverse consequences of caregiving. For

[1] We could further refine this study by attempting to limit children to those who are still in school and by limiting parents to those who are disabled.

example, Keating et al. (1999) found that caregivers who have children under the age of 15 were more likely than other caregivers to have job adjustments as a result of their caregiving duties.[2] They also found that having young children was not associated with lower hours spent in caregiving. Eldercare responsibilities seemed to be added to their parental responsibilities, which may lead to feelings of time crunch.[3] However, being in a sandwich generation also can bring benefits: for example, parents often provide temporary caregiving in times of need — for example, at the birth of a child (Cranswick, 1998).

This paper will examine both the relative size as well as other characteristics of four cohorts who have both living elderly parents and children at home. The cohorts include two mainly historical cohorts, people born in Canada in the 1930s and 1950s, and two projected cohorts, people born in Canada in the 1970s and 1990s. Note that this focus on cohorts means that the main cross-sectional story — population growth — will not be emphasised. A Statistics Canada study found that "over the next few decades, the size of the sandwich generation will increase substantially, but this represents the passage of the baby-boom generation through middle age. The influence of such factors as mortality and fertility is minor in comparison, and would not be much increased even if they were to change significantly" (Smith and Dumas, 1994). However, this paper is mainly interested in examining these comparatively "minor" factors since they may result in huge sociological shifts as the more recent cohorts will have different characteristics than the earlier cohorts. This life cycle view will be derived using the LifePaths model, which will be described in the next section. Unless otherwise stated, all results presented in this paper were simulated using the LifePaths model.

2. The LifePaths Model

The LifePaths model is a longitudinal microsimulation model of individuals and families developed at Statistics Canada. A version can be downloaded from the Statistics Canada website: http://www.statcan.ca/english/spsd/LifePaths.htm. It is a model of individuals and their families with individuals being created at birth and followed until their deaths. LifePaths incorporates

[2] Job adjustment included changing hours of work, coming late, leaving early, missing a day or more of work, and having job performance affected.

[3] However, Keating et al. (1999) found that women caregivers with young children were less likely than other caregivers to feel guilt about their level of caregiving. However, male caregivers with young children felt more guilt.

models of mortality, fertility, nuptuality, inter provincial and international migration, education, work (paid, self-employment, and student), and earnings. It is an overlapping cohort model with the first cohort born in 1872. This year was chosen so that, in the year 1971, LifePaths would have a largely complete and representative set of individuals aged from 0 to 100. As a consequence, starting in 1971 LifePaths produces cross-sectional annual tabulations that can be compared to historical data. The year 1971 is also the first year for which high-quality socio-demographic data were available in the form of a Census with a contemporary design.

The life course of an individual is simulated in LifePaths as a series of events. These events are contingent on the previous history of the individual, and usually have a stochastic component as well. When an event occurs the state of an individual changes, which in turn changes the likelihood of subsequent events. For example, a currently employed individual is at some risk of job loss. The risk of job loss may depend, for example, on the length of time that the individual has held their current job. In the event of job loss, the individual's state changes and they enter the condition of non-employment. This new state may diminish the likelihood that this individual will subsequently become married, and so on.

Two such types of events are fertility and union formation (which is actually made up of multiple events). When one of the overlapping cohorts marries or enters a common-law union, a spouse with appropriate characteristics is created for them. Children are also created when needed. Normally, when they leave the parental home, they are usually no longer in scope for model results and are therefore terminated to save computing time. However, it is possible to continue to follow these children, the second generation, throughout their lives, and examine their children, their children's children, etc., making it a multi-generational model. This paper will take advantage of this feature of LifePaths and instead of focussing on the first generation (the original overlapping cohorts starting in 1872), we instead will focus on the second generation. This allows us to make reference to three generations: the second generation, their parents, and their children.

This leads to a limitation: the generation we will be examining excludes immigrants. Though the LifePaths model does model immigrants in the first generation, the second generation is made up only of people born in Canada and people who were born outside of Canada, and who immigrated as children with their parents. Since in this paper we are mainly interested in the second generation, all immigrants are excluded from the analysis.[4]

[4] People who immigrated as children with their parents were also excluded from the analysis even though the link with their parents still exists.

There has been a lot of time and effort spent on validating the LifePaths model. As it does not start from a database but is instead fully defined by its behavioural equations, LifePaths does not even have the luxury of taking any base year for granted. There is not enough room in this paper to present validation tables or sensitivity analyses given the extensive nature of the LifePaths model with over a century of simulated data ranging from fertility to marriage to employment. Furthermore, many of the simulations presented in this paper cannot be validated against any historical source. For example, there is no historical data available on the presence of living elderly parents; only recent cross-sectional surveys can be used.[5] Two of the cohorts examined are mainly projected, so no validation would be possible. This paper uses mainly *status quo* projections: parameters are largely held constant after a certain date. Though it will be interesting in subsequent work to vary projection assumptions and see the resulting impacts, this paper will deal with the base case exclusively. More details on the projection assumptions used for this paper will be found later in the text.

3. Proportion of Life Spent in Sandwich Situation among Cohorts

Figures 1 and 2 show the proportion of life spent in stages of the life cycle for females and males in each of the selected cohorts.[6] It appears that there has been a large increase in the proportion of life than the more recent cohorts spent as childless adults. Men in the more recent cohorts also spent a greater proportion of their lives as seniors while women only had a small shift, concentrated in the 85 and older age group. This is due to the fact that average age at death for men increased by 14 per cent from the oldest cohort, whose average age at death was 72.8, to the 1990 cohort whose average age at death was 82.8 (Table 1). Women's life expectancy also increased, but at a slower rate (8 per cent).

The proportion of life people spent with children under the age of 25 at home and at least one living parent aged 65 or older has remained constant for all four cohorts hovering around 13 per cent for women and 11 per cent for men. Men are less likely to be in a sandwich situation in LifePaths because children live with their mothers after a marital breakdown. The proportion of life people spent with children under the age of 25 at home and either no living parents or younger parents was highest for the 1930 cohort and has been decreasing. The next section will examine how changes in fertility and mortality led to these results.

[5] Arguably, genealogical data could be created and used for validation.

[6] To be considered a "child" you must be under the age of 25 and still living with your parents, otherwise, you are considered an "adult".

Figure 1: Proportion of Life Spent in Various Stages, Women

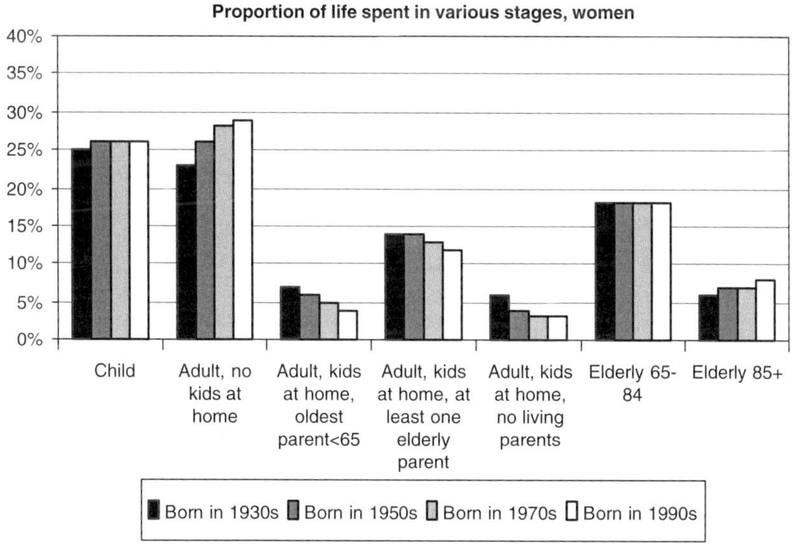

Source: LifePaths Microsimulation Model

Figure 2: Proportion of Life Spent in Various Stages, Men

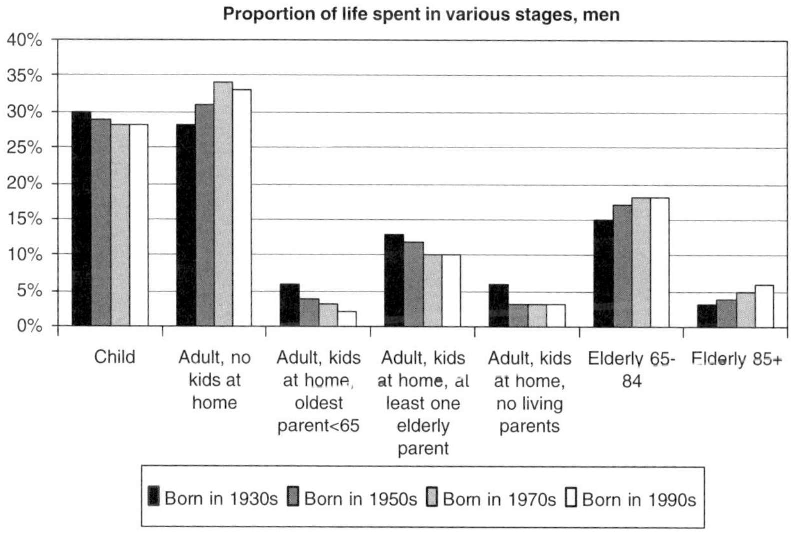

Source: LifePaths Microsimulation Model

Table 1: Average Age at Death

	Women	Men
Born in 1930s	80.1	72.8
Born in 1950s	83.4	77.2
Born in 1970s	85.0	80.4
Born in 1990s	86.5	82.8

Source: LifePaths Microsimulation Model

Figure 3: Proportion with Children at Home by Age of Canadian Born Cohort

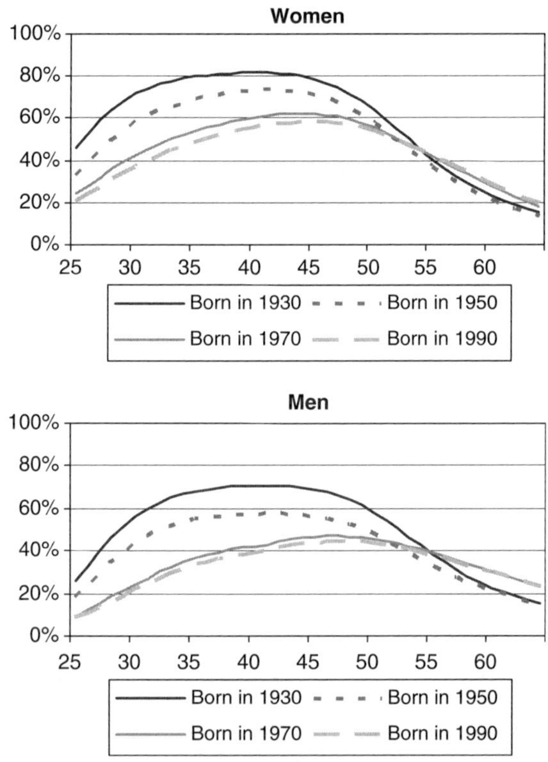

Source: LifePaths Microsimulation Model

4. Fertility and Mortality Rates Go Down

Fertility rates in Canada declined rapidly from the peak of the baby boom in 1960 reaching a below replacement level by 1970 and has remained at a consistently low level ever since. As Figure 3 shows, 82 per cent of women born in the 1930s had a child at home by the age of 39. Women born in the 1990s had a lower probability of having a child at home, 59 per cent, and they reached their peak at an older age, 45.

These 1930 cohort births drove in part the Canadian post-war baby boom, which ended in the mid-1960s. Fertility rates had declined by the time the 1950 cohort had children and kept declining for the later cohorts. Women were having fewer children and they were having them later in life. Women born in the 1930s peaked with an average of 2.7 children living at home, whereas the 1990 cohort peaked with an average of 1.1 children at home (Figure 4).

Fertility in LifePaths is modelled as the decision to have another child. The explanatory variables are the number of previously born children, province of residence, marital status, age at marriage, education, and year of birth. The equations were derived using micro-data pooled on completed fertility from the 1971 through 1991 censuses and the projection assumption

Figure 4: Average Number of Children at Home, by Age of Canadian Born Cohort

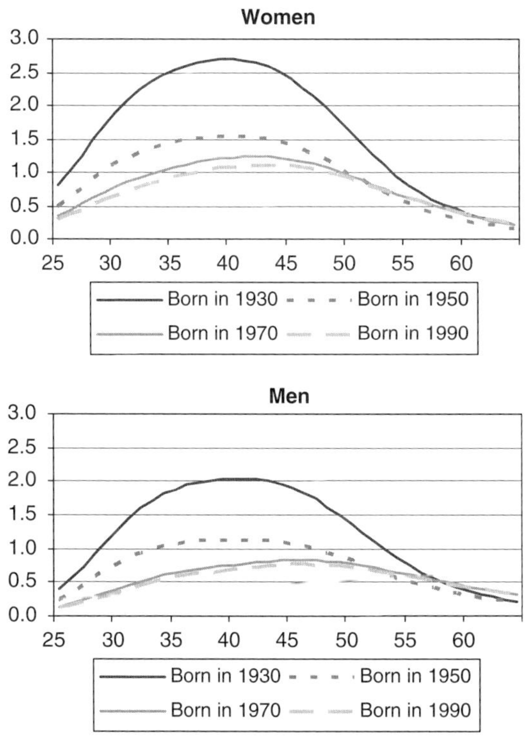

Source: LifePaths Microsimulation Model

is that the fertility rates will remain constant after that — a valid assumption for the recent past. Note that the 1970 and 1990 cohorts though similar, are not exactly the same. This is due to the fact that though the fertility equations may remain constant after 1991, the explanatory variables, such as education and employment status, will change.

Fertility explains how children enter the home, a separate set of equations determine when children leave the family home. According to Canadian censuses, the proportion of young adults who live with their parents dropped between 1971 and 1981 but rose over the 1981–1996 period (Boyd and Norris, 1999). LifePaths estimates the hazard of leaving home by sex, age, and cohort. The hazards which were derived using the Labour Force Survey remain constant after 2001.

The other factor in being part of a sandwich generation is having living parents and is driven by changes in mortality. The probability of dying in LifePaths is based on age, sex, and cohort-specific mortality hazards, which are assessed on the person's birthday. Mortality was projected in LifePaths along with immigration and emigration in order to coincide with Statistics Canada's medium population projections. Figures 5 and 6

Figure 5: Average Number of Living Parents, by Age of Canadian Born Cohort

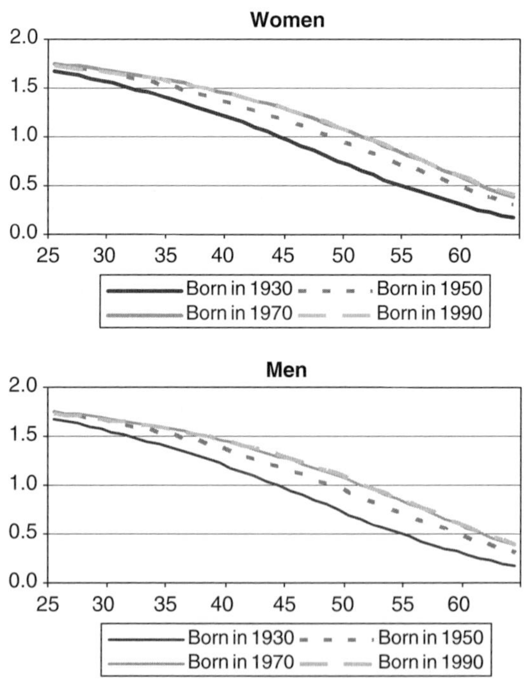

Figure 6: Proportion of Canadian Born Cohort with at least One Living Parent 65 or Older

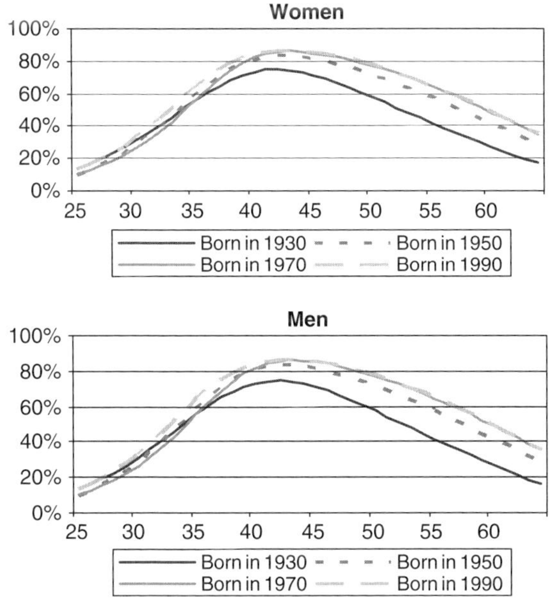

Source: LifePaths Microsimulation Model

indicate that the two projected cohorts are very similar yet different from the historical cohorts which had higher mortality rates. While Figure 5 shows that in their 20s most people had two known living parents, Figure 6 indicates that it is not until their 40s that their parents are likely to have reached the age of 65.[7]

In order to be in a sandwich situation, a person must have at least one child under the age of 25 living at home as well as at least one parent over the age of 65. Figure 7 shows how the combined impact of postponing childbirth and declining mortality rates affect the proportion of people in a sandwich situation by age. Though the different cohorts are spending a similar proportion of their lives in this state, the age distribution of the cohorts are quite different. The more recent cohorts peak at a later age and remain in this

[7] Note that in LifePaths, we do not know or follow the fathers of children who are born to single mothers who are not in common-law unions. Hence these fathers are excluded from the analysis that makes the average number of living parents lower than it would otherwise be.

Figure 7: Proportion of Population with Children <25 at Home and Living Parents 65 or Older, by Age of Canadian Born Cohort

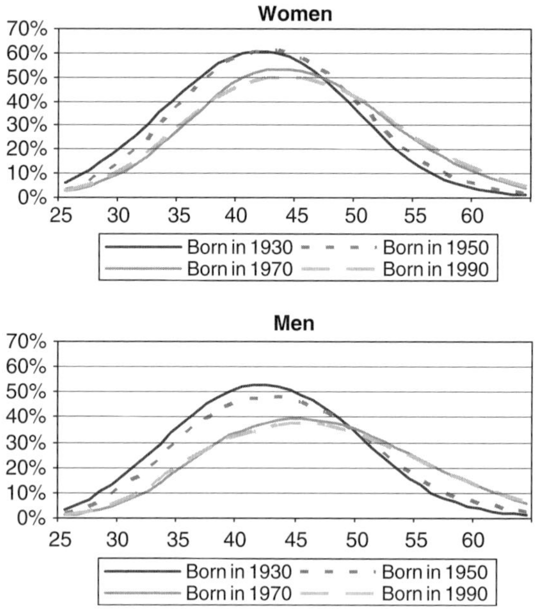

Source: LifePaths Microsimulation Model

situation for longer than did the earlier cohorts. The earlier cohorts peak at younger ages with 60 per cent of women and 50 per cent of men in a sandwich situation by their early 40s. The more recent cohorts peak at slightly older ages and their peaks are about 10 percentage points lower than the earlier cohorts, but they remain in the sandwich generation at older ages.

5. Characteristics of People in a Sandwich Situation

This section of the paper will examine more closely the different characteristics of people who are in a sandwich situation. People will move in and out of the situation as they have children or as their parents either age or die. People in this situation, particularly those with preschool children or with parents over the age of 85 may need to provide more hours of care than others. Figure 8 shows that the proportion of the sandwich generation with parents over the age of 85 is highest for the 1990 cohort due to declines in mortality. Men spent a greater proportion of their time in a sandwich situation with parents over the age of 85: 19 per cent compared to 16 per cent for women for the 1990 cohort, increasing from 6 per cent for both sexes for the 1930 cohort.

Figure 8: Proportion of the Sandwich Generation with a Parent over the Age of 85, by Age of Canadian Born Cohort

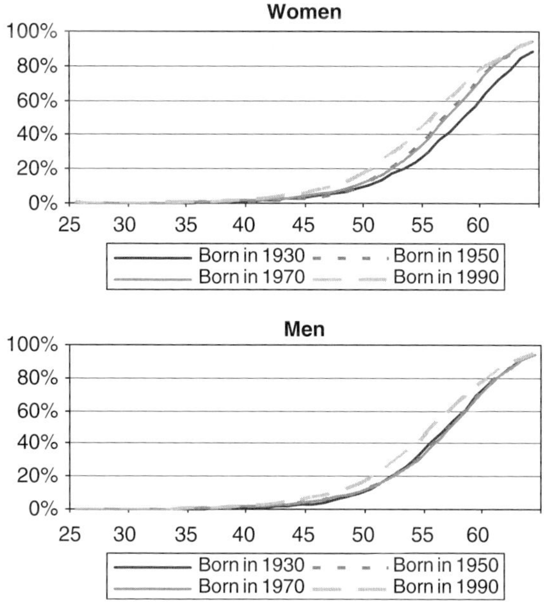

Source: LifePaths Microsimulation Model

Since the more recent cohorts are having their children later in life (e.g., after completing their education to a higher level than in earlier cohorts), it is to be expected that they will also have preschool children at older ages. Figure 9 confirms this and demonstrates that the 1950 cohort spent less of its time in a sandwich situation with preschool aged children than the others. This is mainly due to this cohort having fewer children than the 1930s cohort which resulted in them giving birth to their final children when their parents were still young. Men spent a greater proportion of their time in a sandwich situation with young children when compared to women. This is due once more to the fact that when marital unions broke down, mothers got custody of the children in the LifePaths model.[8] Given increases in divorce rates and the fact that common-law unions, which have historically been less stable,

[8] For example, if a couple where both had elderly parents had a child and then divorced when the child was six, the man would have spent all of his time in a sandwich situation as a parent of a preschooled aged child (since at the divorce, he no longer has a child living at home) but the woman would stay in the sandwich generation until either her child leaves home or until her parents passed away.

Figure 9: Proportion of the Sandwich Generation with a Child <5, by Age of Canadian Born Cohort

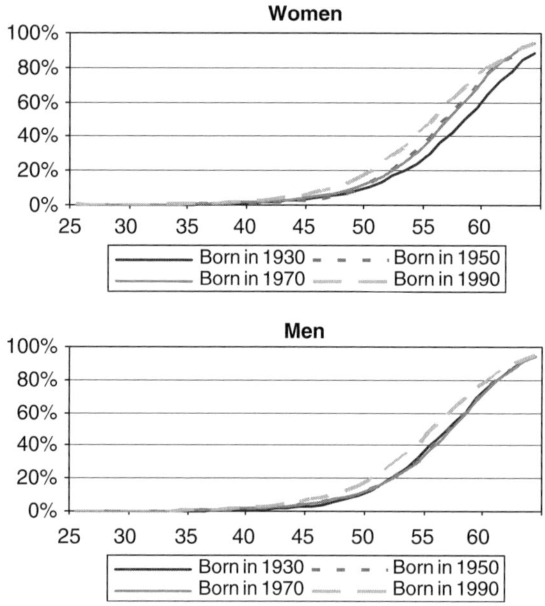

Source: LifePaths Microsimulation Model

Table 2: Marital Status of Sandwich Generation

Women	% Sandwich with spouse (either married or common-law)	% Sandwich legally married to spouse
Born in 1930s	88	86
Born in 1950s	82	68
Born in 1970s	83	28
Born in 1990s	87	19

Source: LifePaths Microsimulation Model

are replacing marriage in many parts of Canada, it might be expected that LifePaths projects a big change in the proportion of people in a sandwich situation who have a spouse.

Table 2 shows that this is not the case and that the proportion of women in a sandwich generation who have a spouse is always greater than

Figure 10: Diagram of Union Formation and Dissolution Transitions in LifePaths[10].

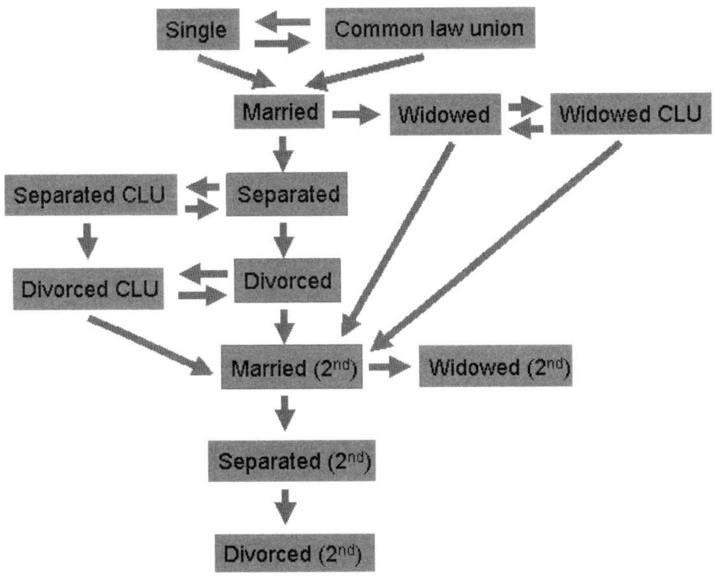

80 per cent.[9] However, this masks the fact that the type of marital union has changed — people in the 1930 cohort were legally married whereas the vast majority of the more recent cohorts were in common-law unions.

LifePaths models marital union formation and dissolution through a series of transitions representing 10 separate events in addition to mortality. The transitions modelled are shown in Figure 10. The equations were derived by combining the Family History Survey, and the 1990 and 1995 General Social Surveys. The events depend on the following states: educational status (e.g., whether the person is currently in school), age, cohort, province (Quebec versus the rest of Canada), pregnancy status, age of children, employment history, common-law union history, immigration, and calendar year (split into three categories representing changes in the divorce regulations).[11] Cohort trends were capped at about birth year 1980 for events up to the first marriage and at about birth year 1975 for events following the first marriage. These caps represent the most recent cohorts for whom meaningful estimates

[9] Men are not shown since the only way that they can have children at home but no spouse is when the mother dies during the marital union. This is a rare event.

[10] CLU = Common Law Union.

[11] Note that not all events depend on every state listed.

Figure 11: Proportion of the Sandwich Generation with a Spouse, by Age of Canadian Born Cohort

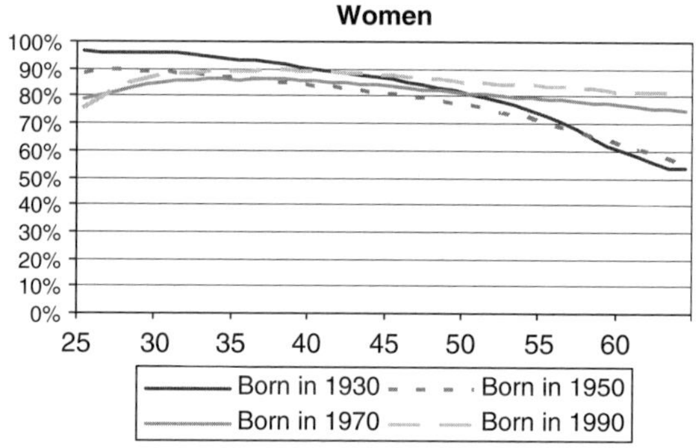

Source: LifePaths Microsimulation Model

were judged possible. Nevertheless, these trend effects represent cohort differences that are maintained throughout subsequent lives (e.g., women born in 1980 may not have completed their fertility until 2030). Otherwise, no parameter projection was made in the model; the behavioural equations were kept constant into the future.

Figure 11[12] shows that the more recent cohorts had a greater probability of having a spouse at older ages, while the earlier cohorts has a greater probability of having a spouse at younger ages. Since the more recent cohorts were also in the sandwich situation at older ages, the overall proportion of time spent with a spouse for those in a sandwich situation did not change much among the cohorts. The spouses are a potential source of support to these caregivers.[13]

Another form of support, especially when it comes to parental care, will come from siblings. Having siblings may mean that parental care may be shared. Figure 12 shows that the average number of siblings for people in a sandwich generation is split among the older and the younger cohort. People born in the 1930s and 1950s have on average four siblings, whereas people

[12] Only women are shown since virtually all men in the sandwich generation are married since they must have children at home. In the LifePaths model, women get custody of children when a marriage or common-law union breaks up. The only way men can be single with children at home is when their spouse passes away, a rare event in these age groups.

[13] Note that having a spouse may also increase the caregiving workload, as parents-in-law may also require care.

Figure 12: Average Number of Siblings for Sandwich Generation, by Age of Canadian Born Cohort

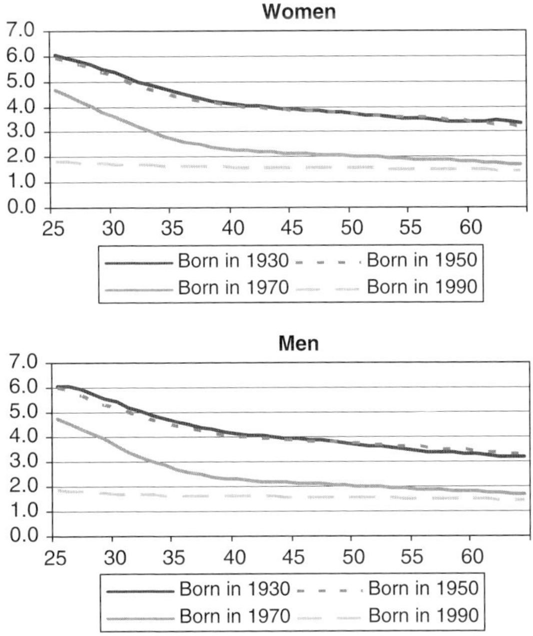

Source: LifePaths Microsimulation Model

born in the 1970s have two, and people born in the 1990s have less than two. Note that siblings here were derived as either full siblings or half siblings who are related to the still living parents; that is why the numbers are much greater than they would be if only full siblings were examined. The more recent cohorts will therefore potentially have fewer people with whom to share elder care. The average number of siblings is much greater for younger people in the earlier cohorts. This is due to the fact that the reason that they are in the sandwich generation is not because their parents delayed fertility as much as it is due to the fact that they were the youngest children born to large families. As Figure 7 showed, there were not many people in the sandwich situation in their 20s.

Finally, Figure 13 shows that the more recent cohorts will also be spending their time in different ways. One of the greatest changes in Canada during this time period was the dramatic increase in women's labour force participation. A much greater proportion of the women in the more recent cohorts are employed compared to earlier cohorts. This means that they will have different responsibilities than their own parents. Williams (2004)

Figure 13: Employment to Population Ratio for Sandwich Generation, by Age of Canadian Born Cohort

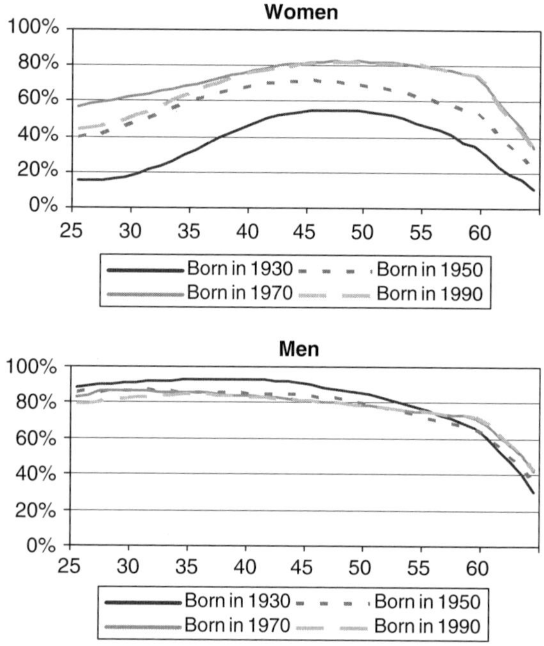

Source: LifePaths Microsimulation Model

showed that caring for an elderly person had an impact on the employment of the sandwich generation and found that "about 1 in 7 sandwiched workers reduced their hours over the previous 12 months, 20 per cent shifted their work hours, and 10 per cent lost income."

6. Conclusion

This paper has examined how four cohorts, people born in Canada in the 1930s, 1950s, 1970s, and 1990s, experience the sandwich situation — simultaneously having children under the age of 25 at home and living elderly parents. The proportion of their lives spent in a sandwich situation did not vary significantly across the cohorts despite changes in mortality and fertility. What did change were the characteristics of the people. This is not the first study to show that an exaggerated importance has been ascribed to the effect of mortality and that changes in fertility have been much more important. As the more recent cohorts delay their fertility, they end up being in a sandwich situation later in life. They have younger children and older parents than did the earlier cohorts, which will lead to different responsibilities. It is not necessarily clear whether many of these changes are negative or positive. For example, the decline in fertility means that the more recent cohorts will have fewer siblings with whom to potentially share parental care responsibilities. However, they will on average have fewer children of their own to make conflicting demands. The net effect of contracting family networks is unclear.

Employment is a potential source of conflict with family obligations, which may become important for the more recent cohorts as women enter the labour force in greater numbers. However, employment is also a source of greater financial resources which may allow for more flexibility in terms of providing formal care. It is not clear whether the anticipated greater labour market activity of sandwiched women makes them less or more able to provide the sort of care that their elderly parents will need or want.

If we had considered only legal marriage, there would have been a dramatic decline in the proportion of people in the sandwich generation with a spouse for the cohorts born after the 1950s. But including common-law unions suggests that, in the future, spouses will be as likely to be available as they were in the past. In fact, at older ages (45+) sandwich generation women born after the 1950s may be more likely to have a spouse present than did the earlier cohorts. Whether this change from marriage to common-law unions will modify the caregiving behaviour of in-laws is a question that has not yet been answered.

On the whole, though LifePaths estimates that the more recent cohorts will have very different experiences living in a sandwich situation than did earlier cohorts, it is not clear what the resulting impact will be. In terms of eldercare as a whole, its also important to note that it is not only adult children with kids who provide care to the elderly. Indeed, in 1996 adult children with or without children only represented about half of the caregivers in Canada. A 1996 study showed that 55 per cent of caregivers for the elderly were adult children but that 20 per cent were "other" family members and 19 per cent were friends.[14] As the size and nature of family networks change, perhaps a greater proportion of informal caregiving will be taken up by friends and other family members.

[14] Friends made up 19.4 per cent of the caregivers and spouses represented only 4.6 per cent. The authors suspect that spouses were underrepresented as people may have considered caregiving to be part of their regular duties as a spouse as opposed to a separate responsibility (Keeting et al., 1999).

References

Boyd, M. and Norris, D. (1999). *The Crowded Nest: Young Adults at Home.* Canadian Social Trends, Statistics Canada Catalogue no. 11-008, 52, pp. 2–5.

Carrière, Y., Légaré, J., Keefe, J., Rowe, G., Martel, L., Lin, X. and Rajbhandary, S. (2003). *Micro-Simulations and the Effect of Changing Family Structure on the Needs for Formal Home Care Services.* Presented at the Canadian Population Society Annual Meeting, Dalhousie University, Halifax.

Cranswick, K. (1998). *Who Needs Short-Term Help?* Canadian Social Trends, Statistics Canada Catalogue no. 11-008, 50, pp. 11–14.

Cranswick, K. (2003). *Caring for an Aging Society.* Statistics Canada Catalogue no. 89-582-XIE.

Cranswick, K. and Thomas, D. (2005). *Elder Care and the Complexities of Social Networks.* Canadian Social Trends, Statistics Canada Catalogue no. 11-008, 77, pp. 10–15.

Keating, N., Fast, J., Frederick, J., Cranswick, K. and Perrier, C. (1999). *Eldercare in Canada: Context, Content, and Consequences.* Statistics Canada Catalogue no. 89-570-XPE.

Lindsay, C. (1999). Seniors: *A Diverse Group Aging Well.* Canadian Social Trends, Statistics Canada Catalogue no. 11-008, 52, pp. 24–27.

Pennec, S. (1997). Four-Generation Families in France. *Population: An English Selection*, 9, 75–101.

Post, W., Van Poppel, F., Van Imhoff, E. and Kruse, E. (1997). Reconstructing the Extended Kin-Network in the Netherlands with Genealogical Data: Methods, Problems, and Results. *Population Studies*, 51, 263–278.

Rowland, D.T. (1984). Old Age and the Demographic Transition. *Population Studies*, 38, 73–87.

Smith, G. and Dumas, J. (eds). (1994). *The Sandwich Generation: Myths and Reality.* Report on the Demographic Situation in Canada 1994: Current Demographic Analysis, Statistics Canada Catalogue no. 91-209E, pp. 111–148.

Watkins, S.C., Menken, J.A. and Bongaarts, J. (1987). Demographic Foundations of Family Change. *American Sociological Review*, 52, 346–358.

Williams, C. (2004). *The Sandwich Generation.* Perspectives on Labour and Income, Statistics Canada Catalogue no. 75-001-XIE, 16(4), pp. 5–12.

Wise, D.A. (1997). Retirement against the Demographic Trend: More Older People Living Longer, Working Less, and Saving Less. *Demography*, 34(1), 83–95.

Wolfson, M. C., Lin, X., Rowe, G., Carrière, Y. and Martel, L. (2003). *Active Life Expectancy in a Multigenerational Family Context.* Presented at the International Conference on Health Policy Research, Chicago.

Chapter 13

A Simulation Model Concerning Future Needs for Long-term Care of Elderly Persons in Sweden

Mårten Lagergren

Stockholm Gerontology Research Centre, Sweden

Abstract

The increasing number of elderly persons to be expected in the coming decades raises serious questions concerning the resources that will be required for provision of long-term care of the frail elderly. Clearly, there is a need for increased resources. However, simplistic calculations based upon the assumption that future needs of care will be proportional to the number of old persons per age group seem to lead to substantially exaggerated results by failing to take into account the positive health development of the elderly. In fact, a simple model earlier developed by the author showed that the expected increase in the period 2000–2030 was reduced from 60% to around 20%, assuming that prevailing health trends should continue. In an effort to corroborate these results and make possible further analysis of different factors pertaining to the estimation of future needs of publicly financed long-term care of frail elderly persons, a new model has been developed. The model also contains a retrospective part, which shows how the consumption of different forms of care services for the elderly in Sweden developed during the period 1985–2000 with respect to the disability, age, gender and marital status of the recipients. Data for the model are derived from different sources— longitudinal studies, local surveys of recipients of care, etc.

1. Introduction

Sweden was one of the first countries in the world to develop an extensive public system of care for frail elderly persons in the 1960s and 1970s. The system follows the general Nordic model aiming at providing low-cost comprehensive services for the elderly and as far as possible enabling old

International Symposia in Economic Theory and Econometrics, Vol. 16

ISSN: 1571-0386 DOI: 10.1016/S1571-0386(06)16013-5

people to live independently with a high quality of life (Lagergren, 2002a, b). Responsibility for the care of the frail elderly rests with three authorities acting at different levels. At the national level, the Riksdag and the Government realize policy goals through legislation and financial control measures. At the regional level, 21 county councils are responsible for the provision of health and medical care. At the local level, Sweden's 289 municipalities have a statutory duty to meet the social service and housing needs of the elderly. Sweden's municipalities and county councils have a high level of autonomy by international standards. Activities in caring services are ultimately controlled by politicians appointed to policy-making assemblies in municipalities and county councils through general elections. The decentralization of responsibility for elderly care makes it possible for local and regional conditions to be taken into account when policies for the elderly are formulated. The national authorities — the National Board of Health and Welfare and the 21 county administrative boards — are responsible for supervision, follow-up and evaluation of municipal and county council caring services.

The so-called Ädel Reform, which came into force on January 1, 1992, made the municipalities comprehensively responsible for long-term service and care for the elderly and people with disabilities. Among other things, it became the duty of municipalities to provide health care in special forms of housing accommodation and in daytime activities. One of the reform's important components was the transfer of financial responsibility for patients in county council hospitals and geriatric departments, whose medical treatment had been completed, from the county councils to the municipalities. This had the simultaneous effect of greatly reducing the number of elderly "bed-blockers" in county council institutions, and expanding municipal housing capacity for elderly in need of care and social services.

The public services for the elderly include, among others, home help services, home nursing and special housing accommodation (formerly: nursing homes, residential homes and group dwelling). Home help services are provided by the municipality and include, for example, cleaning and doing laundry, help with shopping, post office and bank errands, and preparation of meals. Personal care can include assistance with eating and drinking, getting dressed, personal hygiene and moving about. In 2004, 8.5% of persons aged 65 and older were entitled to home help services in ordinary housing. The corresponding figure for those 85 years and older was 27%. Home nursing is in some places provided by the municipalities and in others by the county councils. It can mean both qualified care and highly specialized medical care several times a day, as well as terminal care. About one-third of the persons that receive home help services also receive home nursing care.

A place or apartment in special housing accommodation is granted as assistance under the Social Services Act. In most municipalities today, in order for older persons to qualify for special housing accommodation they must be in very extensive need of care and attention. In 2004, almost 7% of those aged 65 years and older were living permanently in special forms of housing accommodation. The corresponding figure for those 85 years and older was 27%.

The elderly care is heavily subsidized, with the recipient usually paying only a few percent of the actual cost. Each municipality decides its own charges for elderly care and most municipalities have income and delivery related charges. The care and services for the elderly is to the largest part (above 80%) financed by taxes levied by the municipality from its residents. A smaller part of the elderly care is financed by state grants directed to the municipalities. Municipal expenditure on caring services for the elderly in 2004 was estimated at upwards of SEK 80 billion. The biggest item of expenditure, over SEK 53 billion, concerns caring services in special housing accommodation. Expenditure on caring services in ordinary housing totaled some SEK 25 billion.

Up to the year 2000 Sweden used to have the oldest population in the world. The proportion of 80+ years old increased from 3% to over 5% between 1980 and 2000. The rapid increase in the number of old and very old persons and economic pressure due to a severe national economic crisis in the 1990s resulted in public services for the elderly not being able to keep up with the population development (Thorslund and Parker, 1997; Thorslund and Bergmark, 2000). The previous generous allocation of care had to be replaced by a more restrictive approach.

As many other advanced industrial countries Sweden expects the number of elderly persons to increase substantially in the coming decades. The growth in the period 2000–2015 concerns mainly the younger elderly and thus does not have a large effect on the need for elderly care services. The main thrust comes after the year 2020 and the main part of the increase in the period 2015–2030 comes from the oldest age groups.

The expected increase raises serious questions concerning the resources that will be demanded for provision of long-term care of the frail elderly. Clearly, there is a need for increased resources. However, simplistic calculations based upon the assumption that future needs of care will be proportional to the number of old persons per age group seem to lead to substantially exaggerated results by failing to take into account the health development of the elderly (Fölster, 1998). In fact, a simple model co-developed by the author indicated that the expected increase in the period 2000–2030 was reduced from 60% to around 20%, assuming that prevailing health trends according to national surveys should continue (Lagergren and Batljan, 2000; Batljan and Lagergren, 2005).

In an effort to corroborate these results and make possible further analysis of different factors pertaining to the estimation of future needs of publicly financed long-term care of elderly, dependent persons, a new model — the ASIM III-model has been developed. This model consists of two parts: a retrospective part and a prospective part. The retrospective part shows how the consumption of different forms of care services for the elderly in Sweden developed during the period 1985–2000 with respect to age, gender and marital status and degree of disability. The prospective part makes it possible to calculate forecasts for the same development during the period 2000–2030 under different assumptions.

The need for a retrospective part of the model arises from the fact that available official statistics in Sweden are not sufficient for understanding the development of the long-term care system. From official data it is possible to deduce that in the year 2000 a smaller proportion of the elderly received long-term care services compared to 15 years earlier. It is also possible to observe, that the proportion of persons receiving more intensive services has increased. However, since there is no connected measure of the needs development it is impossible to tell whether the reduction and concentration of the services are a reflection of decreasing needs due to improved health and functional capacity among the elderly, or reflect a real decrease in the level of provision of services.

Also, the official statistics are flawed in many ways. The reporting from the municipalities is unreliable, the concepts that are used to describe the service provision are indistinct, and there is no subdivision of the statistics according to the civil status of the care recipients. In fact, as shown by separate studies (Szebehely, 1998) civil status is a very important predictor of care provision as married persons in Sweden tend to receive much fewer public elderly care services than single living. As a result of these statistical deficiencies there has been a severe lack of solid facts to guide the public debate in Sweden concerning the recent developments of the elderly care system. The crucial question: "Who get's what care?" cannot be answered by the official statistics. By combining different data sources the model can provide a clearer picture of the situation and what actually happened.

Calculations concerning the future development of care services needs among the frail elderly have been made in several countries in the last decade (Wittenberg et al., 1998; Singer and Manton, 1998; Zweifel et al., 1999), by the European Union (Bowen and Jackson, 2000) and also by international organisations such as the OECD (Jacobzone et al., 2000). Those predictions that take health development into account have, generally speaking, arrived at much lower estimates of the future needs than those that have omitted this factor. The calculations have, above all, shown that the assumptions you make concerning the development of ill-health and disability among the elderly are extremely crucial for the obtained results. At the same time this development still seems controversial with very different opinions among different researchers. The advantage of using a model that makes it possible to easily calculate the result under different assumptions is that the effect of this controversy can be explored. It is also easy to introduce new data when these become available.

2. Material and Methods — The ASIM III-Model[1]

The retrospective and prospective parts of the model are built according to the same basic structure. The applied approach is to describe the provision of care for different subgroups in the population and then calculate the impact — in terms of costs — of different assumptions concerning the development of these subgroups. In the retrospective part, which covers the period 1985–2000, this description is based on data derived from different sources — longitudinal studies, local surveys of recipients of care, etc. In the prospective part — covering the period 2000–2030-the calculations are based upon different trends that are estimated from earlier developments and prolonged into the future. An important source of data in the future will be the SNAC-study, which started in 2001 (Swedish National Study on Ageing and Care) (Lagergren, 2002a).

The following data sources are used in the model:

The official national statistics on the provision of long-term care,

The national surveys on living conditions (ULF) and different local studies, namely

The ASIM-studies in Solna municipality 1984–1994,

The SNAC study at Kungsholmen, Stockholm in 2001, and the so-called Field Municipalities Surveys in eight Swedish municipalities in 2002.

The basic structure of the ASIM III-model consists of a subdivision of the Swedish population 65 years and above into subgroups according to age (age groups 65–74, 75–84, 85+), gender, civil status (with or without spouse), and degree of ill-health or disability (six classes, cf. below). For each subgroup is denoted the number of persons that receive public long-term elderly care services according to four different levels:

Level 1: Community care: home help <1 h per day,

Level 2: Community care: home help 1–2 h per day,

Level 3: Community care: home help >2 h per day

Level 4: Institutional care in residential home or nursing home.

The prevalence of ill-health or disability for each subgroup (age, gender, civil status) in the population is estimated using the Swedish National Survey of Living Conditions (ULF). These interview surveys have been performed nation-wide in Sweden every second year since the end of the

[1] This model is the third in a series of elderly care services models developed by the author starting in 1985 (Lagergren, 1994).

1970's with a sample size each time of around 3,000 persons between 65 and 84 years (Statistics Sweden, 1999). Among others, participants are asked questions concerning health conditions: subjective health status, restrictions in functional capacity, mobility restrictions. From the answers to these questions a health index with four degrees is constructed — full health, slight ill-health, moderate ill-health and severe ill-health.

The sample size of the ULF surveys does not permit direct estimation of the distribution of ill-health in a local setting such as a municipality. However, using multi-regressional analysis it is possible to estimate the local distribution of ill-health according to ULF in a certain area using age, gender, civil status and income as predictors.

A limitation of the ULF-studies is that there is an upper age limit of 84 years (with the exception of one ULF-survey, 1988–1989). This means that the ill-health distribution of the 85+ age group has to be estimated. This has been done using logarithmic extrapolation over five-year age groups for each of the years 1985, 1990, 1995 and 2000. However, there are reasons to believe that the prevalence of ill-health in the age group 80–84 years is underestimated in the ULF surveys due to non-response. In order to compensate for this an adjustment based upon reasonable assumptions concerning the selectivity with regard to ill-health in the non-response has been introduced. The results have been checked against data from surveys in other countries, among others the US NLTC-survey (Manton and XiLiang, 2001) with satisfactory agreement with regard to increase of disability with age.

The ASIM-data collected in Solna municipality 1984–1994, the SNAC-data from Kungsholmen, 2001 and the Field Municipalities Survey comprise only recipients of care. In these studies all recipients of elderly care living in the area have been registered. The registration involves, among others, provided care services (in same terms as above) and disability measured according to the so-called ASIM index (Lagergren, 1994). This index summarizes information on functional capacity, mobility, incontinence, anxiety and dementia as denoted by the responsible care staff. Using that index a subdivision can be made of the recipients of care into four classes of disability: Low, medium, high–medium and high.

The relation between the ULF-index of ill-health and the ASIM-index of disability has been estimated using data from the SNAC population study (Lagergren, 2002a) and the ULF-index has been imputed in the survey microdata with the help of this relation. Since the ULF-index is a measure of ill-health in the *full population* and the ASIM-disability class only involves *recipients of care* the distributions between index values differ considerably. Thus the estimation shows that all ULF categories except severe ill-health fall into the ASIM "low disability" category. For this reason the ULF category "severe ill-health" has been subdivided into three groups: relatively severe ill-health (= medium disability according to ASIM), severe ill-health

(= high medium disability) and very severe ill-health (= high disability). In this way six ill-health groups have been defined.

Using the ULF-data for Sweden and population data (including income) for Solna (1985, 1990 and 1995) and the field municipalities (2000), regression analysis has been used to arrive at an estimate of the distribution of the elderly population in these municipalities on (ULF-) ill-health groups (six groups, cf. above) per cell (gender, age group, marital status) for each of the years 1985, 1990, 1995 and 2000.

The Solna ASIM-data for 1985, 1990, 1995 and the Field Municipality Survey data from 2000 provide — after imputation of the ULF-index — the local provision of care services per level of ill-health for each sub-group in terms of number of persons on each level of services (cf. above).

Using these data the proportion of persons in each group of ill-health for each cell receiving each level of services in the respective surveys can be calculated. The resulting proportions are aggregated over marital status and ill-health group and compared with the corresponding data from the national official statistics and calibrated to agreement.[2]

The ULF-data for the respective years provide the national distribution of persons per cell and group of ill-health. The final step in order to achieve the national distribution of persons for each year over gender, age-group, marital status, group of ill-health and level of services consists in multiplying the above proportions per level of services with the population data. The result is a series of matrices — one per gender, age group, marital status — for each year 1985, 1990, 1995 and 2000. In each matrix is denoted the number of persons per level of care services and group of ill-health. An example of a matrix of this kind is given in Table 1.

Using standard costs for the respective level of services, the resulting yearly costs per gender, age-group, marital status and class of disability can easily be calculated. These costs are then aggregated and compared with the actual costs for the corresponding year. This has shown good agreement. (If agreement is less than perfect an obvious correction is to adjust the standard cost).

In order to forecast future costs of the care services you need a population forecast (according to gender, age-group and civil status) and assumptions concerning the development of ill-health and disability. The population prognosis is obtained from Statistics Sweden. Figure 1 shows the official

[2] As described above the national data does not provide the level of detail that is given in the local studies (supported with the ULF-data). The calibration assumes that the relative differences between the local areas and the whole country regarding the proportion of persons receiving services at a certain level are the same irrespective of marital status and disability.

Table 1: Example of Model Matrix — The Number of Married Women, Aged 75–84, in 1985 Per Group of Ill-Health and Level of Care Services

	Full health	Slight ill-health	Moderate ill-health	Rel. severe ill-health	Severe ill-health	Very severe ill-health	All groups
Community living without public help	15,323	21,799	14,986	7,486	2,571	1,785	6,3950
Community living, help 1 h/day	79	2,398	4,568	2,881	360	0	1,0286
Community living, help 1–2 h/day	0	0	520	0	0	89	609
Community living, help 2 h/day	0	0	85	262	87	0	435
Total number of community living persons with help	79	2,398	5,174	3,144	448	89	11,331
Institutionalized	0	131	209	787	787	1,931	3,846
Total number of persons with public help	79	2,529	5,383	3,931	1,234	2,020	15,176
Total number of persons	15,402	24,328	20,369	11,416	3,805	3,805	79,126

Figure 1: Population Forecast Per Age Group, 2000–2030

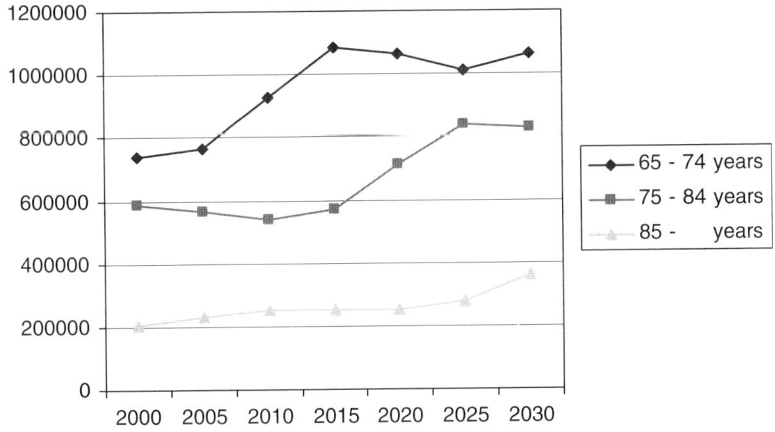

Swedish population forecast per age group and gender for the period 2000–2030. As seen from the figure the number of elderly is expected to increase during the whole period, but in the first two decades the increase is concentrated among the younger elderly. It is not until after the year 2020 that a major increase is expected among the age-group 85+, which is the most relevant when it comes to estimating future needs of aged care services.

There is no official subdivision of the population forecast according to marital status. The development of the proportion of married persons in the period 2000–2030 has been extrapolated (linear regression) per five-year age group and gender from the period 1985–2000. Reduced mortality results in the proportion of married increasing for all age groups except the youngest (65–69). This effect is especially noticeable for the very old. As an example the proportion of married women in the age group 85–89 years increased from 9% to 13% in the period 1985–2000 and is by this calculation method expected to have further increased to 21% by the year 2030. The reason is decreasing mortality among older and very old men.

The default assumption in the model is that the provision of services according to gender, age group, civil status and class of disability is unchanged compared to the year 2000.[3] The development of ill-health (according to ULF) is extrapolated from the development between 1985 and 2000 using logarithmic extrapolation. As will be shown later in this paper these trend extrapolations can be modified in different ways creating different scenarios. The subdivision of the "severe ill-health" group into

[3] This assumption can be adjusted at will.

Figure 2: Development of the Probability of Severe Ill-Health in the Period 2000–2030, Non-Married Men and Women, Aged 75–79 and 85–89 Years, Respectively

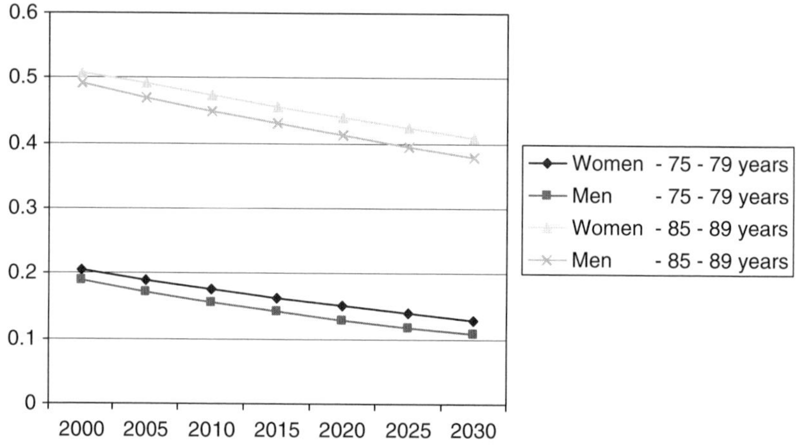

ASIM-disability classes (rather severe ill-health, severe ill-health, very severe; cf. above) is assumed to be unchanged. In Figure 2 shows, by way of example, the calculated development of the probability of severe ill-health for man and women, age group 75–79 and 85–89 years, respectively.

Forecasts are then made for the years 2005, 2010, 2030 simply by multiplying the estimated number of persons in the population per sub-group (gender, age group, marital status, class of disability) each year with the proportion of persons receiving services on the respective levels in the year 2000. Estimates of future costs are then calculated as in the retrospective part of the model using standard costs.

The ASIM III-model is implemented in EXCEL. The above results are aggregated to totals per gender, age group, marital status and class of disability in order to facilitate comparison and analyses of results. Figures showing different aspects of the developments are automatically derived from the calculated data. Different parameters can be used to control priorities with regard to gender, age group, marital status and disability. In this way it is possible to adjust the result to budget constraints and calculate the implications for different sub-groups of the applied priorities.

3. Results

The ASIM III-model can be used for many different types of calculations concerning developments in the period 1985–2000 as well as forecasts for the period 2000–2030. In the sequel a few examples will be given of both kinds of results. One very important issue in the current public debate in Sweden on the development of the public care services for the elderly care concerns the question of which groups of the elderly have suffered reductions in the service level. Figure 3 shows the model estimation of the development in the period 1985–2000 of the proportions of the Swedish elderly population that received care services per degree of ill-health (according to ULF, cf. above).

As shown in Figure 3 the severe service reductions in the years 1985–1995 mainly affected the group with moderate or mild ill-health. Those with severe ill-health were more or less shielded from the reductions. In the period 1995–2000 the service reduction halted and the distribution between the ill-health groups was partly restored. The different developments for younger and older elderly are illustrated by the following Figures 4 and 5.

As can be seen from Figure 4 the model indicates that the sharpest reductions affected the 65–74 group. Figure 5 shows that according to the model the 85+ group was affected in a different way. In 1985 almost all in the 85+ group received services regardless of their level of ill-health. Already in 1990 — before the real crisis set in — this had changed and the model indicates that over the years a much sharper prioritising with regard to ill-health took place. However, the reductions for the most severely dependent, that took place between 1985 and 1995, seem to have been completely restored in the last five-year period.

Another type of application of the model concerns forecasts for the period 2000–2030 under different assumptions. In Figure 6 is shown the projected development of the total costs for the long-term care services for the elderly per age group assuming unchanged health after the year 2000. As shown

Figure 3: Proportion of Elderly Population that Received Care Services Per Degree of Ill-Health, 1985–2000

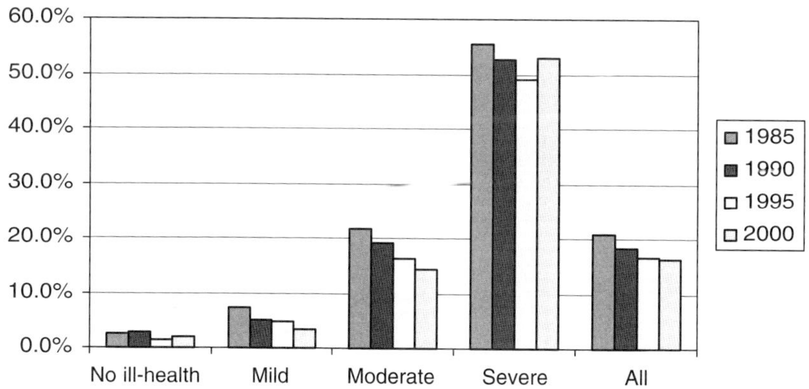

Figure 4: Proportion of Persons in Age-Group 65–74 Received Care Services Per Degree of Ill-Health, 1985–2000

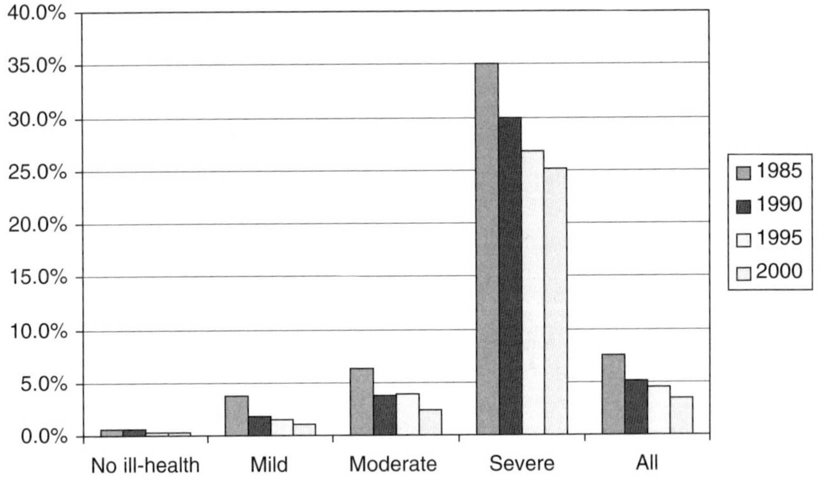

Figure 5: Proportion of Persons in Age-Group 85+ that Received Care Services Per Degree of Ill-Health, 1985–2000

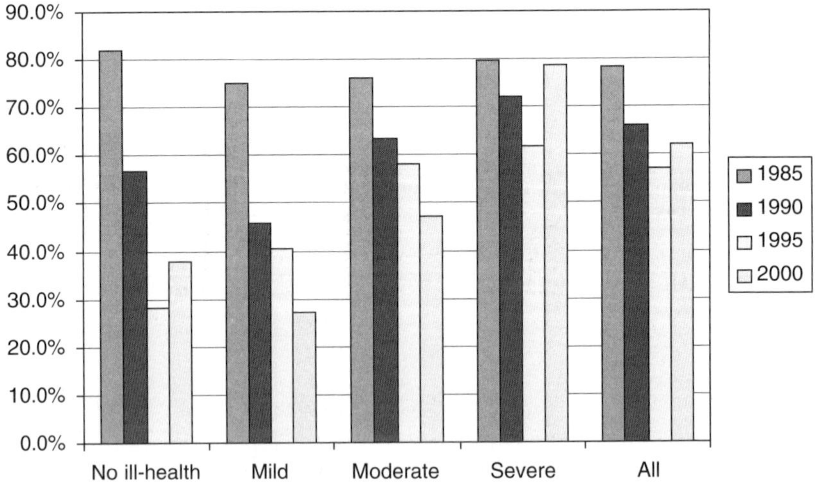

above (Figure 1) the Swedish elderly population is expected to grow considerably in the coming decades. The main thrust comes after the year 2020 and the model shows that the main part of the increase in the period 2015–2030 comes from the oldest age group.

Figure 6: Projected Development of the Total Yearly Costs for the Long-Term Care Services for the Elderly Per Age Group Assuming Unchanged Health After the Year 2000 (millions SEK)

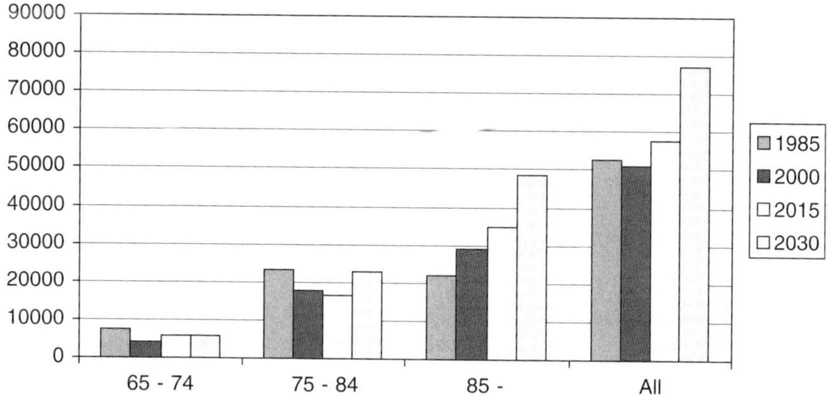

Figure 7: Projected Development of the Total Yearly Costs for the Long-Term Care Services for the Elderly Per Age Group Assuming Unchanged Health Trends After the year 2000 (millions SEK)

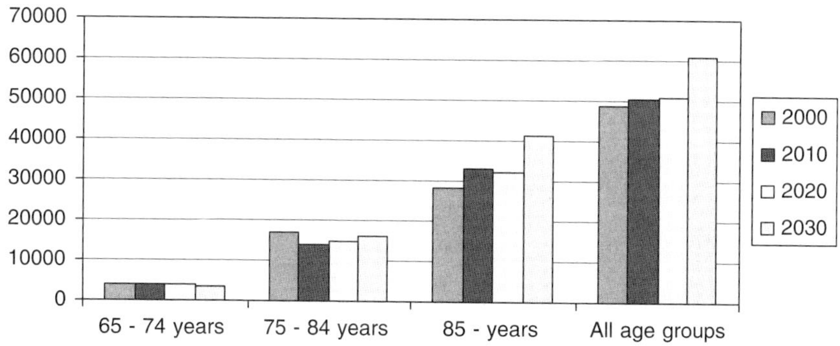

However, assuming unchanged ill-health in the population after the year 2000 is a questionable assumption since according to health surveys the trend since several decades in Sweden as in many other countries is towards improved health among the elderly. Figure 7 shows the development of the same total costs per age group assuming that current health trends persist during the whole period.

As seen from Figure 7 assuming continuing health trends among the elderly results in a much lower expected cost increase. There will still be a substantial cost increase for the 85+ group but this increase is by and large offset by the expected cost decrease in the younger age groups. The total cost increase from 2000 to 2030 in this case amounts to around 25% compared to more than 60% in the former case with unchanged health. Assuming continuing health for another 30 years is probably too optimistic, but the model calculations show clearly the very large impact assumptions concerning the health development among the elderly have on the cost projections.

4. Conclusions

As pointed out above the ASIM III-model serves two purposes: as a tool of analysis for better understanding the development of the elderly care system in the last decades and as an instrument for forecasting future developments of the system under different assumptions. The public system of care for the frail elderly in Sweden has undergone many changes since 1985 (Thorslund and Bergmark, 2000). Partly this has had to do with organizational change — the so-called ADEL-reform mentioned above — and partly with economic pressures due to the severe economic crisis that hit Sweden during the early 1990s. The ADEL-reform moved the responsibility for institutional long-term care from the county councils to the municipalities. As a consequence the housing of the long-term ill elderly improved a lot and more people were able to stay and receive long-term care in their own homes. The economic crisis resulted in a much more strict prioritization. The number of persons receiving public services declined. The model calculations basically confirm the general observations made using official statistics and different local investigations. However, the model makes it possible to look at the development in much more detail and in a much clearer and more systematic way taking health development also in account.

The results of the forecasting part of the model also tally well with earlier, more simple calculations (Lagergren and Batljan, 2000). Again, however, the model facilitates a more detailed look at the development and simplifies the study of the effects of a broad set of different assumptions.

As described above the model uses a combination of different data sets in a novel way. Obviously there are critical issues in the calculation method, which need to be addressed in order to evaluate the reliability of the results. The local data sets from Solna and the Field Municipality Surveys (2000) are judged to be essentially representative of total Sweden. They are calibrated to the national level with respect to gender, age group and level of services, but the distribution of care services according to marital status and class of disability might of course differ in a way that is difficult to foresee. The data sets for the years 1985 and 1990 are pretty comprehensive being based upon three surveys each (1984–1986 and 1989—1991, respectively). The 2000 dataset is of the same order of magnitude — around 5,500 observations. The 1995 dataset, however, is smaller and thus more prone to random variations.

The most critical limitation of the ULF-surveys is that they do not include (except for the year 1988–1989) the age group 85 years and older. As mentioned above the method to extrapolate the distribution of ill-health from the "disability by age" trend in lower age groups — after adjustments for the 80–84 age group has been tested by comparisons with several other surveys and seems to produce acceptable results.

As pointed out above, the ASIM III-model is essentially a tool for analysis. It provides answers under given assumptions to different questions of importance for policy formation in the area of long-term care for the frail elderly. The structure of the model makes it possible to successively improve the basis for the calculations. In this way it is hoped that the model will be able to serve a useful purpose in the coming years of public debate concerning how to meet the growing care needs of the elderly persons in our populations.

The wide range of results produced by alterative assumptions concerning the future ill-health trends shows again how important the health and disability factors are when it comes to estimating future care needs. One obvious conclusion is that there is a need for better data. But perhaps even more important is that this shows very clearly the enormous significance of an effective preventative health policy aimed at the elderly. The care needs of the elderly in the future are to a great extent determined by today's choices of living conditions and lifestyles.

References

Batljan, I. and Lagergren, M. (2005). Future demand for Formal Long-term Care in Sweden. *European Journal of Ageing*, 2(3), 216–224.

Bowen, T. and Jackson, R. (2000). *Scientific and Prospective Evaluation of Final Report for Directorate General V*. European Commission, Brussels.

Fölster, S. (1998); *Kommunerna kan kanske? (Can Swedish Municipalities Do Better?"), In Swedish*. Stockholm, Ministry of Finance, Expert Group on Public Finance (ESO), Ds 1998,15.

Jacobzone, S., Cambois, E. and Robine, J-M. (2000). Is the Health of Older Persons in the OECD Countries Improving Fast Enough to Compensate for Population Ageing? OECD Economic Studies No. 30. OECD, Paris.

Lagergren, M. (1994). *The ASIM system — A Tool for Monitoring, Evaluation and Planning of the Long-Term Care for Elderly and Disabled People*. Doctoral Thesis at Karolinska Institute, Department of International Health and Social Medicine, Kronan Health Centre, Karolinska Institute, Sundyberg.

Lagergren, M. (2002a) SNAC — The Swedish National Study on Ageing and Care. In: Rauner M., Heidenberger K. (eds). Quantitative Approaches in Health Care Management. *Proceedings of the 27th Meeting of the European Working Group on Operational Reasearch (ORAHS)*, Vienna, Peter Lang, Frankfurt am Main.

Lagergren, M. (2002b). The Systems of Care for Frail Elderly Persons: The Case of Sweden. *Ageing Clinical and Experimental Research*, 14, 252–257.
Lagergren, M. and Batljan, I. (2000). *Will There Be a Helping Hand. Annex 8 to The Long-Term Survey 1999/2000*. Stockholm, Fritzes.
Manton, K.G. and XiLiang, G. (2001). Changes in the Prevalence of Chronic Disability in the United States Black and Non-Black Population Above Age 65 From 1982 to 1999. *Proceedings of the National Academy of Sciences*, 11, 6354–6359.
Singer, B.H. and Manton, K.G. (1998). The Effects of Health Changes on Projections of Health Service Needs for the Elderly Population of the United States. *Proceedings of the National Academy of Sciences*, 95, 15618–15622.
Statistics Sweden (SCB) (1999). *The Swedish National Survey of Living Conditions, 1975–1997*. SCB, Stockholm.
Szebehely, M. (1998). Care Supply from the Wife or from the Social Services? In: Everyday life in Social Services for the Elderly, Swedish Council for Working Life and Social Research, Stockholm, pp. 73–88.
Thórslund, M. and Bergmark, Å. (2000). Guest editorial-Solidarity and Welfare Transition. *International Journal of Social Welfare*, 9, 224–227.
Thorslund, M. and Parker, M. (1997). Aging and Social Welfare in Transition. *Scandinavian Journal of Social Welfare*, 6, 150–152.
Wittenberg, R., Pickard, L., Comas-Herrera, A., Davies, B. and Darton, R. (1998). *Demand for Long-Term Care: Projections of Long-Term Care Finance for Elderly People*. University of Kent, PSSRU, Canterbury.
Zweifel, P., Felder, S. and Meiers, M. (1999). Ageing of Population and Health Care Expenditures: A Red Herring? *Journal of Health Economics*, 8, 485–496.

Chapter 14

Providing Income Support Services to a Changing Aged Population in Australia: Centrelink's Regional Microsimulation Model ☆

Anthony King

NATSEM, Australia

Abstract

Centrelink is the organisation with responsibility for delivering income-support services in Australia — and the aged population is an important 'customer segment'. Providing services to this group in an efficient and effective manner requires continuous tailoring of service delivery. For example, service delivery needs to anticipate changing characteristics of the aged population, such as their changing geographic distribution and the changing proportion of 'self-funded retirees'. It also needs to respond to changes in aged people's preferences for the way in which they deal with Centrelink in the context of new and evolving possibilities for interaction.

The chapter will describe how a sophisticated regional microsimulation model, the Customer Service Projection (CuSP) Model (jointly developed by Centrelink and NATSEM), is providing a projections tool to assist Centrelink in responding to these changing demands, preferences, and opportunities in the delivery of services to the aged population.

1. Introduction

The most important element of Australian retirement incomes is the Age Pension, a means-tested income support payment available to males 65 years and

☆ *This is an abridged version of the paper presented to the 'International Conference on Population Ageing and Health: Modelling our Future', Canberra, 7–12 December 2003.*

International Symposia in Economic Theory and Econometrics, Vol. 16

ISSN: 1571-0386 DOI: 10.1016/S1571-0386(06)16014-7

more and females 62 years and more[1]. About 80 per cent of the population over these qualifying ages receives the Age Pension (Treasury 2002b, p 8).

Centrelink is the agency with responsibility for delivering the Australian government's income-support services, and Age Pensioners account for over a quarter of the customers receiving these services. Age Pension customers do not, however, generate a commensurate share of the Centrelink service delivery effort. Age Pensioners are typically in receipt of the payment for a long period, experience relatively little change in their circumstances, and are not subject to any form of labour market activity or disability testing as is done for other customer groups. Accordingly, the level of their interaction with Centrelink is low compared to that of other income-support customers, such as those receiving income support while looking for work. Still, because of their large numbers, providing income-support services to Age Pensioners amounts to a major part of Centrelink's role.

With Age Pensioners making up a significant part of Centrelink's customers, the ageing of the Australian population will clearly have important implications for future demands on Centrelink operations.

However, it is more than just an issue of the rapid projected growth in Australia's aged population. There are other factors that may have a bearing on the implications for Centrelink — factors that may affect the number of Age Pensioners and/or the manner and intensity of their dealings with Centrelink. Besides this need to take account of the interaction of a range of factors, if it is to continue to provide services to a changing Age Pensioner population in an efficient and effective manner, Centrelink also needs information at the small-area level. The implications may vary markedly from one part of the country to another, with consequent important implications for the deployment and organisation of Centrelink resources.

Addressing this issue therefore requires a capacity to generate small-area projections of the numbers and characteristics of Centrelink customers. To meet this type of information need, and with aims of more efficient/effective service delivery and higher customer satisfaction, Centrelink embarked in 2000 on a Regional Microsimulation Modelling Project. Centrelink is undertaking this project in partnership with the National Centre for Social and Economic Modelling (NATSEM) at the University of Canberra. The core microsimulation model for the project, the Customer Service Projection (CuSP) model, has been developed by NATSEM.

This chapter describes the nature of the CuSP model and demonstrates the potential use of a regional microsimulation model in a service-delivery

[1] Over the period from 1995 to 2014, the qualifying age for women to receive Age Pension is being gradually increased from 60 to 65 years. At the time of writing, the qualifying age was 62 years.

application with two scenarios about the Age Pensioner population that have been developed for illustrative purposes. The scenarios cover selected aspects of the changing Age Pensioner population over the period to 2012. One scenario incorporates a number of factors that will have a bearing on the number of Age Pensioners in future years. A second scenario adds an element of possible change in the average intensity of interactions between Centrelink and Age Pension customers.

It should be stressed that these are illustrative scenarios that have been developed for the purposes of this chapter. The scenarios only cover selected aspects of Age Pension futures for Centrelink, are implemented in the CuSP model at a broad level, and abstract from much of the detail and complexity that enter into actual use of the model in Centrelink research.

An overview of the CuSP model is provided in Section 2. Section 3 provides an account of the development of the illustrative scenarios of selected aspects of the changing Age Pension population and the way they have been incorporated in the model. An indication of the nature of the model output is then provided in Section 4 with summary results for the two illustrative scenarios. Concluding comments are made in Section 5.

The modelling for the analysis reported here draws on detailed data from Centrelink and the Australian Bureau of Statistics (ABS). It should be noted that these data have been used by NATSEM in either a confidentialised or aggregated form that does not allow the identification of individuals.

2. The CuSP Model

2.1 The Task for the CuSP Model

The aim of the CuSP model is to provide a tool that can generate small-area projections of

- Centrelink customer numbers and characteristics; and
- Associated channel use ('channels' are the methods of contact available between Centrelink and its customers).

The time horizon for the projections is generally five years into the future,[2] and the projections need to be made under scenarios that can capture alternative views about the future environment. The model needs to be able to accommodate changes in the demographic and economic environment,

[2] For the illustrative application described in this chapter, projections have been generated 10 years out.

Figure 1: CuSP Model — Overall Structure

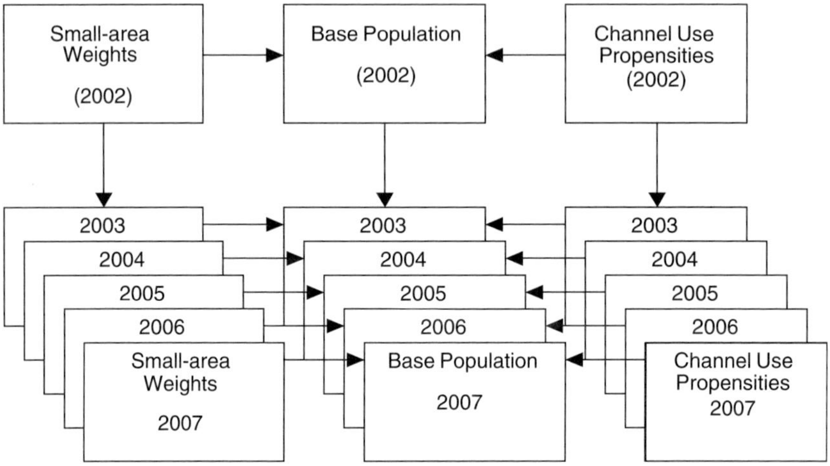

changes in government policy, changes in service delivery directions, and changes in customer behaviour.

2.2 Structure of the CuSP Model

Essentially, the model involves the generation and linking of three datasets based on common characteristics between cohort groups (Figure 1).

1. A base population file (which includes a pool of detailed records for individuals).[3]
2. Small area weights (which specify the prevalence of each individual in the pool in each small area).
3. Channel use propensities (which specify expected channel use given a person's characteristics).

Application of the weights to the base population file gives the estimate of the numbers and characteristics of Centrelink customers in each small area. Application of the channel use propensities to the customer estimates then gives the estimate of channel use. These three datasets are produced for the base year (2002 at the time of writing) and then each is updated for the projection years.

[3] These records are based on ABS survey data of real, but unidentifiable, Australians.

The model draws together the following data from Centrelink, the ABS, and other sources.

- Amalgamated Centrelink customer data;
- Amalgamated Centrelink channel use data;
- Small-area data from the Census of Population and Housing;
- Detailed data on population characteristics from the ABS Household Expenditure Survey; and
- Various data for the construction of projection scenarios.

and also incorporates elements of two established NATSEM models:

- STINMOD — a 'microsimulation' model which allows the detailed identification of entitlements to income support; and
- MarketInfo — a 'regional microsimulation' technique that is used to generate a detailed picture of the characteristics of the population in small areas. MarketInfo is a joint commercial product of NATSEM and MDS Market Data Systems.

2.3 Elements of the CuSP Model

The main features of the elements of the CuSP model shown in Figure 1 are described here, with more detail available in King et al. (2002).

The Base Population

The base population for CuSP-02b[4] is a detailed representation of the Australian population at June 2002. It is based on the confidentialised unit record data[5] from the ABS' 1998–1999 Household Expenditure Survey (HES), with a sample of almost 14,000 people aged 15 years and more. The HES data is updated and enhanced using STINMOD to provide a population sample that is representative of the Australian population at June 2002, and that has more detail on income support entitlements than is available in the original HES.

Small-Area Weights

Each person in the HES sample has a weight that reflects his/her prevalence in the Australian population. In this step, corresponding sets of weights are

[4] CuSP-02b is the second version of the CuSP model produced with a 2002 base year.

[5] Unit record data are the detailed confidentialised data available on separate records for each individual in the sample survey.

generated which reflect the cases' prevalence in the population of small areas. This is done by applying the MarketInfo techniques to updated small-area data from the census.

The core of MarketInfo is custom-written multi-vector reweighting software. The MarketInfo techniques have an established reputation in commercial applications — such as market identification — and have also increasingly been used in socio-economic analyses (Lloyd et al., 2000; Lloyd et al., 2001). MarketInfo 2001 updates the small area data from the Australian census and links it with the unit record data from the ABS 1998–1999 HES to produce a set of weights for the HES for each small area.

The areas used in the CuSP model are 'postal areas', which are an ABS approximation of Australia Post postcodes. This geographic unit is used because it relates to the address information in Centrelink administrative data, though there are some difficulties in the correspondence between postcodes and postal areas. The current version of the model, CuSP-02b, operates with almost 2,400 postal areas, with an average population of about 8,400 people in each postal area.

The link in MarketInfo between the small-area census data — the tabular socio-demographic profiles available from the census — and HES data is provided by a selection from the limited set of household and personal characteristics that are common to both datasets. From 16 common characteristics such as age, sex, marital status, labour force status, income, and housing tenure, 68 reweighting target variables are used.

The final step in the creation of the 2002 small-area weights is their benchmarking to June 2002. This adjusts the small-area weights in line with three types of June 2002 small-area data: detailed customer data from Centrelink, and small-area demographic and labour force data from the ABS. The GREGWT multi-vector reweighting package, developed by the ABS, is used for this step.

Channel Use Propensities

The third element of the CuSP model is a file of channel use 'propensities'. Channel use propensities measure the average likelihood of a Centrelink customer with given characteristics using a particular access channel over a 12-month period. Channel use propensities are specified for each channel and by customer characteristics. Accordingly, these propensities provide the important link between the number and characteristics of customers and the associated channel use that is generated. More information on the channel use propensities and their calculation is provided in Section 2.6.

2.4 How Projections are Made?

Given the three component parts of the CuSP Model for June 2002 — base population, small-area weights, and channel use propensities — projections are then made by adjusting each of these datasets to reflect particular aspects of the future environment. For example:

- Changes in the size of the population and its demographic and labour market structure at the postal-area level can be incorporated by changing the small-area weights. This changes the assumed number of people of a given type in the area.
- Changes in the income-support system, or the impacts of earnings and CPI growth on means testing, can be simulated in the base population by using the 'outyears' facility of STINMOD.
- Changes in channel use propensities — which may stem from changes in the options made available by Centrelink, changes in Centrelink requirements, or possible behavioural changes on the part of customers — are handled by altering the channel use propensities dataset.

A particular projection scenario can thus range from a simple scenario involving change in just one aspect of the future environment through to a more complex scenario that combines changes in many aspects of the future environment. Scenarios can also be specified at different levels of geographic detail. For example, different labour market prospects can be specified for particular parts of the country.

Once a projection scenario has been designed, the required amendments are made to the CuSP model elements (base population, weights, and propensities), and running the model then generates:

- the projected number and characteristics of customers;
- the amount of associated channel use;
- for each of the 2,378 postal areas; and
- for the base year and each of the projection years.

2.5 Customer Types

An important aspect of the CuSP model is the extent to which different groups of customers are identified. The importance of this flows particularly from the marked variations in channel use between different customer groups (see Section 2.6).

In CuSP-02b, customers are grouped according to

- age (13 groups: 15–19, 20–24, … , 70–74, 75 years and more);
- sex;
- customer type (13 groups); and
- region (2,378 postal areas).

For the illustrative application of the CuSP model reported in this chapter, the customer population was confined to Age Pensioners. Age Pensioners amount to 27.3 per cent of the customers in the CuSP-02b base population.

2.6 Channel Use Propensities

What are Channel Use Propensities?

Channel use 'propensities' provide the link in the CuSP model between the projected number and type of Centrelink customers, and the channel use that they generate. The term 'propensity' has a specific meaning in CuSP, as it relates total channel use over a 12-month period to the number of customers at a single point in time during that period. Thus, given a certain number of customers of a particular type at a point in time (say June 2004), the channel use propensities specify the amount of channel use that would be expected to be generated by that type of customer over the corresponding 12-month period (say, January–December 2004).

Examples of the channels covered by the CuSP model include mail from Centrelink to customers, telephone calls from customers to Centrelink Call Centres, 'internal appointments' (appointments held in Centrelink offices), 'call-back appointments' (arranged telephone calls from Centrelink to customers), certain e-mail from customers, and 'drop-ins' (cases where a customer visits a Centrelink office without an appointment). Not all forms of channel use are modelled in CuSP currently. For example, Centrelink currently receives a large volume of incoming mail and fax correspondence from customers, and reporting of casual earnings and payment enquiries are now available to some customers over the Internet. The extension of the model to capture these and other contact channels is being examined for future versions of CuSP.

How the Propensities are Calculated

The channel use dataset covers all instances of use of each channel over a 12-month period, with key customer characteristics recorded alongside each instance of channel use. The channel use propensities in the CuSP model are periodically updated as new data become available, with the propensities in CuSP-02b based on channel use over the period from January to December 2002.

The channel use propensities are specified separately by customer type, age, and sex. These groups are further broken down by location, with distinction between areas classified by their degree of accessibility/remoteness using the ARIA+ index,[6] and by regions within metropolitan areas. Different levels of geographic disaggregation do, however, apply to the different channels depending on judgement about the level of disaggregation that is justified with the particular data.

The reason why the channel use propensities in the CuSP model are specified with a high degree of disaggregation is the considerable variation in channel use between different groups of customers. For a start, they are affected by the different reporting requirements attached to each payment, such as the general requirement that Newstart Allowance customers submit fortnightly applications for continuation of payment. Channel use propensities are also influenced by customers' channel use preferences and constraints. For example, those with easy access to a Centrelink office are more likely to choose to visit the office than are those with more difficult access.

2.7 Use of the CuSP Model

The CuSP model has been used by Centrelink to explore the service delivery implications that arise from a range of factors that affect the customer population and its interactions with Centrelink. This is done at both the national and small-area levels. In the latter case of area analyses, the consideration of CuSP output alongside other forms of small-area information and intelligence has proved a useful form of validation for the model.

3. Illustrative Age Pension Scenarios

This section provides an account of the development of the illustrative scenarios of selected aspects of the changing Age Pension population, and the way they have been incorporated in the model.

---

[6] The ARIA+ index is the accessibility/remoteness index for areas developed by the National Centre for Social Applications of Geographic Information Systems (GISCA), at the University of Adelaide, on behalf of the (then) Department of Health and Aged Care.

3.1 Selected Aspects

As was noted in Section 1, there are a range of factors that can be expected to have a bearing on the number of Age Pensioners and the intensity of their contact with Centrelink (channel use) over the period to 2012. These factors can be grouped under two broad headings.

1. Factors that affect the number of Age Pensioners.
2. Factors that affect the extent to which Age Pensioners use particular Centrelink access channels.

Under the first heading, the most obvious factor is population growth and ageing — the simple increase in the number of people in the older population as a result of past fertility, overseas immigration, and continuing increases in life expectancy. As the Australian population continues to age, with fastest growth among the older age cohorts, Age Pension customers can be expected to make up a growing share of Centrelink customers. This will be tempered somewhat by the current phasing-in of an increased Age Pension qualifying age for women which will attain parity with the male qualifying age of 65 years in 2014. Any continuation of recent trends in labour market participation rates for older Australians would also see a moderating effect on the future number of Age Pensioners. Still, the picture is likely to be dominated by the underlying demographic developments, with a strong increase in the number of Age Pensioners in the coming years.

There is, however, another important factor at play. Age Pension is just one element, albeit the major element, of the Australian retirement income system. Other elements include occupational superannuation and various forms of private saving. Superannuation coverage of the workforce expanded in the post-World War 2 period, though it was not until the early 1990s that coverage became practically universal through the introduction of the Superannuation Guarantee. While the effects of the Superannuation Guarantee on retirement incomes will not be fully felt until the system matures from the 2030s, the effects of increasing superannuation coverage over the earlier period are already apparent. They are manifest in higher private incomes and asset holdings among older Australians.

With the Age Pension subject to means testing through incomes and assets, this growth in the level of private incomes and assets of older Australians has two implications for the population of Age Pensioners. First, an increasing proportion of older Australians will have a level of private incomes and/or assets that preclude an entitlement to Age Pension — though this effect is likely to be relatively modest because of the degree of generosity in means testing. More importantly, the growth in private incomes and assets can be expected to lead to the need for increasing effort in application of the means tests. Moreover, as the complexity and variety of retirement income products has increased, so has the corresponding complexity of applying the means tests. This aspect of a growing intensity of required dealings between Centrelink and Age Pension customers and, in particular, of increasing intricacy in application of the means tests, is referred to as increasing 'complexity'. It has the potential to markedly affect the extent to which Age Pensioners use the Centrelink access channels.

Another factor with a possible impact on the use of access channels is any shift in the duration of payment structure of the Age Pensioner population. Other Centrelink research has revealed, for example, that channel use is more intense at the start of payment receipt than for those who have been in receipt of a payment for some time. With any change in the rate of growth of the Age Pensioner population, the proportion of new customers will change with resulting impacts on average channel use.

Channel use levels and patterns could also change with any change in aged people's preferences for the way in which they deal with Centrelink, particularly in the context of new and evolving possibilities for interaction. Centrelink is continually researching how best to service customers in the future — for example, looking at which channels are best for which processes, and the scope for self-service, new technologies, and streamlined processes.

Finally, there is always the possibility of policy change, which could change the requirements made on Age Pensioners and alter channel use accordingly.

In summary, the following factors could all play an important role in determining the level and patterns of Centrelink channel use by Age Pensioners over the period to 2012.

1. Demographic increase
2. Increasing Age Pension qualifying age for women
3. Increase in labour force participation
4. Increased complexity
5. Changing duration structure
6. Changing customer preferences
7. Changes to Centrelink service delivery
8. Policy change

Only the first four of these aspects are, however, incorporated in the illustrative scenarios developed for this chapter. This selection is based on ease of modelling for an illustrative application and, for the same reason, the fourth aspect — increasing complexity — is modelled in a highly simplified manner.

The four aspects covered have been used to construct two future Age Pension scenarios.

1. Base scenario
2. Increased complexity scenario

The base scenario incorporates the effects of demographic change (size of the population by age, sex, and geographic distribution), the increasing Age Pension qualifying age for women, and an assumption about increased labour force participation. The increased complexity scenario adds to the base an assumed change in the complexity structure of the Age Pension population.

The assumptions about the four elements of these scenarios, and the manner in which they are incorporated in the modelling, are set out in the remainder of this section.

3.2 Population Size and Age Structure

With eligibility for Age Pension principally tied to reaching a given age — currently 62 years for females and 65 years for males, the fundamental driver of the future Age Pension population is clearly the future size of the older age cohorts in the population.

The basic feature of the ageing Australian population is the shifting age structure, with a growing share of the population in the older age groups. Over the coming 10 years, while the total Australian population is projected to increase by around 10 per cent, the older age groups are projected to increase at notably higher rates — at around 35 per cent for the population aged 60 years and more. Within this aged population, there are quite different growth prospects for particular age groups. The size of the 60–64 year old and 65–69 year old age groups is projected to increase by around 50 per cent, as the 'baby boomer' generation moves into these age groups. The number of 70–74 year olds are in fact projected to decline over the initial part of the projection period, before increasing to levels around 20 per cent higher than 2002, while the numbers of Age Pension customers aged 75 or more increase steadily over the projection period.

The implications for the population of Age Pension customers are rapid growth, together with some shift in the age structure toward younger Age Pensioners.

3.3 The Qualifying Age for Age Pension

The first step beyond simple age–sex projection of the future number of Age Pensioners concerns a change in women's qualifying age for Age Pension.

Figure 2: Number of Age Pensioners: Actual (1989–2002), Projected (2003–2012)

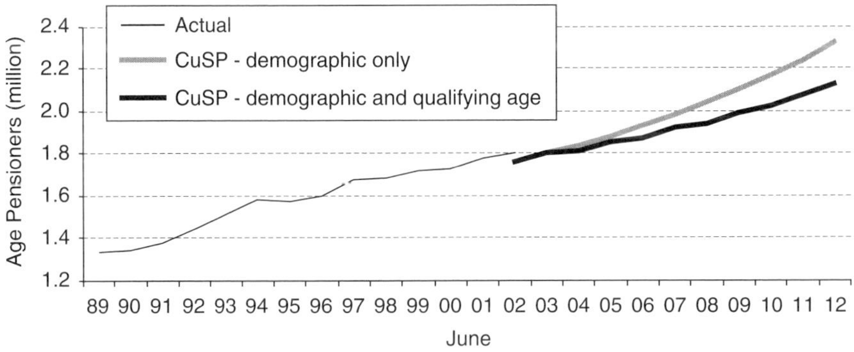

Source: Department of Family and Community Services (2001, Table 2.3) and Centrelink for historic data; CuSP-02b for projections
Note: The apparent discontinuity between the actual and projected series is due to the exclusion from the CuSP model of overseas recipients of Age Pension.

The phasing-in of an increase in women's qualifying age from 60 to 65 years means that, over the period from 2002 to 2012, the proportion of 60–64 year old females who will qualify for Age Pension will fall dramatically — from around 60 per cent in 2002 to just around 10 per cent by 2012. With the rapid growth in the size of this age cohort, the raising of women's Age Pension qualifying age has a dramatic impact on the projected numbers of Age Pensioners (Figure 2).

Taking account of women's increasing Age Pension qualifying age reduces the projected numbers of Age Pensioners in 2012 by about 8 per cent — though it still leaves projected Age Pension numbers rising at a rapid rate, with a 21 per cent increase from around 1.8 million in 2002 to around 2.1 million by 2012.

The changing qualifying age for women will also have an impact on the age structure of the Age Pension population. The effect of this, together with the effect of the different growth rates projected for particular age cohorts, will see in particular a rapidly diminishing share of 60–64-year olds, and a growing share of 65–69-year olds.

3.4 Labour Force Participation

Any change in labour force participation rates (LFPRs) among the older age groups is likely to have an effect on the numbers of Age Pensioners. Two sources of data on projected LFPRs provided the basis for the participation rate scenarios used in this exercise. These were projections prepared by the ABS in 1999 (Australian Bureau of Statistics, 1999) and projections

Table 1: Summary of Labour Force Participation Rate Assumptions

Sex/age group	CuSP under constant labour market structure (with adjustment for Age Pension eligibility age) (%)		Increased labour force participation rate assumption	
	June 2002	June 2012	June 2012 change from CuSP (% points)	June 2012 (%)
Females				
60–64 years	23.3	30.5	+3.4	33.9
65–69 years	10.1	10.1	+1.8	11.9
70–74 years	3.4	3.4	0	3.4
75+ years	1.6	1.7	0	1.7
Males				
65–69 years	22.2	22.3	+1.8	24.1
70–74 years	11.3	11.2	0	11.2
75+ years	4.1	4.0	0	4.0

Note: Rounded to one decimal point.

prepared by Treasury for the 2002 Intergenerational Report (IGR) (Treasury, 2002a). Both sets of projections were based on long-term trend analysis and, as such, did not capture the impact of the increasing Age Pension eligibility age for women. Accordingly, further modification to the projections was made to allow this.

The two LFPR scenarios are specified in Table 1. Under the first scenario of 'constant labour market structure', the proportions of employed, unemployed, and those not in the labour force are held constant for groups defined by age, sex, customer type, and location. The second scenario of 'increased LFPRs' is implemented in a linear manner across the 10-year period from 2002 to 2012, and by increasing full-time employment, part-time employment, and unemployment by the same factor (i.e., the relative shares of these three labour force states are unchanged).

The overall effect of incorporating this LFPR scenario in the projection of the number of Age Pensioners is slight, with the growth rate to 2012 falling from 21 to 20 per cent. The impact is, of course, more marked on those particular age groups assumed to experience an increase in LFPRs.

3.5 Complexity

The fourth element being introduced into the Age Pension projections under these illustrative scenarios is the issue of 'complexity'. This is a reference to the intensity of required dealings between Centrelink and Age Pension customers and, in particular, a reference to the intricacy of applying the means tests. Receipt of the Age Pension is subject to both an income test and an assets test and, as the importance of private retirement income components and the complexity and variety of retirement income products has increased, so has the corresponding complexity of applying the means tests. Examples of this are the increased incidence of customers with accumulation of assets in, or receipt of income from, complex sources such as trusts, companies, small business, and real estate. The required channel use for an Age Pension claimant without any private income or assessable assets will accordingly be considerably less than that for a claimant who has a portfolio of different assets and various private income streams.

For this illustrative application, a simple indicator of complexity is used. The indicator includes the following three classes (in order of assumed increasing complexity):

1. Full-rate customers: Customers who have no private income or assets, or whose private incomes and assets are not enough to reduce their entitlement to full-rate Age Pension.
2. Part-rate income-tested customers: Customers whose Age Pension entitlement is reduced through application of the income test.
3. Part-rate assets-tested customers: Customers whose Age Pension entitlement is reduced through application of the assets test.

Channel use propensities in 2002 for Age Pensioners showed clear differences in propensities between these three complexity classes. Channel use by part-rate customers was markedly higher than for full-rate customers. Among part-rate customers, there were further differences between income-tested and asset-tested customers, though the relativities varied across channels. A change in the complexity structure of the Age Pensioner population can, accordingly, be expected to result in a noticeable change in projected channel use.

Developing the Increased Complexity Scenario

An illustrative increased complexity scenario is specified here in terms of

1. the proportion of Age Pensioners who are receiving a part-rate pension; and
2. among part-rate pensioners, the proportion whose entitlement is reduced due to application of the assets test.

There are a range of issues that might be brought to bear in projecting the future proportion of part-rate Age Pensioners, and the proportion whose rate

Table 2: Illustrative Scenario of Increasing Complexity among Age Pensioners

Complexity indicator class	Males (%)		Females (%)	
	2002	2012	2002	2012
Full-rate	64.7	55.4	68.5	66.0
Part-rate (income-tested)	26.4	25.1	24.6	21.2
Part-rate (asset-tested)	8.9	19.5	6.9	12.8
Total	100.0	100.0	100.0	100.0

Source: Department of Family and Community Services, 2003; Treasury, 2002b

is reduced by the assets test. It should properly be a major exercise, though the approach adopted here — simple linear extrapolation — is not intended to be more than an illustrative first cut at addressing the issue. The available basis for the projections scenario includes historical data since 1989 for these two proportions, and some broad long-term projections of the shift in the proportion of part-rate Age Pensioners (Department of Family and Community Services, 2003, Commonwealth Treasury, 2002b). The increasing complexity scenario, derived by linear extrapolation, is summarised in Table 2.

It is also likely that the expected increase in older people's private incomes and assets that underlies this scenario of increased complexity would also have some impact on the number of Age Pensioners. In some cases, the level of income or assets would be such as to remove all entitlement to Age Pension, rather than to cause a shift from a full-rate to a part-rate pension. This effect is not modelled here, and the STINMOD projections of entitlements do not take into account asset accumulation issues. However, this is arguably not a grave omission because at least a part-rate pension can still be received with significant levels of private income or assets.

4. Projected Channel Use under Illustrative Scenarios

To provide a taste of the nature of the output and capabilities of the CuSP model, this section provides some summary output from the modelling of the two illustrative Age Pension scenarios developed in the previous section. As was noted in that section, these scenarios only incorporate selected aspects of Age Pension futures, and treat complexity in a simplified manner.

The two illustrative scenarios are

1. Base scenario
2. Increased complexity scenario

The base scenario incorporates the effects of demographic change (size of the population by age, sex, and geographic distribution), the increasing Age

Table 3: Summary of Illustrative Scenario Content

	Base scenario	Increased complexity scenario
Demographic change	✓	✓
Increased AP qualifying age for women	✓	✓
Increased labour force participation	✓	✓
Increased complexity	X	✓

Pension qualifying age for women, and the assumption about increased labour force participation. The increased complexity scenario adds to the base the assumed change in the complexity structure of the Age Pension population, as was set out in Section 3.5. This involves an increasing proportion of part-rate Age Pension customers and, among those who are part-rate, an increasing share who are assets tested. The content of the two scenarios is summarised in Table 3.

The results of the CuSP model simulations under these two scenarios are presented here in two parts — looking first at the aggregate Australia-wide results and, second, at some distributional outcomes across the country.

It is important to note that the projections presented in this section are based on current channel use patterns by Age Pension customers in CuSP and have been designed to be for illustrative purposes. Centrelink is constantly changing the way services are being delivered to customers to ensure more efficient and effective service delivery.

4.1 Aggregate Australia-Wide Outcomes

The overall channel use outcomes under the two scenarios are presented in Table 4, with the results shown limited to those five channels covered, of which Age Pensioners make significant use. The number of Age Pensioners (under both scenarios) is projected to increase by 20 per cent over the period from 2002 to 2012 (see Section 3.4). Under the base scenario, channel use is projected to grow at slightly lower rates of between 16 and 19 per cent. This is a likely reflection of changes in the age and sex distribution of the Age Pension population. There is not much difference in the projected growth rates for the five channels shown under the base scenario.

The picture of channel use growth, however, is quite different under the increased complexity scenario. In this case, there is considerable variation in the projected growth rates for the different channels — ranging from a low of 21 per cent for drop-ins and incoming calls to a high of 37 per cent for internal appointments. The varying prospects for the different channels are a result of the different degrees of difference in channel use propensities for,

Table 4: Projected Growth in Channel Use by Age Pensioners under Illustrative Scenarios, 2002–2012

Channel	Growth in channel use from 2002 (%)	
	Base scenario	Increased complexity scenario
Outgoing mail	19	25
Incoming calls	16	21
Internal appointments	17	37
Drop ins	18	21
Callback appointments	16	32

Source: CuSP-02b model

Figure 3: Illustrative Contributions to Projected Growth in Channel Use by Age Pensioners: 2002–2012

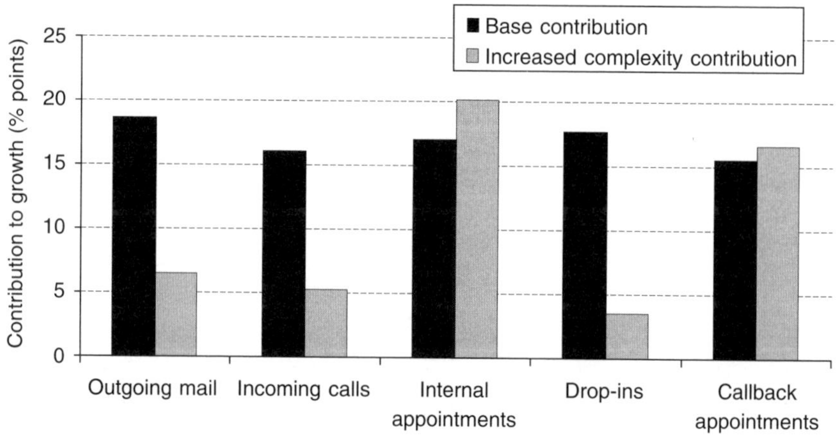

Source: CuSP-02b model

particularly, full-rate and part-rate customers. The propensity to have internal appointments, for example, is considerably higher for part-rate than full-rate Age Pension customers.

Projected channel use growth under the base scenario can broadly be seen as growth that flows from an increasing Age Pension customer population. Growth under the increased complexity scenario also includes growth that would flow from possible increasing complexity in Age Pension customers' dealings with Centrelink. Comparison of the outcomes under the two scenarios allows the relative contributions of these two sources of channel use growth to be examined (Figure 3).

Figure 3 compares the relative contributions of customer numbers and increased complexity in projected growth in channel use to 2012. For outgoing mail, incoming calls, and drop ins, the major source of growth is customer numbers, though increased complexity still adds a significant component. For internal appointments and callback appointments, on the other hand, increasing complexity is as important a source of channel use growth as is the increase in customer numbers. Indeed, with internal appointments, increased complexity emerges as the major source of growth. Possible increases in complexity can clearly have an important impact on projected channel use.

4.2 Regional Outcomes

The Australia-wide results presented above are in fact the aggregated model outcomes for 2,378 postal areas across the country. A distinctive feature of the CuSP model is its small-area disaggregation in reflection of Centrelink's need for information on outcomes for small areas. So, how much geographic variation is there in these implications for Centrelink of the changing Age Pensioner population? It is impossible to present the detailed model output in this chapter and, instead, some indicators of the extent of geographic variation are provided.

Table 5 provides summary measures of the distribution of selected growth rates to 2012 across the 2,378 postal areas. Looking first at the projected rate of growth in Age Pensioner numbers, Table 5 shows a broad dispersion. The median figure is 15 per cent, though 25 per cent of postal areas are projected

Table 5: Distribution of Projected Growth Rates across Postal Areas of Selected Age Pension Characteristics: Growth Rate from 2002 to 2012 under Illustrative Scenarios

	Growth in number of Age Pensioners (%)	Growth in number of internal appointments made by Age Pensioners (%)		Difference in internal appointment growth rate due to increased complexity (% points)
		Base scenario	Increased complexity scenario	
Mean	22	19	39	20
Bottom 10% cut-off	−4	−9	7	12
Bottom 25% cut-off	4	6	18	16
Median	15	11	31	20
Top 25% cut-off	32	27	48	23
Top 10% cut-off	50	47	71	27

Source: CuSP-02b application

Figure 4: Distribution of Postal Area Growth Rates in the Number of Internal Appointments Made by Age Pensioners, 2002–2012 under Illustrative Scenarios

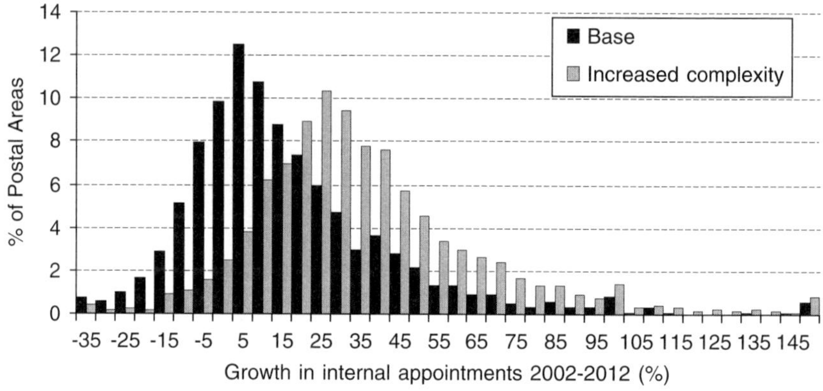

Source: CuSP-02b application

to experience a 4 per cent or less rate of growth, and 25 per cent are projected to experience growth rates of 32 per cent or more.

Similar spreads in growth rates are evident in the projected numbers of internal appointments by Age Pensioners (Table 5 and Figure 4), though the distribution under the increased complexity scenario is, as expected, shifted to the right of the base scenario, and also appears slightly more dispersed. Under the increased complexity scenario, the median projected growth rate among postal areas for internal appointments is 31 per cent. But 25 per cent of postal areas are projected to experience growth of 48 per cent or more, and 10 per cent to experience growth of 71 per cent or more.

The model output was also analysed to examine the degree to which projected growth in Age Pensioner numbers may be a good indicator of projected growth in channel use. For most postal areas (about 85 per cent), their positions on these two distributions of growth rates were close (in the same decile or an adjoining decile). However, for a significant minority of postal areas (around 15 per cent), their projected customer growth rate would not be a good indicator of projected growth in channel use.

5. Overview

The growing and changing Australian aged population has important implications for Centrelink. The simple increase in the size of the aged population will lead to a rapid increase in the number of Age Pensioners, though the changing structure of the Age Pensioner population and a number of other factors could also play important roles.

Analysis of selected aspects of the implications for Centrelink of the changing Age Pension population have been used here to illustrate the capabilities of a regional microsimulation model in a service delivery application. The capabilities include the ability to explore the interactions between a range of factors, and to do so at a small-area level. While the analysis reported here was restricted to selected aspects and subject to a number of simplifications, the CuSP model has been designed to incorporate considerable detail and flexibility. Actual applications have, for example, included variations in channel use propensities according to policy developments under consideration, and geographical variations in assumed labour market prospects.

An important feature of this type of model is the capacity to conduct sensitivity analysis under alternative scenarios in order to assess the sensitivity of outcomes to particular aspects or the relative magnitudes of various sources of change. In this regard, some useful observations can be made by comparing the outcomes under the illustrative scenarios developed here, despite their being partial scenarios and the modelling partly simplified. Under the illustrative scenarios modelled, a 20 per cent growth in the number of Age Pensioners is projected from 2002 to 2012. This is largely driven by demographic change, though with a significant moderating influence from the increasing Age Pension qualifying age for women, and a slight tempering through assumed increases in labour force participation.

If patterns of channel use remained at current levels, projected growth in channel use associated with Age Pensioners would be at a similar rate. However, increasing rates of channel use are expected because of increasing complexity in the application of means testing as the level of private incomes and assets among older Australians continues to increase. Under the increased complexity scenario modelled here, channel use by Age Pensioners is projected to grow faster than customer growth. The actual picture varies across the various access channels and also across geographic areas — features which can be identified in considerable detail with use of a regional microsimulation model.

Acknowledgement

The author would like to acknowledge the substantial and valuable input from Centrelink in this research. However, the views expressed in this chapter are those of the author and do not necessarily reflect those of Centrelink. The assistance provided by Carol Farbotko and Elizabeth Taylor of NATSEM is also gratefully acknowledged.

References

Australian Bureau of Statistics. (1999). *Labour Force Projections: 1999 to 2016*. ABS Cat. no 6260.0, Australian Bureau of Statistics, Australia.

Department of Family and Community Services. (2001). *Income Support and Related Statistics: A 10-year Compendium, 1989–1999*. Occasional Paper no 1 Department of Family and Community Services, Canberra.

Department of Family and Community Services. (2003). *Inquiry into Long-Term Strategies to Address the Ageing of the Australian Population over the Next 40 Years*. Commonwealth Department of Family and Community Services Submission to the 2003 House of Representatives Standing Committee on Ageing, Occasional Paper no 8, Department of Family and Community Services, Canberra.

King, A., McLellan, J. and Lloyd, R. (2002). *Regional Microsimulation for Improved Service Delivery in Australia: Centrelink's CuSP Model*. Paper presented to the 27th General Conference of the International Association for Research in Income and Wealth, Stockholm.

Lloyd, R., Given, J. and Hellwig, O. (2000). The Digital Divide: Some Explanations. *Agenda*, 7(4), 354–358.

Lloyd, R., Harding, A. and Hellwig, O. (2001). Regional Divide? A Study of Incomes in Regional Australia. *Australasian Journal of Regional Studies*, 6(3), 271–292.

Treasury. (2002a). *Intergenerational Report 2002–03*. 2002–2003 Budget Paper no 5, Australian Government, Canberra.

Treasury. (2002b). *Inquiry into Superannuation and Standards of Living in Retirement*. Submission by the Commonwealth Treasury to the Senate Select Committee on Superannuation, Commonwealth Treasury, Canberra.

Part IV: Health Human Resources Modelling

Chapter 15

Building Policy-Relevant Health Human Resource Models

Anil Gupta and Kisalaya Basu

Applied Research and Analysis Directorate, Health Policy Branch, Health Canada, Canada

Abstract

Health Human Resource (HHR) policy-developers are increasingly relying upon modellers to provide timely relevant information — e.g., the Canadian Advisory Committee on Health Delivery and Human Resources has made modelling a key priority. In anticipation of Health Canada's need for HHR modelling, the Microsimulation Modelling and Data Analysis Division (MSDAD) has completed a 2-year program of work to develop HHR models. This paper provides an overview of the physicians and nurses demand and supply forecast models developed by MSDAD. Given the worldwide concern about HHR and the common problems in building policy-relevant models, the lessons distilled from the MSDAD process will prove useful to those facing similar challenges elsewhere in the world.

1. Introduction

The demand for health care services changes as the population both increases and ages, but in a manner that may be somewhat unpredictable. For example, the overall healthier lifestyles of today's baby boomers may smooth their age-related health care needs, implying that the disease prevalence of the next generation of elderly may well differ from the current elderly (Denton et al., 1993, 1995).

A study (UK study, 1997) suggests that the demand for health care will rise significantly and grow faster than long-term historical trends because of (1) demographic changes, (2) medical advances (new treatments and tests),

International Symposia in Economic Theory and Econometrics, Vol. 16

ISSN: 1571-0386 DOI: 10.1016/S1571-0386(06)16015-9

(3) rising expectations, for example, public desire for higher quality health care and (4) political initiatives such as the reduction in waiting time.

This paper presents the Health Human Resource (HHR) demand and supply forecast model for physicians and nurses developed by MSDAD at the Applied Research and Analysis Directorate, Health Canada.

2. Understanding the Demand and Supply Process of HHR

Hospitals are the principal institutions within the health system to provide intervention-based services. Most HHR are located within hospitals. However, hospitals alone do not constitute the health system. Different segments of the health system perform different roles when engaged in health care interventions. Consequently, to understand properly the interaction between patients and the providers of health care, a thorough mapping of the structure of the health care system where medical intervention can take place is essential.

The health system can be broadly categorized into five areas: (1) ambulatory care, (2) acute care, (3) long-term care, (4) home care and (5) laboratories and other supporting services.

The majority of health care expenditures can be attributed to these categories. If a model can capture the main aspects of the patient–system interaction, the model can be extended to predict the effect of changes to patient loads on specific components within the system. Figure 1 illustrates the potential patient flow among the health system categories (Caceres, 2001).

3. Establishing Utilization of HHR

Once the different segments of the health care system are defined, the major inputs into the provision of health services (i.e., HHR) are populated within each subsection of the health system. Likewise, patients are the major output in the system and are subdivided by each subsection of the health system. The result is a relationship showing the base level of patient utilization of HHR.

For hospitals, HHR are assigned to different functions within each of the segments of the institution. For example, patients visiting the operating room will use a certain amount of surgical specialist services as well as nursing and other support services. Consequently, hospital resource data, such as that found in the Annual Hospital Survey previously compiled by Statistics Canada, will assist in establishing the level of HHR used in a given hospital area. These data can be compared against hospital admission and

Figure 1: Patient Flow Diagram within Health System

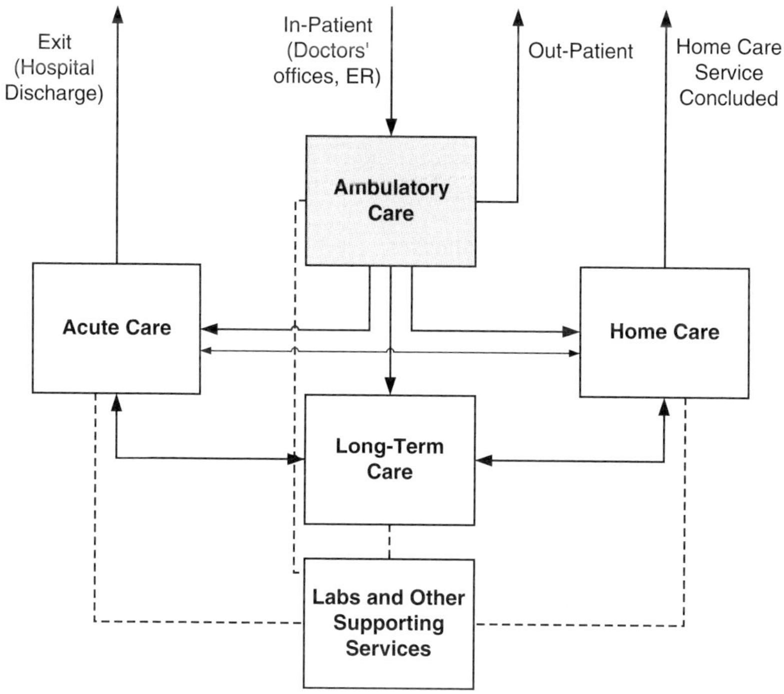

discharge data to verify patient and HHR levels within each hospital area. Figure 2 presents the interconnection among population, health status, patients and the HHR within each segment of the health system.

Note that we have only identified three components of the health system (acute care, home care and long-term care). Other components (such as primary care) can be incorporated in Figure 2. By subdividing the health care system into subcomponents, not only HHR but also all health resources (including technology) used in the provision of health care services can be analysed individually. These health system subcomponents also permit other economic issues to be studied such as substitution across HHR types, and between HHR and other resources such as diagnostic equipment and drugs. Before such scenarios can be contemplated, the subcomponent base must be developed first (Caceres, 2001).

4. MSDAD Models Overview

The MSDAD in Health Canada is building a set of models to project future HHR supply and demand. The HHR demand and supply models

Figure 2: Overall HHR Demand Model Structure

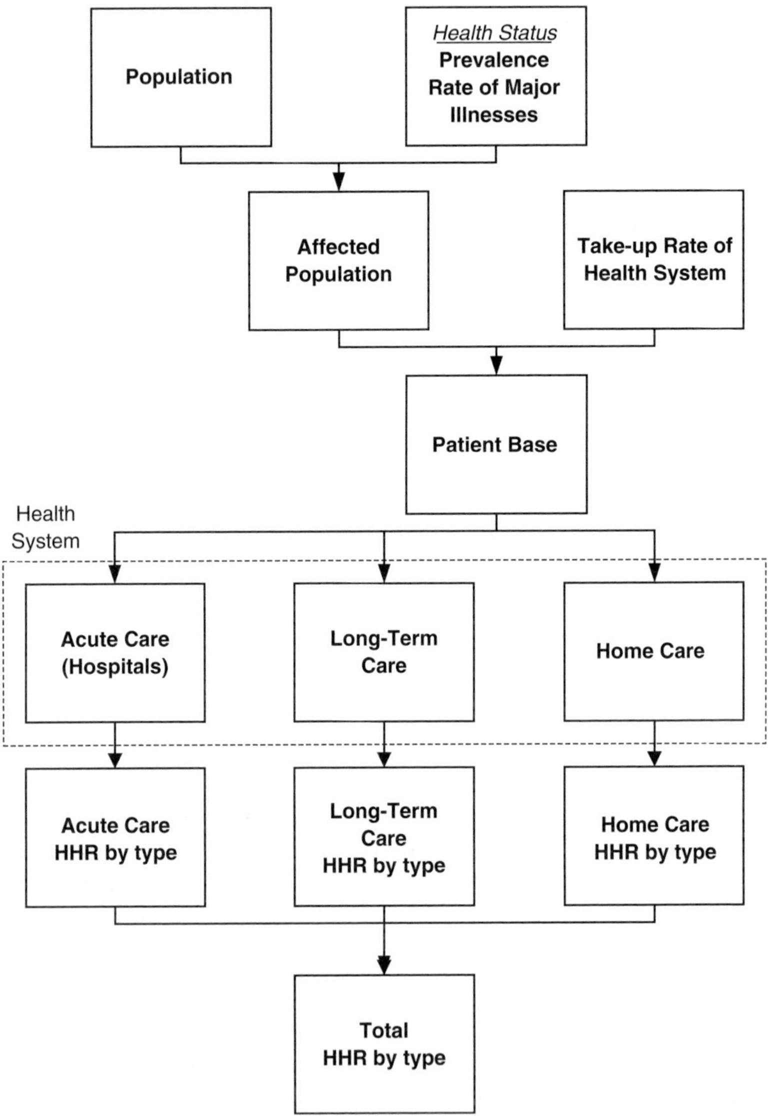

for physicians and nurses are tools that aim, through available datasets, to project future HHR requirements, as well as the employment among physicians and nurses based on current trends. The model has three main purposes:

- Understand and quantify those factors that affect the demand and supply of physicians and nurses in Canada;
- Calculate the perceived shortage to aid in identifying the areas of health policy that must be addressed and
- Develop policy scenarios with specific parameters to aid the government in addressing future HHR challenges.

5. Projection of Physician Demand and Supply

In the next two subsections, we discuss the methodologies and the data used to build utilization-based HHR demand models for physicians for Nova Scotia and the physician supply model for Canada. In spite of their limitations, these models can serve a very useful purpose in understanding the future HHR requirement of the provinces. In the subsequent section we use the results of these models to understand the future challenges in Nova Scotia. It is reasonable to believe that the general scenarios for other provinces could be developed with little modifications.

5.1 Projection of HHR Demand Model for Physicians: Data and Methodology

Conceptual Model

The two most often utilized measures of physician human resource are counts of active physicians and full-time equivalent (FTE) measures. The use of physician counts or physician population ratios for policy analysis and resources planning purposes is flawed since it implicitly assumes that physician resources are homogeneous — that all physicians are equal in terms of workload and productivity. While the FTE is a better measure than the count of active physicians, there are several methodologies to measure FTE. Basically, FTE methodologies rely on measures of physician payment or income as proxies for workload and employ various statistical manipulations or assumptions to estimate effective physician resource stock (Kralj and Weinkauf, 1997).

The methodology used to calculate FTE in our model is similar to the one used by the Canadian Institute for Health Information (CIHI) to calculate the FTE. Here, we first calculate the income of each unique physician using Nova Scotia's Physician Billings Data and then we calculate the 40th and 60th percentile income levels for each of the 40 specialties. The following formula calculates the FTE_{jk}, which is the FTE of physician k of specialty j. P_{jk} is the income of physician k of specialty j. The 40th and 60th percentile income levels of physician specialty j are $P_{\alpha,j}$ and $P_{\beta,j}$, respectively. Log is used to shorten the right-hand tail of the distribution.

$$\mathrm{FTE}_{jk} = \begin{cases} \frac{P_{jk}}{P_{\alpha,j}} & \text{if} \quad P_{jk} < P_{\alpha,j} \\ 1 & \text{if} \quad P_{\alpha,j} \leq P_{jk} \leq P_{\beta,j} \\ 1 + \log\left(\frac{P_{jk}}{P_{\beta,j}}\right) & \text{if} \quad P_{jk} > P_{\beta,j} \end{cases} \tag{1}$$

Now, j specialty is divided into three broad categories of specialties. They are as follows:

1. General Practitioners (GP)
2. Medical Specialty (MS)
3. Surgical Specialty (SS).

The model assumes the constant prevalence of diseases and utilization rate by age and gender and projects the requirement of FTE physicians for the period 2000–2025. The Figure 3 flow chart shows the mechanism of the projection.

Data Sources

Nova Scotia's physician billings data has been used to calculate the FTE of physicians by four broad categories of specialty in the base year. The variables used in the Physician Demand model are Physician's ID (scrambled), physician's specialty, amount paid to the physician for each service, patient ID (scrambled),

Figure 3: Summary Depiction of the Physician Forecast Model

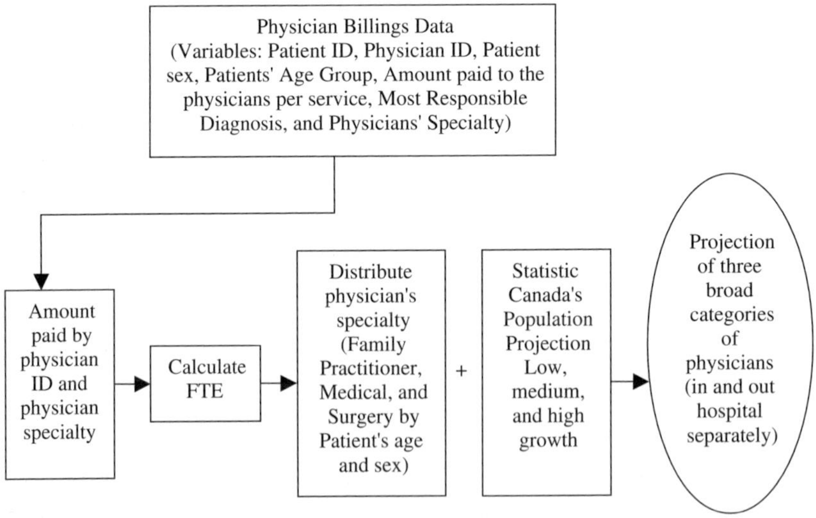

patient's age, patient's sex, primary diagnosis of the patient, a variable indicating whether the service was performed inside or outside the hospital.

The model accommodates three options for the population projection of Nova Scotia — the Statistics Canada's high, medium and low growth population projection for Nova Scotia to project the future FTE requirements of physicians.

How the Model Works

The Physician Demand Model for Nova Scotia is a Microsoft Excel and Visual Basic-based application. It calculates the FTE of Physicians by physician specialty, patient age, patient sex, most responsible diagnosis (MRD) and hospital status for any given population projections of Nova Scotia. The model incorporates the method described earlier to calculate FTE. All of the information in the model is stored in Excel spreadsheets in the background in order to protect the data. However, the user is allowed access to the data through a customized Pivot Chart that allows him to display any combination of the above categories. The user is also able to graph any combination of the data categories as well.

The model is rendered more flexible by allowing the user to change the base FTE requirements of physician specialty for three categories: age group, sex and MRD. This allows potential changes to the HHRs market under study. The model also allows any two data sets to be evaluated together to reflect their differences.

5.2 Health Human Resources Supply Model for Physicians (HHRSM)

Conceptual Model

The HHRSM is based on a stock/flow approach to express changes in employment. This section presents broadly the conceptual underpinnings of this approach, as well as establishing dimensions and variables for the HHRSM. It is important to note that the MSDAD model does not predict behavioural responses to changes in, say, income.

The individual employment changes (such as new entrants or retirements) contribute to the change in employment stock from year to year. For the sake of simplicity, let us consider only the family physicians P at this time. Stock of family physicians at time t, distributed by single year age cohort i, sex category j is denoted by

$$S^P_{i,j,t} = S^P_{i-1,j,t-1} + N^P_{i,j,t} + (I^P_{i,j,t} - E^P_{i,j,t}) - R^P_{i,j,t} - D^P_{i,j,t} \tag{2}$$

where S represents the stock of physicians, N the new entrants as physician, I the immigrants, E the emigrants, R the retirements and D the death. It is to be noted that S is stock, while N, I, E, R and D are flows. Now the total number of family physicians at time t can be expressed as

$$\begin{aligned} S_t^P &= \sum_i \sum_j S_{i,j,t}^P \\ &= \sum_i \sum_j S_{i-1,j,t-1}^P \\ &+ \sum_i \sum_j \left[N_{i,j,t}^P + (I_{i,j,t}^P - E_{i,j,t}^P) - R_{i,j,t}^P - D_{i,j,t}^P \right] \end{aligned} \quad (3)$$

This is to note that for family physician we have

$$I_{i,j,t}^P = A_{i,j,t}^P + \alpha L_{i,j,t} + \beta(1-\alpha) L_{i-3,j,t-3} \quad (4)$$

where A^P represents family physicians returning from abroad, L the landed immigrant physicians, α the proportion of landed immigrant physicians with *arranged employment* and β the proportion of landed immigrant physicians *without arranged employment* becoming family physicians after 3 years. (Note that we assume that for Medical Physician $I_{i,j,t}^D = A_{i,j,t}^D$ and for Surgical Physician $I_{i,j,t}^G = A_{i,j,t}^G$). The stock at period t_1, which is the sum of the stock at period t_0 and other positive and negative flows at period t_1, becomes the stock at the beginning of period t_2.

Data Sources

The Southam Medical Database (SMDB) is used to identify the stocks and the information about the medical students is obtained from Canadian Post-MD Education Registry (CAPER). The immigration and emigration information are obtained from Citizenship and Immigration Canada (CIC). The Labour Force Survey (LFS) was the primary source used to obtain the retirement rate of the physicians. In some cases, data were not available and, thus, were imputed based on reasonable assumptions. Imputation was done mostly for flow data. The following flow chart (Figure 4) illustrates the stock and flows of the base period t_1 and how the data are fed into the model as well as the sources of the data. It also shows how some of the variables are imputed based on some simple assumptions.

Family Physicians

Family physicians include general practitioners, emergency family medicine, emergency medicine, public health, addiction medicine, family medicine and community medicine. But, family practice and general practice are the major ones. In 1999, family physicians constitute 51.26 per cent of the total number of physicians.

Figure 4: Flow Chart for HHR Physician Supply Model

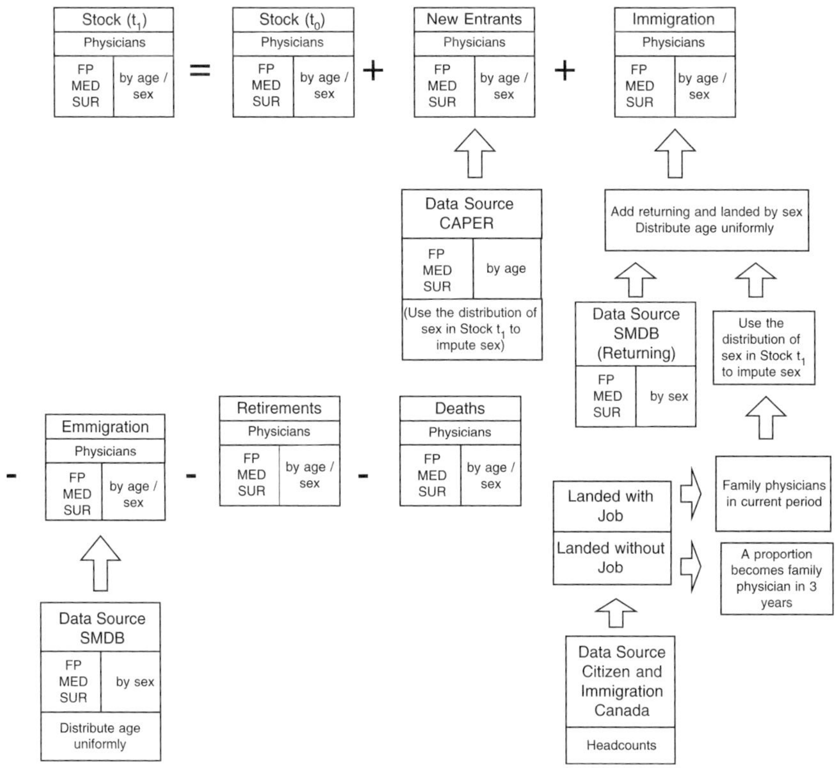

Stock

The stock for family physicians is extracted from Southam Medical Database (SMDB). Only active physicians were considered as available for employment. Family physicians registered with the Canadian Medical Association (CMA), but not active at the time were excluded. These are retirees, semi-retirees, temporary retirees, temporarily not in practice, on leave of absence, on sabbatical, in active military duty and deceased.

New Entrants

The data from CAPER for the family physician new entrant categories are available only by age and not by sex. The distribution of family physicians stock by sex for the year 1999 is used to calculate the family physicians new entrants in 1999 by age and sex.

Immigration and Emigration

Immigration includes the number of physicians who returned from abroad, as well as landed immigrant physicians who arrived in the country with or without prior arranged employment. Citizenship and Immigration Canada categorizes individual landed immigrants by their occupation. Data for physicians returning from abroad by sex and specialty is available from SMDB.

For the physicians who are landed immigrants, the total number is available by employment status. All the physicians with arranged employment are assumed to be family physicians and a fraction of the physicians without arranged employment are assumed to become family physicians in 3 years. The distribution of family physicians stock in 1999 across gender is used to calculate the family physicians landed immigrants in 1999 by sex.

The family physicians returning from abroad and landed immigrants with arranged employment are summed up to get the family physician immigration for 1999 by sex. Physicians who moved abroad are available by sex and specialty (CIHI, 1999).

It is assumed that both immigration and emigration occurs only between ages 30 and 64. Based on this assumption, we distribute the numbers equally across ages.

Retirements

The probability of retirement at each age starting from age 40 is calculated based on the assumption that the average age of retirement is 63. To calculate these probabilities, first the data from LFS for the employment of the entire labour force from 1976 to 1999 are plotted to estimate the parameters of a fitted logistic curve in order to obtain the probability of retirement at different ages. These probabilities by age are applied to the previous year's stock by age to get the actual retirement by age. Figure 5 shows the probability of retirement by age for three different average ages of retirement.

Deaths

There are no mortality rate data specific to physicians. Therefore, the mortality rate for the general population was used to calculate deaths. It is assumed that the mortality rate does not change in the future.

How the Model Works

The HHRSM simulator allows the projection to be disaggregated by three specialties — family, medical and surgical — and by age and sex. The base year for projection is 1999. The model projects up to year 2020.

Figure 5: Probability of Retirement by Age in Canada, 1976–1999

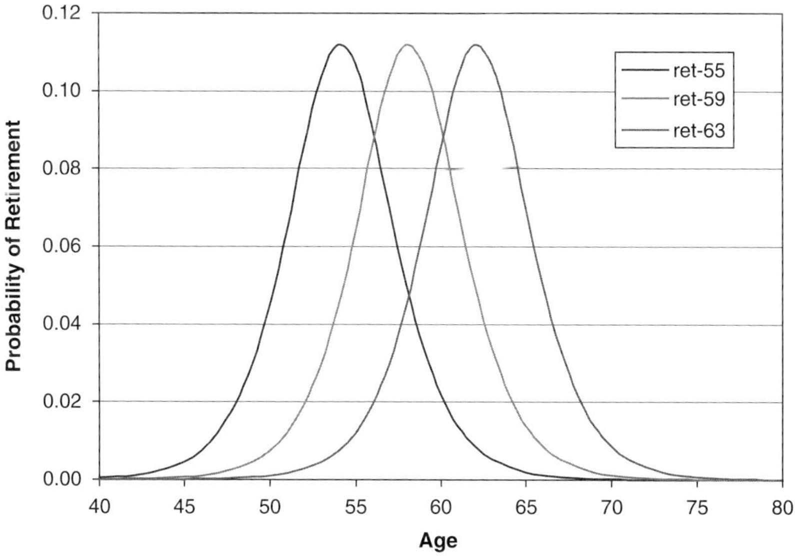

New Entrants

There are various ways the number of new entrants can be fed into the model: (1) entering the number of new entrants for all the projection years; (2) entering the number of new entrants for the base year 1999 and an annual growth rate; (3) entering the number of students enrolled in the 1st year MD program in all the projection years and (4) entering the number of students enrolled in the 1st year MD program in any of the projection years, the initial value in that particular year, and the annual growth rate.

The model can calculate the new entrants from the number of new students entered in the MD program. An MD title is received after 4 years of education. Before receiving an MD 3 per cent (default value based on analysis of CAPER data) of the students drop out. Further, based on statistics from CAPER, at the beginning of the 5th year, 39 per cent go into family residency, 43 per cent go into medical residency and the remaining 18 per cent go into surgical residency.

Residency is completed after 2 years for the family physicians, after 4 years for medical specialty and after 6 years for surgical specialty. During the residency training 1 per cent (default) drop out.

It takes 5 years from first entering into practice for any physician to be considered an *experienced physician*. During these 5 years, 3 per cent (default) of the physicians from each specialty drop out. The default values are coded as parameters in the model and are thus available to the user to modify like any other parameter in the model.

The entered numbers are distributed by age, sex and specialty based on the previous year's distribution. The full-time equivalencies (FTE) are calculated by age, sex and specialty based on the base year's FTE by age, sex and specialty. The model produces both the headcounts and FTE.

Immigration and Emigration

For the immigration and emigration (1) the default 1999 value can be changed for every consecutive year; (2) the growth rate can be incorporated to an initial value for the consecutive years; and (3) the initial value can be changed to the consecutive years based on any specific mathematical function. The entered numbers are distributed by age, sex and specialty based on the previous year's distribution. The full-time equivalencies (FTE) are calculated by age, sex and specialty based on the base year's FTE by age, sex and specialty.

Retirement

Retirement is calculated based on the distribution of age in the last period stock. The average default retirement age in the model is 63 years but that can be changed to be between 50 and 75.

Deaths

Death rate is calculated based on the mortality rate of the general population in the base year and applied on the previous year's stock.

6. Projection of Nurses Demand and Supply

In the next two subsections, we discuss the methodologies and the data used to build utilization-based provincial HHR demand models for nurses and nurses supply models for Canada. In spite of their limitations, these models can serve a very useful purpose in understanding the future HHR requirement of the provinces.

6.1 Health Human Resources Demand Model for Nurses

The MSDAD, Health Canada, has first built, in collaboration with Alberta Health and Wellness, a HHR demand model to project the future in-hospital Registered Nurses (RNs) requirements for Alberta for 2000–2030

(Wall and Basu, 2003). Later, MSDAD used the methodology to build similar models for all provinces.

The model employs two basic assumptions: (1) RNs utilization is proportional to total Resource Intensity Weight (*RIW*) in a nursing function (Basu et al., 2003) and (2) a full-time RN is equivalent of 0.9 FTE and a part-time RN is equivalent to 0.6 FTE. These numbers have been independently validated using 1998 cross-sectional Public-Use Microdata File (PUMF) for the Survey of Labour and Income Dynamics (SLID), which is a collection of income, labour and family variables on adult persons in Canada (Basu and Wall, 2003).

The model uses the base-year (1999–2000) relationship between the demographic/clinical characteristics of inpatients (i.e., age, sex, MRD, case-mix and case-complexity) using Discharge Abstract Data, and the full-time equivalence RNs who provide the care. The need for FTE RNs is estimated using CIHI Registered Nurse Database (RNDB), which is an annual registry of all RNs eligible (i.e., registered) to practice by nursing function and employment status. The sensitivity of projections of future requirements for RNs takes into account scenarios of possible changes in population, medical need for active inpatients and RN staffing within each nursing function.

Data

The Registered Nurses Database (1999) published by CIHI is used to calculate the FTE of RNs by several nursing functions. RNDB provides the headcounts of RNs by full-time and part-time and by nursing functions. For our purpose we concentrate on the RNs working in nursing functions within direct care units of the hospitals. We exclude such areas as administration, education and research.

Discharge Abstract Data was used to determine the base year utilization in terms of demographic/clinical characteristics of active care inpatients (i.e., age, sex and MRD). The model links the relative need for nursing and other resources (case-mix and case-complexity), and the full-time equivalence (FTE) RNs who provide such nursing care.

The model also uses Statistics Canada's both low and high growth projections of population to project to 2025.

Logic and Structure of the Model

Figure 6 shows how RNs are assigned to the direct care nursing units using RNDB data, and how they are linked to the patients using enhanced Discharge Abstract Data (DAD) by MRD group, age and sex.

Figure 7 starts with the RNDB-DAD dataset with RNs head counts by full-time (FT), part-time (PT) and nursing functions. The head-counts of

Figure 6: Estimating Expected RN-Use (Headcounts) by Acute Care Nursing Function and Patient Age-Gender Group

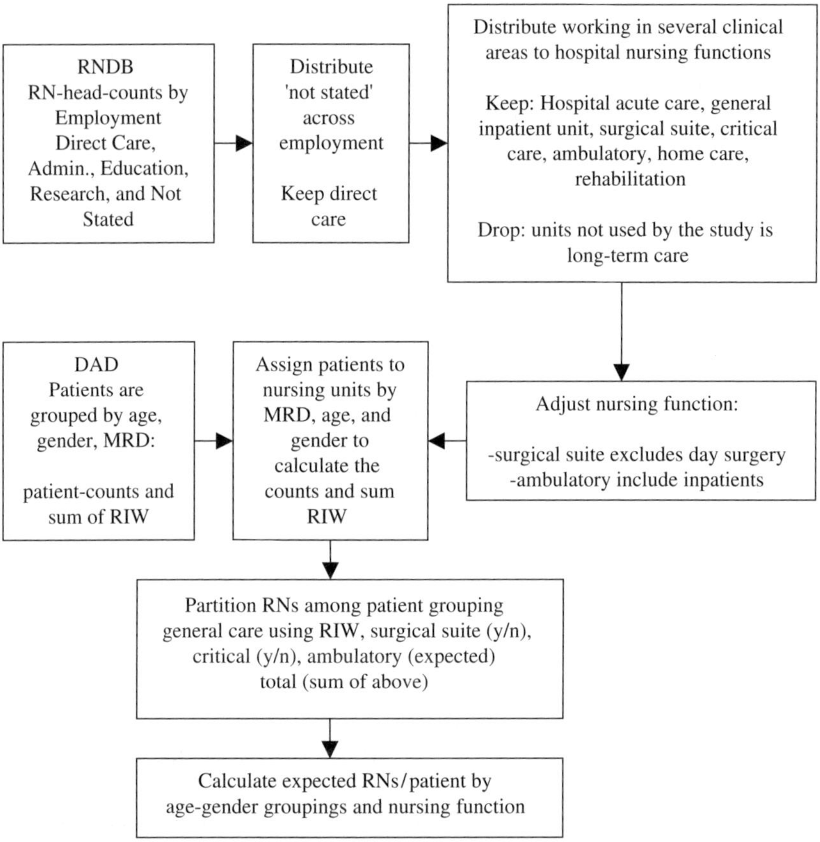

FT and PT RNs are then used to estimate the FTE of RNs. The relationships between FT and FTE, and between PT and FTE are obtained from CIHI and are then validated by MSDAD using the Survey of Labour and Income Dynamics. Using those relationships, we obtain the FTE of RNs by nursing functions. The nursing functions are: (1) medical/surgical, (2) psychiatric/mental health, (3) paediatric (patients age less than 16: except for Oncology), (4) maternal/newborn, (5) oncology, (6) critical care (CC), (7) operation room/recovery room (OR/RR), (8) rehabilitation, (9) ambulatory care and (10) home care.

The *RIWs* for each patient is added by nursing function. The RIW is a relative value assigned to each patient upon discharge, according to the amount of resources he or she used. It is assumed that RNs utilization is

Figure 7: RNs Demand Projection Model for Provinces

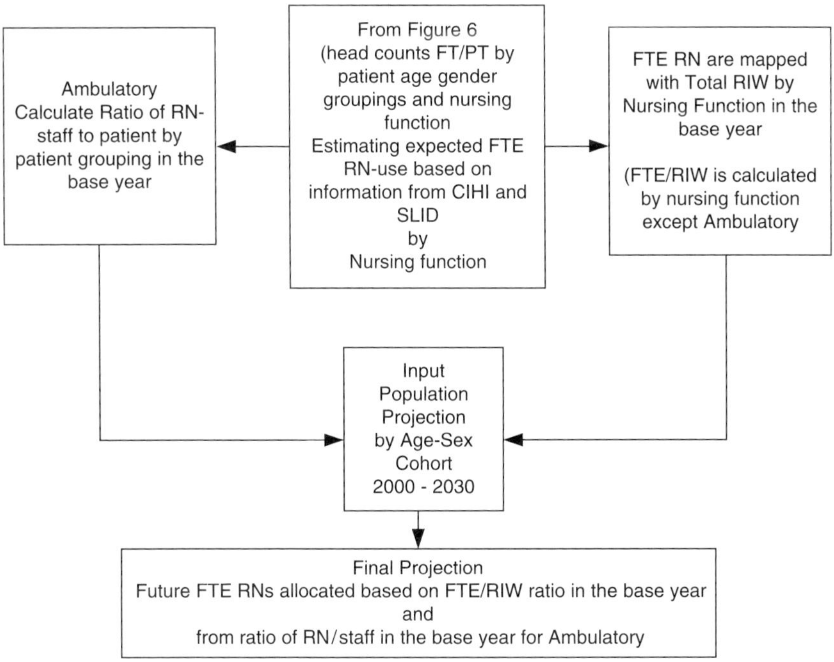

proportional to total *RIW* in each of these nursing functions. This allows us to estimate the change in demand for these RNs over time, i.e., not all nursing functions are equal.

We use the ratio of RNs to patients by patient grouping in the base year for the nursing function ambulatory care as the *RIW* is not available for those patients. We assume that the ratio of RNs to patients will remain constant in the subsequent years, that is, practice mix and technology remain constant. Figure 7 shows the process in detail.

6.2 Health Human Resources Supply Model for Nurses

Conceptual Model

The HHRSM is based upon a stock/flow approach to express changes in employment. The supply model for nurses is conceptually the same as the physicians' except that the landed immigrant nurses are assumed to get a nursing job immediately upon arrival.

Data

The model uses RNs Data for 1999.

Stock

The stock data for RN in Nova Scotia is extracted from Registered Nurses Database (RNDB), 1999 (CIHI, 2000). The stock data is available only by 5-year age group starting from 20–24 to 70–79. The "fit-curve" method is used to get the data for single years from ages 20 to 80. In 1999, 4.63 per cent of RNs were male and 95.37 per cent were female. These percentages are then applied to the single values to get RN stock data by age and sex.

New Entrants

The number of first-time takers of the RN examinations in 1999 (Source: Canadian Nurses Association, 2002) is used to determine the number of new entrants. The number is divided by 15 (as it is assumed than new entrants are between the ages 23 and 37) to get the new entrants data for each age. The female to male ratio of 9:1 is applied to this data to get the new entrants by age and sex.

Drop-Out Rates

The default dropout rates used for the students enrolled in the RN program are 10 per cent for the 1st and the 2nd year, 5 per cent for the 3rd and 4th year and 10 and 5 per cent, for the 1st and the 2nd year of practice, respectively.

Immigration

The data on RNs who became landed immigrants in 1999 are available by employment status (RNDB, 1999) (Source: Special request, Citizenship and Immigration Canada, 2000; RNDB, 1999, p. 26). This number is divided by 30 (as it is assumed that the immigration occurs between the ages 30 and 59) to get the immigration for each age. The female to male ratio of 9:1 is applied to this data to get the immigration by age and sex.

Emigration

Data for Canadian emigrants admitted as permanent residents to the USA by occupation including nurses are available from 1993 to 1997 (Source: United States Immigration and Naturalization Service, 2000; RNDB, 1999, p. 26). The data are not available after the 1997 data year (RNDB, 2000, p. 24 line 28). So, the 1997 number is used for 1999 as well. Again, this number is divided by 30 (as it is assumed that the emigration occurs between the ages 30 and 59) to get the emigration for each age. The female to male ratio of 9:1 is applied to this data to get the emigration by age and sex.

Retirement

The probability of retirement at each age is calculated based on the assumption that the average age of retirement is 63. To calculate these probabilities, first the data from Labour Force Survey (LFS) for the employment of the entire labour force from 1976 to 1999 are plotted to estimate the parameters of a fitted logistic curve in order to obtain the probability of retirement at a different age.

Deaths

There is no mortality rate data specific to RNs. Therefore, the mortality rate for the general population is used. The mortality rate is multiplied by single-year age of stock from the previous year to obtain the number of deaths by age and sex.

7. Illustrations of Models

Now we illustrate some results from our models. One of the most important reasons as envisaged in Figure 8 is that the population is ageing. The population of Nova Scotia like the rest of Canada is ageing. In the next 25 years the population above 65 years will double, and in 10 years it will grow by 50 per cent. Since the elderly population uses a disproportionately larger amount of HHR, the demand for HHR will grow faster than the population. As discussed earlier, to meet the demand for HHR in, say, 2015, we need to plan now. This is particularly so because the HHR will also be ageing, so the gap between the demand and supply will be growing if no action is taken right now.

Figure 9 shows the requirements of both in- and out-hospital FTE physicians and in-hospital RNs per 100,000 populations by age group in Nova Scotia. The figure illustrates that the requirement for RN's increases faster than the requirement of physicians ages 35–84. Beyond 84 years, the requirement for RNs decreases and the requirement for physicians increases significantly. Therefore, as the population ages as envisaged in Figure 8, it is expected that the prevalence of the diseases that are by and large associated with old age will increase over the time horizon.

Figure 10 compares the requirements of physicians for Neoplasm in Nova Scotia when there is a shock that reduces the prevalence of Neoplasm by 40 per cent in 2010 and 2015 with the baseline requirements (no change).

Figure 8: Elderly as a Fraction of Population Over Time: Nova Scotia

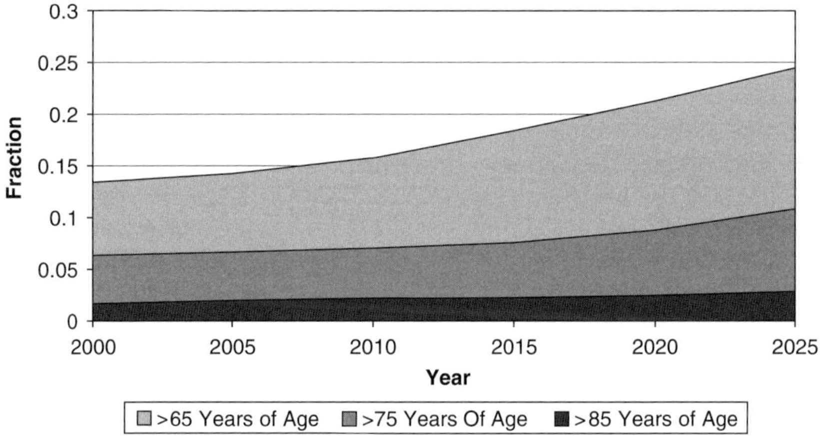

Figure 9: Requirement of HHR/100,000 Population by Age Group in Nova Scotia

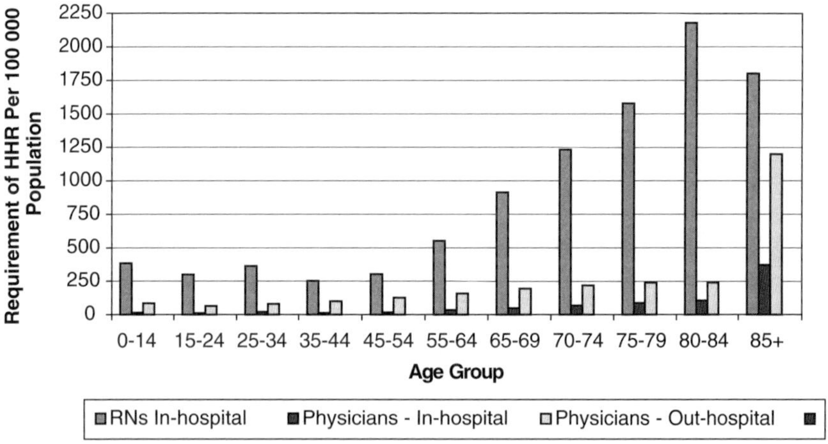

The model can also project the requirements of physicians when shocks are introduced by age, sex, MRD and physician specialty, or any combination of these categories.

Figure 11 shows the projection of RNs by hospital function till 2026. This projection uses Statistics Canada's Medium Growth Population Projection. The model is capable of incorporating any shock unrelated to demographic change for any nursing function and at any time. The figure shows the projection of in-hospital RNs by nursing functions, such as paediatric

Figure 10: Projection of Physician's Requirement for Neoplasm when Shock Changes the Demand in Nova Scotia

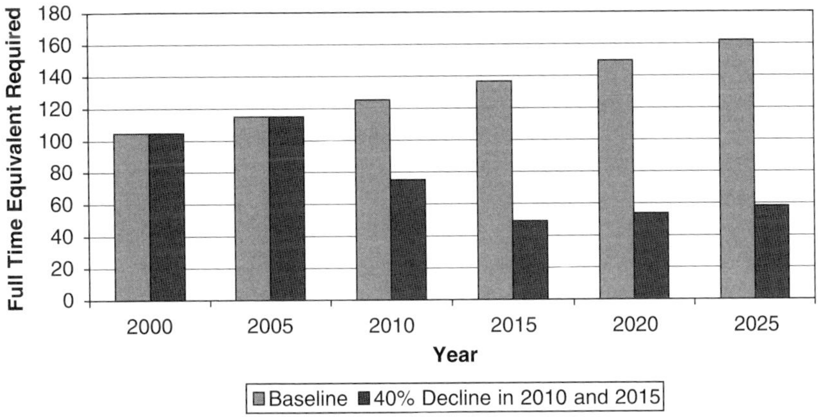

Figure 11: Demand for RN FTE per 100,000 Population in Canada

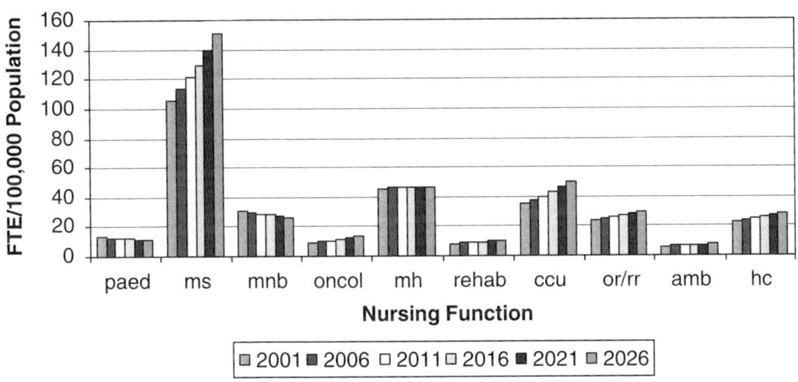

(patients under 16: except for oncology), medical/surgical, maternal/newborn, oncology, psychiatric/mental health, rehabilitation, critical care, operation room/recovery room, ambulatory care and home care in Canada.

7.1 Future Challenges

The demand for both physicians and RNs will increase considerably in Nova Scotia over the next 25 years as depicted in Figure 12. Using Statistics Canada's High Growth Population Projection, the requirement for active in-hospital RNs will increase by 1.18 per cent annually, the requirement for

Figure 12: Demand for Physicians and RNs per 100,000 Population in Nova Scotia

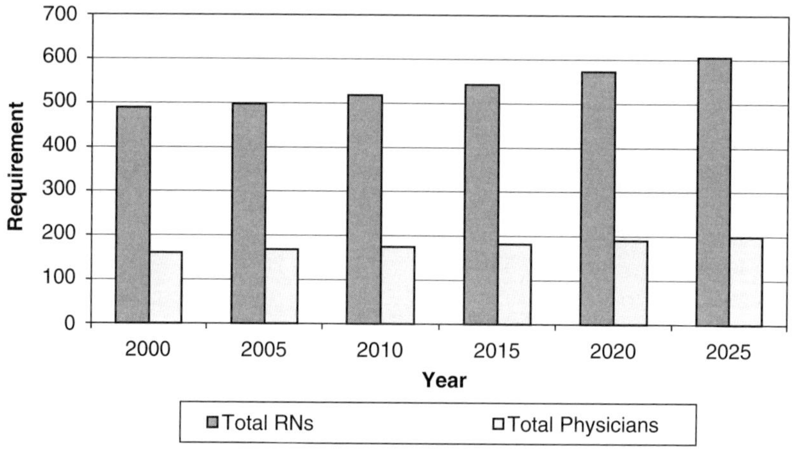

Figure 13: Supply of Physicians and RNs per 100,000 Population in Nova Scotia

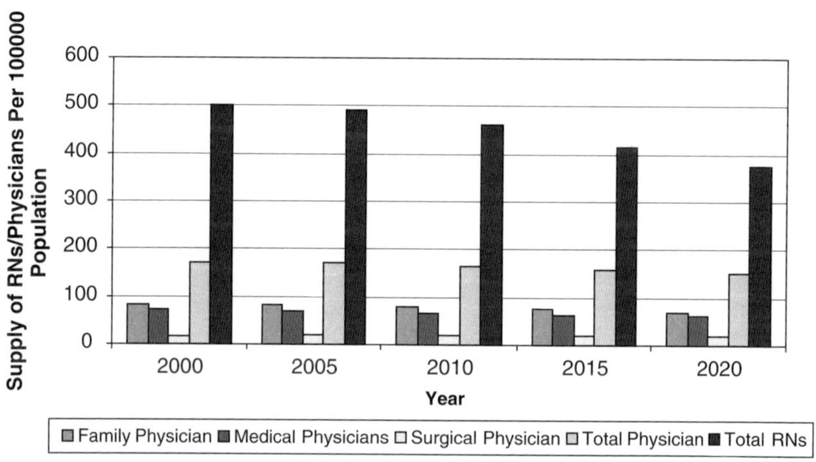

in-hospital physicians will increase by 1.49 per cent annually, and the requirement for out-hospital physicians will increase by 1.10 per cent annually over the next 25 years.

Figure 13 shows that the supply of both physicians and nurses will decrease in Nova Scotia if the current flow of new entry, immigration, emigration, retirement and the death of physicians and nurses exist for the next 25 years. So we have an increasing requirement for physicians and nurses and a decreasing supply of physicians and nurses. Since the population aged above 65 requires disproportionately more nurses than physicians, the demand for nurses will be much greater than the demand for physicians due to the ageing population.

8. Conclusions

The demand models for physicians and nurses described in this paper are based on utilization data. The models assume that the incidence rates of diseases remain constant. However, the models parameterize the rates of incidence, thus allowing for changes to it. Further, the physician forecast model projects the requirements for three broad categories of physician specialties for both in- and out-hospital environments. The nursing forecast model forecasts the in-hospital RN requirements by hospital functions.

The supply models for physicians and nurses are based on an inflow–outflow approach. In many respects, the approach to supply modelling is elegant in its simplicity. It is complex in the sense that it is demographically rich in terms of detail relating to sex, age and specialty.

As the population ages over the next two decades the requirement for both physicians and nurses will grow faster than it has during the last two decades. The production of physicians and nurses requires specific training that spans over several years. Therefore, to meet the requirement of future physicians and nurses it is necessary to determine the number of physicians and nurses required to train today so that they may be available at the appropriate time.

A specific program should be established that would help the immigrant physicians and nurses to acquire the necessary supplementary training that will equip them with necessary skills to serve the Canadian population. A potential problem may arise due to the proximity to the United States. The population in United States is also ageing. As a result, the requirement of both physicians and nurses will grow in the United States and at the same time more of the physicians and nurses will retire in the next two decades. Under this circumstance, the Canadian HHR market has to be competitive with that of the United States both in terms of the working conditions and the salary structure. This will also create pressure on the cost of health care in Canada.

References

Basu, K., Paré, S. and Wall, R. (2003). *Simulating the Components of Resource Intensity Weight: A Good Proxy for Allocating Health Human Resources across Inpatients?* Longwoods Publishing, HRResources.ca.

Basu, K. and Wall, R. (2003). Estimating the Full Time Equivalence of Part-Time and Full-Time Registered Nurses. *Microsimulation Modelling and Data Analysis Division (MSDAD Working Paper)*.

Caceres, J. (2001). *Health Human Resources Model: Projection Tool for Health Policy*. Canadian Health Economics Research Association Conference, Toronto, Canada.

Denton, F.T., Gafni, A. and Spencer, B.G. (1993). The SHARP Computer System — A Tool for Resource Planning in the Health Care Sector, in Malek, M., Rasquinha, J. and Vacani, P. (eds), *Strategic Issues in Health Care Management*, John Wiley and Sons, pp. 45–56.

Denton, F.T., Gafni, A. and Spencer, B.G. (1995). The SHARP Way to Plan Health Care Services: A Description of the System and Some Illustrative Applications in Nursing Human Resource Planning. *Socio-Economic Planning Science*, 29(2), 125–137.

Kralj, B. and Weinkauf, D.K. (1997). Measuring Physician Human Resource Supply: An Appraisal of Current Methodologies and Potential Alternatives, Department of Economics, Ontario Medical Association. Unpublished Manuscript.

UK Study. (1997). Planning the Medical Workforce, Medical Workforce Standing Advisory Committee: Third Report.

Wall, R. and Basu, K. (2003). Registered Nurses Projection Model for Alberta 2000–2030: A Methodology. *Microsimulation Modelling and Data Analysis Division (MSDAD Working Paper)*.

Chapter 16

What is Behind HRSA's Projected U.S. Supply, Demand, and Shortages of Registered Nurses

Marilyn B. Biviano, Steve Tise and Timothy M. Dall

National Center for Health Workforce Analysis, Bureau of Health Professions, Health Resources and Services Administration, and The Lewin Group

Abstract

An adequate supply of nurses is essential to achieving the nation's goals of ensuring access to affordable, high-quality healthcare. The adequacy of nurse supply varies geographically throughout the nation, with a general consensus that at the national level there is currently a moderate shortage of registered nurses (RNs). The HRSA state-based RN supply and demand models provide projections of future U.S. supply and demand for RNs and allow for sensitivity analysis of many relevant policy variables, such as nursing wages, local nursing training program "production" of nurses, projected patient demographics, and employment trends in major sectors (such as hospitals). The findings of our analysis suggest that the current shortage of RNs will continue to grow in severity during the next two decades if current trends prevail, and that some states face a more severe shortage than do other states. The growth and aging of the population, along with the nation's continued demand for the highest quality of care, will create a surging demand for the services of RNs over the next two decades. At the same time, the supply of RNs remains flat as many RNs are approaching retirement age and the nursing profession faces difficulties attracting new entrants and retaining the existing workforce.

1. Background

The mission of the National Center for Health Workforce Analysis (NCHWA) in the Bureau of Health Professions (BHPr), Health Resources and Services Administration (HRSA), is *to collect, analyze, and disseminate health workforce information and facilitate national, state, and local workforce planning efforts*. To meet this mission as it pertains to the nurse

International Symposia in Economic Theory and Econometrics, Vol. 16

ISSN: 1571-0386 DOI: 10.1016/S1571-0386(06)16016-0

workforce, NCHWA collects data on the nurse workforce through its quadrennial sample survey of registered nurses (SSRN) and maintains two models to project the supply of and demand for registered nurses (RNs): the nursing supply model (NSM) and the nursing demand model (NDM). In this paper we provide a brief overview of these two models; describe the data, methods and assumptions used to project RN supply and demand; present findings from the models; and discuss the limitations of these and other models and methods to forecast demand for health workers.[1]

In 2000, RNs comprised the single largest health care profession with almost 1.9 million full-time equivalent RNs, accounting for 20% of the nation's health care workforce, and equal to 678 RNs per 100,000 population. RNs provide a significant amount of health care and while approximately half of all RNs are employed in hospitals, they can be found in almost every sector of the economy from large businesses, to schools, to industrial settings.

2. Nursing Supply Model

The NSM produces annual, state-level projections of RN supply through 2020. The NSM tracks nurses by age, state and highest level of educational attainment (i.e., diploma or associate degree, baccalaureate degree, and graduate degree). Starting with the number of licensed RNs in 2000, the NSM adds the estimated number of newly licensed RNs, subtracts the estimated number of separations, and tracks cross-state migration patterns to calculate an end-of-year estimate of licensed RNs by state (Figure 1). The end-of-year estimate becomes the starting value for the next year's projections.

The model projects the number of licensed RNs and then applies labor force participation rates to estimate the number of RNs active in the health workforce and the number of full-time-equivalent (FTE) RNs employed in healthcare. In computing FTE RNs, nurses who work full time are counted as 1 FTE, while nurses who report working part time or for only part of the year are counted as 0.5 FTEs.

The NSM has three major components: (1) modeling new graduates from nursing programs, (2) modeling the location and employment patterns of the current licensed nurse population, and (3) modeling separations from the nurse workforce. For each of these components, we describe the data, assumptions, and methods used to project future RN supply.

---

[1] Additional Information on these models, projections from these models, and the data and assumptions is available in other reports: *Projected Supply, Demand, and Shortages of Registered Nurses: 2000–2020* (NCHWA, 2002).

Figure 1: Overview of the Nursing Supply Model

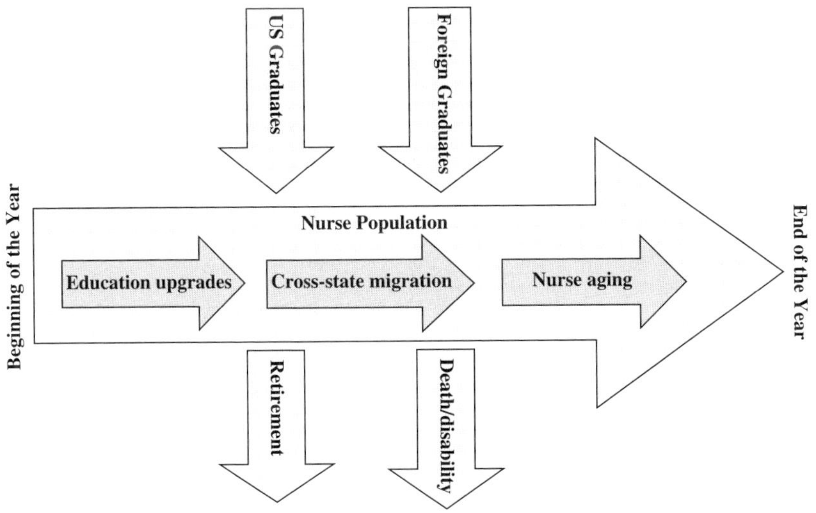

2.1 New Graduates from Nursing Programs

RNs typically enter the nurse workforce prepared at the diploma, associate, or baccalaureate level. (Some RNs enter at the masters degree level, but are modeled here as BSN graduates who upgrade their education.) Data on the number of first-time candidates taking the National Council Licensure Examination for Registered Nurses (NCLEX-RNs), as published by the National Council of State Boards of Nursing, suggest that in 2000 approximately 71,100 RNs graduated from U.S. nursing programs. Approximately two-thirds of these graduates were prepared at the diploma or associate level, with the remaining one-third prepared at the baccalaureate level or higher. The number of graduates in 2000 shows a continuing decline compared to earlier years (e.g., there were approximately 76,300 graduates in 1999 and 83,000 graduates in 1998). The literature discussing reasons for this trend is extensive (see, for example, Buerhaus et al., (2000); Seago et al., (2001)), but reflects increasing professional opportunities outside of nursing for women, stagnant pay, and more onerous working conditions for many in nursing, and a decline in pubic perception of the attractiveness of the nursing profession.

Baseline projections of the number of new nursing school graduates are based on the assumption that the nursing profession will continue to attract its current share of the applicant pool. The population of women age 20 to 44 is used as a proxy for the size of the applicant pool, and the population projections used in the NSM come from the Census Bureau's middle series population projections.[2] Combining state-level NCLEX-RN data with state-level estimates of the number of women age 20 to 44 creates a separate applicant pool share for each state. Over time, each 1% increase (decrease) in the size of the applicant pool is assumed to cause a 1% increase (decrease) in the number of RN graduates for that state. Under the baseline scenario, the number of new nurse graduates is relatively constant through 2020 at the national level. The number of nurse graduates of each education type (E) in each state (S) and year (Y) is expressed mathematically:

$$\text{Graduates}_{\text{E,S,Y}} = \left(\frac{\text{PopW}_{\text{S,Y}}}{\text{PopW}_{\text{S,2000}}}\right) \times \text{Graduates}_{\text{E,S,2000}}$$

The NSM software was built with algorithms to model the impact on the number of nursing graduates resulting from changes in RN compensation, working conditions, teaching capacity, and tuition costs. However, the research has yet to be completed for modeling the relationship between the number of nurse graduates and those determinants that reflect the attractiveness of nursing as a career (Figure 2).

In addition to graduates from U.S. nursing programs, the NSM assumes net immigration of 3,500 RNs per year from foreign countries.

2.2 The Licensed Nurse Population

The Current Licensed Nurse Population

The NSM tracks the population of licensed RNs, or "bodies," regardless of whether the RN is providing nursing services. The NSM applies estimated labor force participation rates to the projections of licensed RNs to project the nurse supply (defined as number of nurses employed or seeking employment in nursing) and FTE supply (defined as the FTE number of nurses providing nursing services).

The model starts with the number of licensed RNs in each state, tracked by age and education level, as estimated using the 2000 National Sample Survey of RNs. The education level and age composition of the licensed RN

[2] The Census Bureau's projections were developed prior to the 2000 Census and underestimated the U.S. population in 2000. Consequently, we adjusted the Census Bureau projections to reflect this undercount. Men continue to constitute a small percentage of the RN workforce, doubling from approximately 2.7% in 1980 to 5.4% in 2000. (BHPr, 2001) As the proportion of RNs who are male grows, the NSM might need to add a gender component to track difference in labor force participation patterns and retirement rates between male and female RNs.

Figure 2: National Baseline Projections of Annual Nursing School Graduates

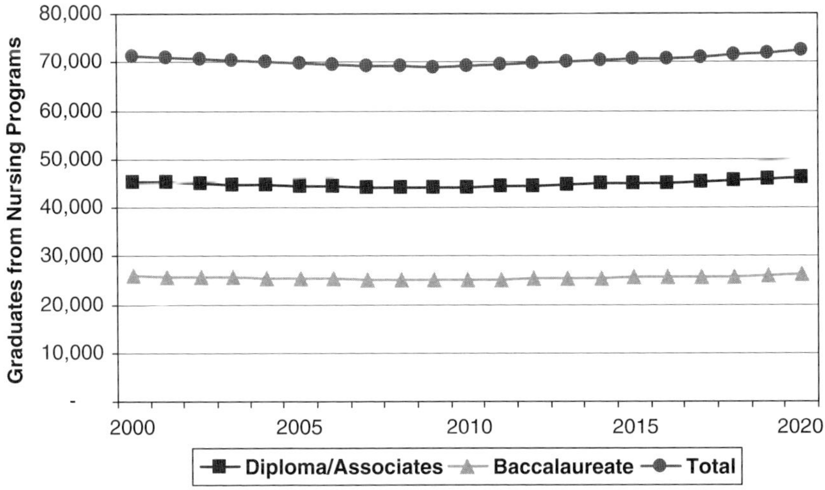

population has important implications for the current and future supply of RNs as labor force participation, cross-state migration, and retirement patterns vary systematically by age and education level.

Over time, the nurse population has continued to age due to the large number of baby boomer nurses, increasing difficulties in attracting new entrants to the profession. Also, the average age of new entrants is increasing (Figure 3).

Labor Force Participation

The RN supply is defined as the licensed RN population who provide nursing services or are seeking employment in nursing. The supply estimate excludes RNs who are licensed but not working in the nursing field (e.g., retired RNs who retain a license, RNs who have temporarily left the workforce, and licensed RNs employed in non-nursing positions). Responses to the NSSRN are somewhat subjective, with individual respondents determining whether they are employed in a nursing position. The NSM applies national rates of labor force participation, by RN age and education level, to the projected licensed RN population in each state to project nurse supply (Figure 4).

In a recent survey of approximately 7,300 licensed nurses (ANA, 2001), 672 respondents who were not currently working in a nursing position stated reasons for their decision not to work in a nursing position. Approximately 25% found their current position more rewarding professionally, 20% cited better

Figure 3: Trend in Age Distribution of the RN Population

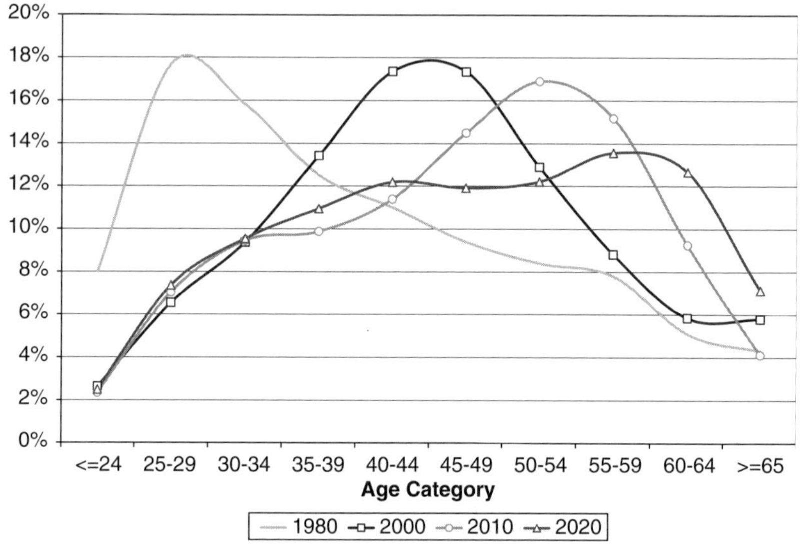

Figure 4: Labor Force Participation Rates of Licensed RNs, by Age and Highest Educational Attainment

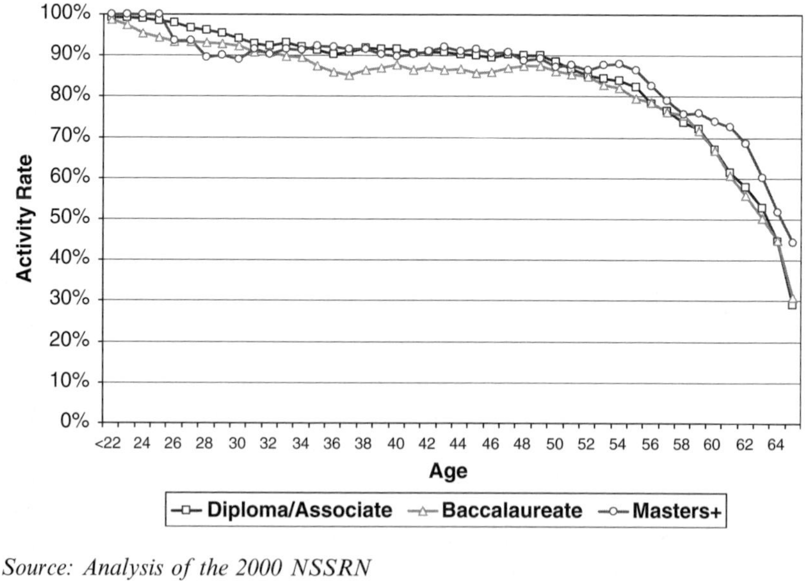

Source: Analysis of the 2000 NSSRN

salaries in their current position, 20% reported more convenient work hours in their current position, and 18% cited personal safety concerns with working in a healthcare environment. If these estimates are representative of the entire licensed nurse workforce, then of the approximately 136,000 licensed RNs in 2000 employed in non-nursing positions (BHPr, 2001), an estimated

- 34,000 would find their current position more rewarding professionally,
- 27,000 would cite better salaries in their current position,
- 27,000 would report more convenient work hours in their current position, and
- 24,000 would cite personal safety concerns with working in a healthcare environment.

Only 70% of nurses in 2000 report being satisfied in their current position, which is significantly lower than U.S. workers in general (85%) and professionals in particular (90%) (BHPr, 2001). Job satisfaction among RNs was lowest in nursing homes and hospitals, and highest in nursing education. Thus, of the approximately 2.2 million RNs employed in nursing in 2000, an estimated 672,000 were dissatisfied with their work.

The NSM software contains algorithms that allow the user the potential to model changes in labor force participation rates over time based on projected changes in RN compensation and working conditions. There exists a paucity of research, however, identifying appropriate measures of working conditions and the impact of changes in these factors on RN labor force participation.

The NSM also projects the FTE supply of RNs by applying FTE labor force participation rates that vary by RN age and education level (Figure 5). The FTE supply counts RNs who are working full time in nursing as 1 FTE, and RNs working part time as 0.5 FTEs.

Cross-State Migration Patterns

Nurses migrate between states for better career opportunities, because of change in location of spouses' employment, and for many other reasons. Some states are net exporters of RNs — i.e., more RNs leave than enter the state in a given year — while other states are net importers. The NSM estimates the number of RNs who will leave or enter the state each year by applying migration probabilities that vary by RN age, education level, and state. We estimated these migration probabilities by estimating a probit model using data from the 1992, 1996, and 2000 NSSRN. The NSSRN asks survey participants in which state they resided at the time of the survey and one year prior to the survey. Nurses who change states between the survey date and the preceding year are identified as cross-state migrants. The probit model

Figure 5: FTE Labor Force Participation Rates of Licensed RNs, by Age and Highest Educational Attainment

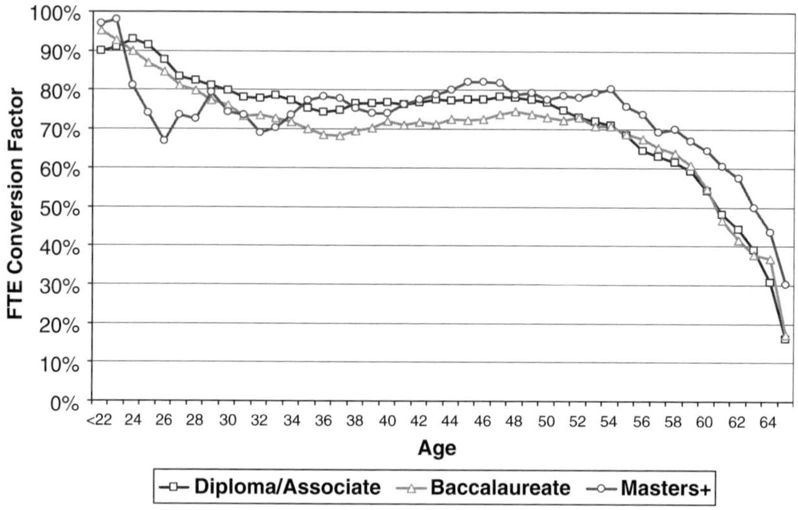

Source: Analysis of the 2000 NSSRN

estimates the probability of leaving (or entering) a particular state as a function of RN age, education level, and state of residence. The model first estimates the number of nurses leaving each state by age and education level. Then, the model allocates this pool of migrating nurses to each state based on immigration probabilities that vary by state, RN age, and RN education level.

RNs prepared at the masters level or higher are more likely to migrate than are RNs prepared at the baccalaureate level, who in turn are more likely to migrate than are RNs with a diploma or associate degree (Figure 6). The analysis also shows significant variation across states in migration patterns. Younger RNs are more likely to migrate across states than are older RNs, reflecting factors such as greater transience among professionals early in their career as they seek employment after graduation.

Change in Educational Attainment

Some RNs will continue their schooling and thus move to a higher education category during the year. The NSM tracks two types of education upgrades: RNs prepared at the diploma or associate level who earn a baccalaureate degree, and RNs prepared at the baccalaureate level who earn a masters or higher degree. The probability that an RN will upgrade his or her education level varies by age, as shown in Figure 7, and was estimated using a probit model and data from the 1992, 1996, and 2000 NSSRN.

Figure 6: Probability of Cross-State Migration, by Age and Education Level

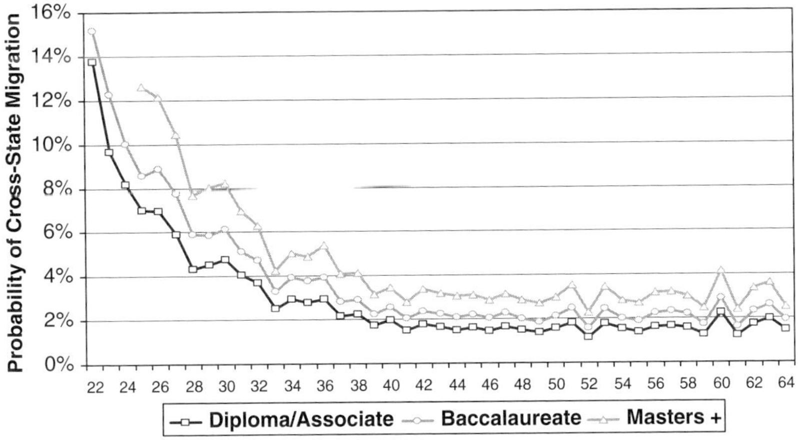

Source: Analysis of the 1992, 1996 and 2000 NSSRN
Note: Probability of immigration and emigration varies by state.

Figure 7: Percentage of RNs Who Upgrade their Education, by Age

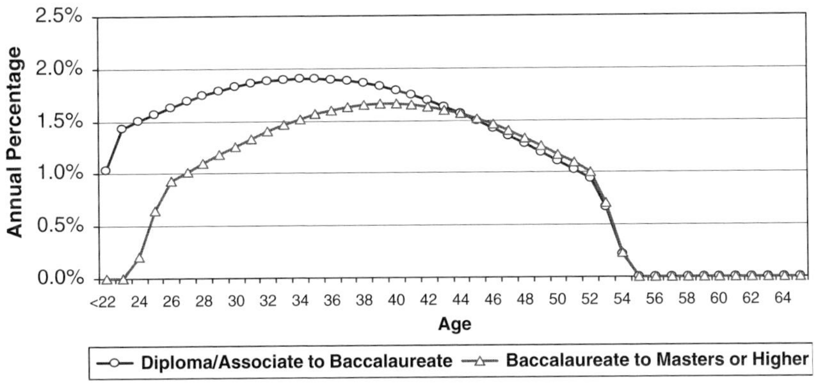

Source: Analysis of the 1992, 1996, and 2000 NSSRN
Note: An analysis of the NSSRN found that very few nurses age 55 and older upgrade their education, and the drop in probability of education upgrade for nurses in their early 50 s reflects this transition to a zero probability

2.3 Permanent Separation from the Nurse Workforce

Reasons why RNs permanently leave the workforce and do not renew their license include retirement, mortality, disability, and other factors. The NSM contains one set of attrition rates that combines all reasons for failing to renew one's license. These rates do not, however, reflect temporary departures from the nurse workforce that are captured through the use of labor force participation rates as described previously.

We constructed separation rates (Figure 8) by combining mortality rates for women obtained from Minino et al. (2002) and estimated rates of attrition for reasons of disability and retirement using data from the 1998, 1999, 2000, and 2001 March surveys of the Current Population Survey (CPS). The CPS collects data on respondents' age, gender, education level, and workforce participation. These workforce departure rates were constructed based on data for all college-educated women in the U.S. There exists a paucity of information on workforce separation rates for RNs, and in particular, the number of RNs who fail to renew their license after changing careers. (The NSSRN only surveys those nurses with an active license.) Anecdotal evidence suggests that many RNs who leave nursing retain their license even when they have no intent of returning to nursing. Nurses who change careers but continue to renew their license are accounted for in our labor force participation and FTE supply rates.

Figure 8: Workforce Separation Rates for College-Educated Women

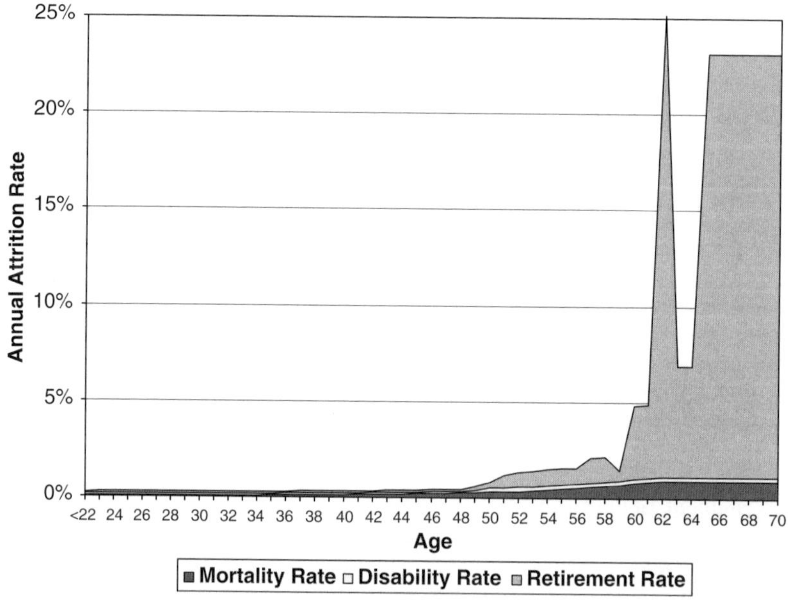

Source: Analysis of the 1998–2001 CPS files; mortality rates from Minino et al. (2002)

2.4 Nursing Supply Projections

Baseline Projections

The NSM baseline projections reflect the level of RN supply that is most likely to occur if current trends continue. At the national level, the number of licensed RNs is projected to remain relatively constant at about 2.7 million nurses between 2000 and 2020. The number of licensed RNs is projected to increase slightly through 2012, but then to start declining as the number of retiring RNs exceeds the number of new graduates. The number of RNs who are active in nursing is projected to remain between 2.1 and 2.3 million during this period, while the FTE supply of RNs is projected to decrease slightly from 1.89 million in 2000 to 1.81 million in 2020. At the state level, there is substantial variation in the growth (or decline) of the RN population between 2000 and 2020 based on the number of new RN graduates in each state, net cross-state migration, and attrition from the RN population (Table 1).

To assess the sensitivity of the model to key determinants of RN supply, we projected supply under alternative scenarios where we vary key assumptions.

Scenario 1: Change in Output from Nursing Programs

Under the baseline projections, the year-to-year percentage change in the number of graduates from nursing programs in each state is directly proportional to percentage change in the size of the states' female population age 20–44 (which as discussed previously is used as a proxy for the size of the pool of nursing school candidates). The NSM uses state-level estimates of

Table 1: Baseline RN Projections: 2000–2020 (In thousands)

	2000	2005	2010	2015	2020	% Change 2000–2020
Licensed RNs	2,697	2,752	2,795	2,781	2,705	0
RNs providing nursing services or seeking employment in nursing	2,249	2,303	2,305	2,250	2,163	−4
FTE RNs providing nursing services	1,891	1,943	1,941	1,886	1,808	−4

Figure 9: FTE Supply Implications of Changes in Projected Number of New Graduates from U.S. Nursing Programs. (Additional information on the Registered Nurse Demand Model is available in the section, Model 17, pages 527–531.)

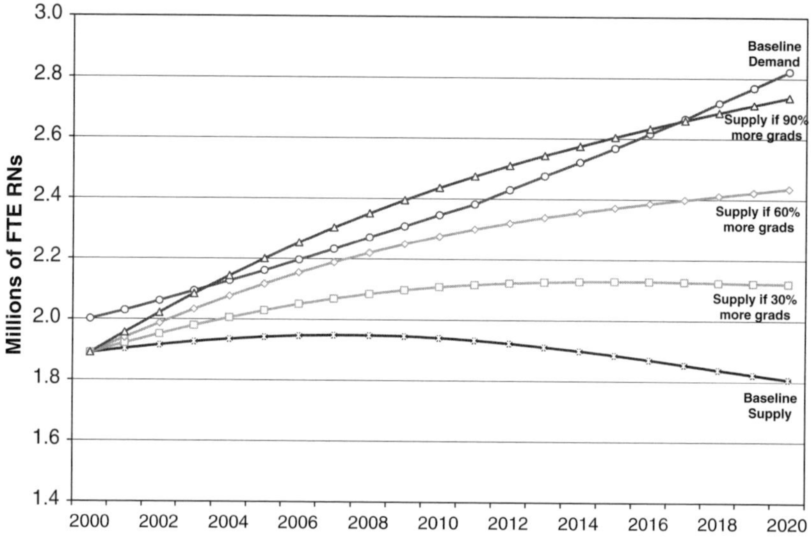

new RN graduates in 2000 as the starting point for the projections. Figure 9 shows projections of the FTE RN supply under alternative scenarios where the number of graduates from U.S. nursing programs, relative to the baseline projections, is 30%, 60%, and 90% higher year after year. Over time, the difference in projected total FTEs between each scenario grows such that by 2020 the difference in totals FTEs, relative to the baseline projections, is +314,000, +628,000, and +929,000 for, respectively, the +30%, +60% and +90% scenarios. *To meet projected growth in demand for RN services, the U.S. needs to graduate approximately 90% more nurses from U.S. nursing programs relative to the baseline graduate projections.*

Scenario 2: Change in RN Wages

If wages for nursing services increase relative to wages in alternative occupations then, all else being equal, nursing becomes a more attractive career. In the short run, an increase in wages for nursing services would increase the FTE RN supply by motivating

- Licensed RNs not practicing nursing to return to nursing,
- Part-time RNs to work more hours, and
- RNs to delay retirement or leave retirement.

The short-term percentage increase in FTE RN supply attributed to each 1% increase in wages for nursing services is referred to as *short-term wage elasticity of supply*.

In the long run, an increase in wages for nursing services will also attract new entrants to the nursing workforce (assuming there are no constraints on nursing school capacity). Because of the time to recognize an increase in RN wages and the time to train new nurses, a delay of several years is expected between the time that RN wages increase and any increase in new entrants to the nursing profession. The *long-term wage elasticity of supply*, consequently, is larger than the short-term wage elasticity of supply.

There exists a paucity of research that estimates the wage elasticity of supply for nurses, and the few studies that have been published report a large range of elasticity estimates. One challenge when assessing the validity of these estimates for modeling the supply of RNs is to distinguish between short-term and long-term wage elasticities, and to distinguish between market wage elasticities and wage elasticities specific to a particular provider (e.g., if one hospital increases RN wages then that hospital will draw nurses away from other hospitals). Sloan and Richupan (1975) obtained wage elasticity estimates for RN labor force participation that ranged from 0.18 to 2.82. Using a sample of Norwegian nurses, Askildsen et al. (2002) estimate wage elasticities for labor force participation ranging from 0.253 to 0.843. For comparison, a review of the literature assessing the military's ability to recruit finds most pay elasticity estimates in the 0.5–1.5 range (Hogan et al., 1995).

For this scenario, we assume annual growth in RN wages, relative to wage growth in alternative occupations, of 0% (the assumption in the baseline projections), +1%, +2% and +3% annually between 2000 and 2020.[3] The wage growth rates have a compounding effect over time, so a 1% growth rate over a 20-year period means that by 2020 wages of RNs would have increased, relative to other occupations, by 22%. We assume that each 1% increase in wages increases the number of RN graduates by 0.8% and increases labor force participation rates by 0.3%. By 2020, relative to the baseline projections, the number of FTE RNs is +228,000 (+13%), +518,000 (+29%), and +886,000 (+49%), respectively, for the scenarios with 1%, 2%, and 3% annual growth in real wages (Figure 10).

The baseline demand projections, which are discussed in more detail later, assume that RN wages will grow at the same rate as wages of LPNs and other healthcare occupations. If RN wages were to rise faster than, say, LPNs, then employers of nurses would have a financial incentive to

[3] An annual survey of RN salaries finds that RN hourly earnings increased by nearly 7%, on average, between 2002 and 2003 (Robinson and Mee, 2003).

Figure 10: Projected FTE RN Supply Under Alternative Wage Growth Scenarios

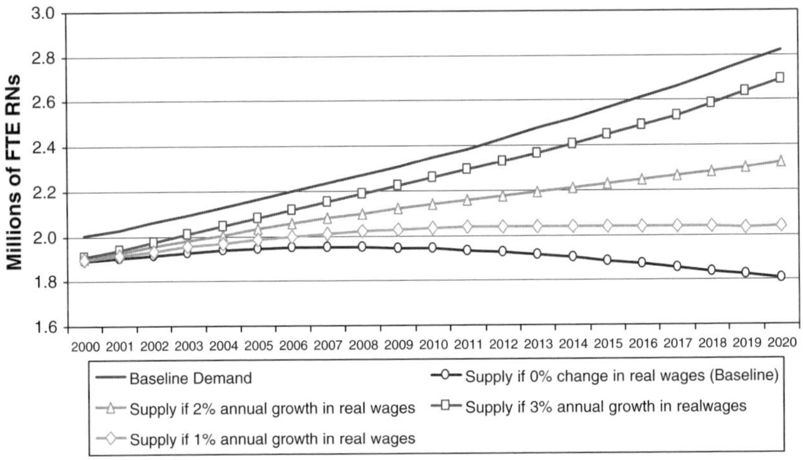

Note: Projections assume wage elasticities of 0.8 for new graduates and 0.3 for FTE labor force participation rates.

substitute lower-cost LPNs for higher-cost RNs, where feasible. *Assuming each 1% real increase in RN wages increases the number of new RN graduates by 0.8% and increases FTE activity rates by 0.3%, then a continuous 3% annual increase in RN wages would still result in a shortfall of approximately 100,000 FTE RNs but would prevent the shortage from growing more severe.*

Scenario 3: Change in RN Retirement Patterns

The rate at which RNs permanently separate from the RN workforce varies by age and education level, with high rates of departure between age 62 and 65 as nurses qualify for Social Security and Medicare benefits. Using the NSM, we project RN supply if each RN were to work an additional four years before retiring. Delays in average retirement age might occur as a result of (1) government policies delaying eligibility for Social Security and Medicare, (2) a healthier population able to remain longer in the workforce, or (3) improvements to RN working conditions that increase the propensity that nurses will remain active in the workforce. Compared to the baseline projections, delaying retirement by an average of four years would increase the FTE supply of RNs by nearly 158,000 (9%) in 2020. Still, such an increase has only a modest effect on alleviating the projected, growing RN shortage (Figure 11).

Figure 11: Impact of Changing Retirement Patterns on FTE Supply of RNs

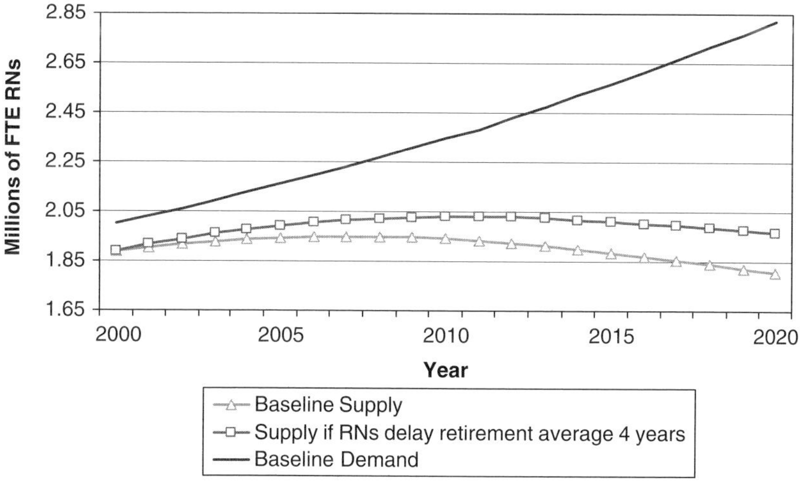

3. Nursing Demand Model

The NDM projects state-level demand for FTE RNs, licensed practical nurses (LPNs) and vocational nurses, and nurse aides (NAs)/auxiliaries and home health aides through 2020. The NDM projects demand for RNs (which is the focus of this paper) in 12 employment settings. Nurse demand is defined as the number of FTE nurses that employers are willing to hire given population needs, economic considerations, the healthcare operating environment, and other factors.

Changing demographics are a key determinant of projected demand for FTE RNs in the baseline scenario. The U.S. Census Bureau projects a rapid increase in the elderly population starting around 2010 when the leading edge of the baby boom generation approaches age 65 (Figure 12). Because the elderly have much greater per capita healthcare needs compared to the non-elderly, the rapid growth in demand for nursing services is especially pronounced for long-term care settings that predominantly provide care to the elderly.

In addition to state-level Census Bureau projections of changing demographics, the NDM projects nurse demand as a function of changing patient acuity, economic factors, and various characteristics of the healthcare operating environment.

The NDM contains two major components: (1) the data and equations to project future demand for healthcare services, and (2) the data and equations to project future nurse staffing intensity.

The model first extrapolates expected utilization of healthcare services by combining national healthcare utilization patterns and state population

Figure 12: Population Growth: 2000 – 2020

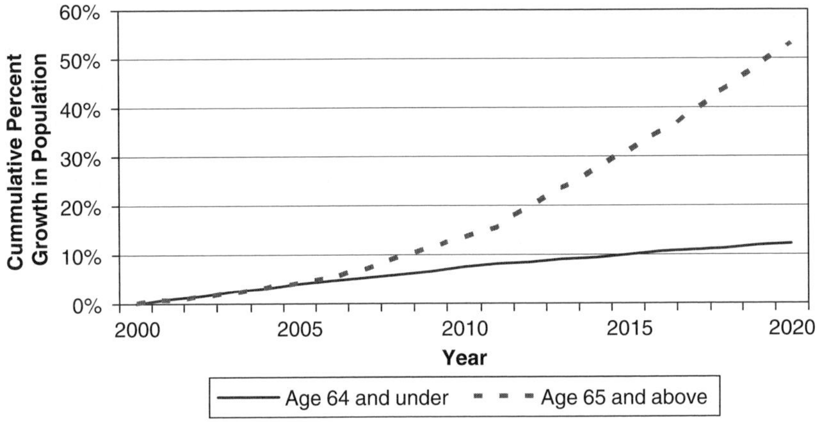

projections by age and gender. Then, the model adjusts the healthcare use extrapolations for each state to account for factors that cause healthcare use to deviate from their expected levels (e.g., state-level variation in managed care enrollment rates).

The model next projects nurse staffing intensity (e.g., FTE RNs per hospital inpatient days) as a function of current staffing intensity and trends in major determinants of nurse staffing intensity (e.g., average patient acuity). Combining projected healthcare utilization (e.g., inpatient days) with projected nurse staffing intensity (e.g., FTE RNs per inpatient day) produces projections of demand for FTE RNs by setting, state, and year. We describe the data, assumptions, and methods used to estimate demand for healthcare services and nurse staffing intensity, and we present our findings. A more complete description of the NDM is available in other reports.[4]

3.1 Modeling Demand for Healthcare Services

The demand for nurses is derived from the demand for healthcare services. To accurately project the future demand for nurses, therefore, one must first project the demand for healthcare services. The NDM projects demand for healthcare services for 6 of the 12 employment settings in the NDM. (For five settings, demand for RNs is projected using RN-per-population

[4] NDM Development and Baseline Projections (NCHWA, forthcoming), NDM User's Guide (NCHWA, forthcoming), and The Nursing Demand-Based Requirements Forecasting Model (Fritz, 1999).

ratios. Demand for nurse educators is projected assuming that nurse educators remain a fixed proportion of total RN demand in each state.) Measures of demand for healthcare services projected by the NDM include inpatient days, outpatient visits, and emergency visits to short-term (ST) hospitals; inpatient days at long-term (LT) hospitals (e.g., psychiatric, rehabilitation, and all other hospitals); nursing facility residents; and home health visits.

The NDM uses a two-step process to make state-level projections of demand for healthcare services for each of the six settings modeled. The first step applies national per capita utilization rates for 32 population subgroups to Census Bureau population projections for each state and year.[5] The 32 population subgroups are defined by eight age categories (ages 0–4, 5–17, 18–24, 25–44, 45–64, 65–74, 75–84, and 85 and above), by gender and by metropolitan or non-metropolitan location.

Multiplying each per capita utilization rate by its respective state-level population projection creates a state-level extrapolation of the *expected* demand for healthcare services that controls for differences across states and over time in demographics. (Step 2 adjusts these extrapolations based on trends in the healthcare operating system and other factors.)

The following equation describes this step, where $\mathbf{EU_{S,H,Y}}$ is the expected level of healthcare utilization in state **S** in healthcare setting **H** in year **Y**. The variables **P** and **R** are, respectively, the size of the population in state **S** and the national per capita healthcare utilization for each age category (**a**), by gender (**s**) and by metropolitan or non-metropolitan location (**l**). The first component of this equation is a calibration factor to ensure that base year estimates of *expected* healthcare utilization equal estimates of *actual* utilization.[6]

[5] To estimate per capita use of healthcare services, we use the 1996 Health Cost Utilization Project (HCUP) database for hospital inpatient services, the 1996 National Hospital Ambulatory Care Survey (NHAMCS) for hospital outpatient and emergency services, the 1997 National Nursing Home Survey (NNHS) for nursing facilities, and the 1995 National Home and Hospice Care Survey (NHHCS) for home health.

[6] Estimates of actual utilization of healthcare services come from multiple sources. The American Hospital Association (AHA) provides state-level estimates of inpatient days, outpatient visits and emergency visits. The American Health Care Association (AHCA) provides state-level estimates of residents in nursing facilities. State-level estimates of home health visits were constructed using data from the Centers for Medicaid and Medicare Services (CMS) and other sources.

$$\mathrm{EU}_{\mathrm{S,H,Y}} = \left(\frac{\mathrm{AU}_{\mathrm{S,H,1996}}}{\sum_{\mathrm{l=urban}}^{\mathrm{rural}} \sum_{\mathrm{s=female}}^{\mathrm{male}} \sum_{\mathrm{a=1}}^{8} \mathrm{P}_{\mathrm{a,s,l,S,1996}} \times \mathrm{R}_{\mathrm{a,s,l,H}}} \right) \times \left(\sum_{\mathrm{l=urban}}^{\mathrm{rural}} \sum_{\mathrm{s=female}}^{\mathrm{male}} \sum_{\mathrm{a=1}}^{8} \mathrm{P}_{\mathrm{a,s,l,S,Y}} \times \mathrm{R}_{\mathrm{a,s,l,H}} \right)$$

Step two adjusts up or down these initial extrapolations of healthcare utilization in each state and year based on projected changes in the healthcare operating environment, economic considerations, and other factors. The utilization adjustment factor differs by state, year, and setting, and is calculated using projection equations whose parameters describe the relationship between healthcare utilization and various exogenous variables.

$$\begin{aligned}\text{Projected Utilization} &= \mathrm{EU}_{\mathrm{S,H,Y}} \times \mathrm{Adjustment}_{\mathrm{S,H,Y}} \\ &= \mathrm{EU}_{\mathrm{S,H,Y}} \times (\beta_0 + \beta_1 \times X_1 + L \\ &\quad + \beta_{\mathrm{k}} \times X_{\mathrm{k}})\end{aligned}$$

We estimated these parameters using multiple regression analysis and a panel data set consisting of state-level data for the period 1996–2000. The dependent variable in the regression equations measures the degree to which actual utilization (AU) of healthcare services deviate from expected utilization (EU) in a given state and setting during the period included in the regression analysis as described in Step 1.

The actual regression equations contain the logged form of the dependent and many of the exogenous variables. Taking the logged form of these variables has two major advantages over the unlogged form. One, using a logged form ensures that the model will not project a negative value of the dependent variable. Two, the coefficients of logged exogenous variables can be interpreted as "elasticities" that represent the percent change in the dependent variable for each 1% change in the exogenous variables (holding constant the other variables in the model). Having the coefficients in a common metric (e.g., elasticities) allows one to more easily compare the magnitude and precision of coefficients between variables, across regression equations, and with empirical findings in the literature. The HMO variable and the region dummy variables are the only variables not in log form.

Selection of the exogenous variables used in the healthcare utilization regressions, as well as those used in the staffing intensity regressions, was based on both theory and empirical analysis.

Several factors complicated the selection of exogenous variables in the

$$\mathrm{Adjustment}_{\mathrm{S,H,Y}} = \left(\frac{\mathrm{AU}}{\mathrm{EU}}\right)_{\mathrm{S,H,Y}}$$

regressions. First, in a few cases an exogenous variable is not statistically significant, though the factor that this variable reflects is presumed essential for developing a dynamic model (e.g., the HMO variable in the equation to estimate RN staffing patterns in hospital inpatient settings). A determination was required whether to include these variables with low statistical significance. In a few cases, variables deemed important that had a level of statistical significance between 0.05 and 0.2 were included in the final regressions. The coefficients on these variables are unbiased despite the lack of precision. These coefficients were closely scrutinized and compared with other findings from this analysis and from the literature to help ensure their reasonableness.

A second complication is that some of the exogenous variables that theory suggests are determinants of the dependent variable — and thus should be considered for inclusion in the equation — are correlated. For example, HMO enrollment rate is correlated with population density, and both HMO enrollment rates and population density might affect healthcare utilization and staffing intensity. (An example of how population density might affect nurse-staffing patterns is that healthcare providers in metropolitan areas might benefit from economies of scale that might not be realized in rural areas.) Multicollinearity among the exogenous variables means that their independent effects might not be precisely estimated even though the estimated effects are unbiased. Also, the stepwise regression approach might result in one variable forcing a correlated variable from the equation. Preliminary regressions were estimated to test the robustness of the regressions with respect to the inclusion or exclusion of correlated variables, and the results helped determine which variables to include or exclude from the final regression specifications.

A third complicating factor is that some regressions contain data from multiple years, and observations from the same state are not completely independent which means there is some heteroskedasticity in the data. Heteroskedasticity can result in underestimates of the coefficient standard errors, which in turn overstates the statistical significance of the coefficients[7]

[7] Preliminary analyses to control for heteroskedasticity included the estimation of "difference-in-differences" models, using regression analysis, to control for state fixed effects. In these regressions, both the dependent and exogenous variables are transformed so that the estimate for each state in a particular year is that years' deviation from the state's multi-year average. One important limitation of the difference-in-differences approach is that it eliminates cross-state variation in the dependent and exogenous variables, which is an important source of information for estimating the relationship between healthcare use and its determinants. For example, HMO enrollment rates vary substantially across states, but in a given state may change little over the few years included in the regression analysis. Many of the exogenous variables that were statistically significant in the difference-in-differences models are the same variables used in the NDM's final projection equations.

The dependent and exogenous variables in the equations are estimates based on hospital census data and surveys of patients and healthcare providers. The concern that estimates for smaller states are less precise than estimates for larger states led to the decision to weight each observation in the regression by the square root of the states' population.

Multiple regression analysis provides estimates of the relationship between healthcare use and its determinants. Note that the regressions predict the relationship between healthcare utilization and its determinants *after* adjusting for differences in the demographic composition by age category, gender, and urban or rural location.

3.2 Modeling Nurse Staffing Intensity

Nurse staffing intensity is defined as the number of FTE nurses divided by some measure of workload specific to the setting being modeled (e.g., FTE nurses per 1,000 inpatient days at ST hospitals). The NDM calculates base year values of nurse staffing intensity for each state and setting by dividing estimates of RN employment by estimates of healthcare utilization. Thus, in nursing facilities, base year estimates of employed FTE nurses per resident are used as the staffing intensity measures.

We use 1996 as the base year for several reasons. First, the importance of the SSRN in estimating base year RN supply and demand limits the base year to a year in which the SSRN was conducted (e.g., 1992, 1996, 2000). Second, indications that the current nurse shortage has grown more severe in recent years suggests that an earlier year (e.g., 1996 vs. 2000) might produce nurse staffing intensity estimates that reflect a market where there was a relative equilibrium between nurse supply and demand. We make one exception to the argument that nurse employment in a setting is the best measure of nurse requirements. In hospitals, we estimate that RN demand was approximately 7% higher than RN employment in 1996. The lower than demanded number of RNs employed in hospitals reflects the rapid and significant changes taking place in the hospital sector during the early and mid 1990s when hospitals were downsizing in response to the rapid rise in managed care and hospital consolidations. We arrive at this 7% estimate by comparing RN staffing intensity in hospitals using SSRN and American Hospital Association (AHA) data for 1992, 1996, and 2000.

After establishing base year nurse staffing intensity, the NDM then projects future nurse staffing intensity. For four employment settings, nurse staffing intensity is measured as a nurse-to-population ratio (because of data limitations) that is assumed constant over time. Demand for nurse educators is calculated as a constant fraction of total demand for RNs. For 7 of the 12 employment settings modeled, future nurse staffing intensity is projected as a function of changes in exogenous variables (X) such as average patient acuity levels, economic considerations, and characteristics of the healthcare operating environment. The projection formula is specified:

$$\frac{\text{FTE RNs}_{\text{S,H,Y}}}{\text{Workload Measures}_{\text{S,H,Y}}} = \delta_{S,H}(\beta_0 + \beta_1 \times X_1 + \cdots + \beta_k \times X_k)$$

where the parameters β represent the estimated relationship between nurse staffing intensity and its determinants and δ an adjustment factor so that the base year projections equal actual nurse staffing intensity in the base year. The parameters were estimated using multiple regression analysis with state-level data from 1996 through 2000 (although most regression equations were estimated using a subset of these years based on data availability).

Both theory and empirical analysis helped determine which exogenous variables to use in the projection equations. Also, as with the healthcare utilization regressions, the dependent variable and most of the exogenous variables enter into the regression equation in a log form. Also, the equations were estimated using a stepwise regression that results in a parsimonious model but that overstate the significance statistics often used to assess how robust are the regression findings.

Nurse Wages

The ratio of RN to LPN wages is used to estimate the degree to which employers substitute lower-cost LPNs for higher-cost RNs as RN wages rise relative to LPN wages.[8] In the baseline projections, we assume that this ratio stays constant over time. The regressions do not simultaneously control for nursing supply, which could bias the wage elasticities (ε) toward zero. The size of the estimated elasticities, however, appear reasonable based on a priori expectations and a comparison with the literature. Demand for RNs is less responsive to changing relative wages in doctors' offices ($\varepsilon = -0.64$) and inpatient settings at ST hospitals ($\varepsilon = -0.65$) compared to home health ($\varepsilon = -1.06$) and LT hospitals ($\varepsilon = -1.20$).

The wages elasticity estimates from this analysis are comparable to the few -studies in the recent literature that report wage elasticities. Lane and Gohmann (1995), in their analysis of nurse shortages, estimate the wage-

[8] The ability of healthcare providers to substitute lower-cost nurses for higher-cost nurses is not simply an economic phenomenon, but also reflects legal and quality considerations. RNs receive special training that enables them to provide certain services that LPNs cannot provide. Thus, there is only a limited range in which substitution could be made without jeopardizing health care delivery quality.

elasticity of nurse demand by simultaneously estimating a supply and demand equation.[9] The authors combine both RNs and LPNs in their analyses. They estimate nurse own-wage elasticity in ST hospitals to be approximately −0.9.

Spetz (1999) estimates a demand equation for RNs using hospital-level data for short-term, general hospitals in California during the period 1976–1994. To control for the endogeneity of nurse wages, Spetz uses an instrumental variables approach to estimate the RN demand curve which she compares to a demand curve estimated using OLS. As expected, her estimate of wage elasticity from the OLS regression ($\varepsilon = -0.194$) is less elastic than the estimate obtained using the instrumental variables approach ($\varepsilon = -2.778$) when she models the daily services units of California hospitals. Similarly, when she estimates demand equations for the medical-surgical units of California hospitals the wage elasticity estimates are less elastic from the OLS regression ($\varepsilon = -0.342$) than from the instrumental variables regression ($\varepsilon = -3.653$). Spetz also finds that an increase in LPN wages is associated with a statistically significant rise in RN employment in daily service units of hospitals, but the converse is not true.

As discussed previously in the context of RN supply, in the short-term wage demand elasticities are typically smaller than long-term wage elasticities. In the short term, employers might have few options to replace RNs as they become relatively more expensive. In the long term, employers can changing nurse staffing practices and adopt new technologies that alter how RNs are used.

- *HMO enrollment rates.* An increase in HMO enrollment rates produces mixed effects on staffing intensity. The HMO variables in the regressions are not logged so the interpretation of the coefficients is different from the other variables. An increase in the HMO enrollment rate by 1 percentage point increases RN staffing intensity in ST hospital inpatient, ST hospital outpatient, and home health by 0.30, 0.67, and 0.97%, respectively. An increase in the HMO enrollment rate by 1 percentage point decreases RN staffing intensity in doctor's offices by 0.51%.
- *Possible reasons why HMO enrollment rates affect nurse-staffing patterns.* One, HMOs decrease inpatient days in ST hospitals through efforts at

[9] Lane and Gohmann estimate nurse supply and demand simultaneously using two approaches: (1) a two stage least squares model, and (2) a "switching" model that relaxes the assumption that the market for hospital nurses is in equilibrium. The authors report an own-wage elasticity of demand of −1.14 when using the two stage least squares model, but they believe the estimate of −0.92 from the switching model to be more accurate.

preventive care and efforts to channel patients with less-severe problems to less expensive settings. This reduction in inpatient days might be raising the average acuity level of patients who are admitted to the hospital, which results in higher RN staffing per 1,000 inpatient days. Two, the efforts of HMOs to reduce costs could contribute to their adopting technologies or substituting between different types of healthcare professionals. As discussed previously, HMO enrollment rates are correlated with other variables such as the percent of population in urban area. Consequently, the coefficient on the HMO enrollment rate variable could be capturing some of the relationship between staffing intensity and other factors correlated with HMO enrollment rates. In both regressions where HMO enrollment rate affects staffing intensity, the variable percent of population in urban area is also included.

- *Hospital inpatient and outpatient surgeries.* Changes in technology can have a mixed effect on the demand for healthcare services and staffing intensity. One measure used in the NDM that reflects, in part, technological advances is the percentage of hospital-based surgical procedures performed on an outpatient basis. Improvements in technology and medical procedures that shift some surgical procedures from an inpatient to an outpatient setting could affect nurse-staffing intensity in both the inpatient and outpatient setting. If patients with less severe health problems are shifted from an inpatient to an outpatient setting, then average patient acuity in both settings could rise. This situation could result in greater staffing intensity per inpatient day and per outpatient visit while decreasing overall nurse demand. Each 1% increase in the proportion of hospital surgeries performed in an outpatient setting increases staffing intensity for FTE RNs per 1,000 ST hospital inpatient days by 0.64%. As discussed previously, a 1% increase in the proportion of hospital-based surgeries performed on an outpatient basis reduces ST hospital inpatient days by 0.47%, increases outpatient visits by 1.64%, and increases home health visits by 1.86%. Surprisingly, the net effect of a 1% increase in this surgery variable causes virtually no change in overall demand for RNs — it just shifts where the RNs are providing services.
- *Healthcare reimbursement rates.* A rise in average Medicare and Medicaid payments for services is associated with greater staffing intensity. Part of this increase might be due to greater patient acuity, and part might be due to the ability of healthcare providers to purchase nursing services. A 1% increase in average Medicare payments per home health visit increases demand for RNs by 1%. A 1% increase in average Medicaid daily rates for nursing facilities increases staffing intensity of RNs in nursing facilities by 0.34%.
- *Percent of population uninsured.* The rate of uninsured in the population could increase the level of uncompensated care provided by healthcare providers. A 1% increase in the proportion of the population that is uninsured decreases RNs per 1,000 ST hospital inpatient days by 0.37% and decreases RNs per 1,000 visits to doctor's offices by 0.21%. RN per 1,000

inpatient days in LT hospitals rises by 0.3% for each 1% increase in the rate of uninsured, although the reason for this positive relationship is not readily surmised.

- *Percent of population medicaid eligible.* A 1% rise in the proportion of the population that is Medicaid eligible decreases RN staffing per 1,000 emergency department visits by 0.19%. As discussed in the previous section, a 1% rise in the percent of the population that is Medicaid eligible increases demand for emergency department services by 0.29% so the net effect of a 1% rise in this variable is to increase demand for RNs in emergency departments by 0.05%.
- *Per capita personal income.* As the population grows wealthier, the demand for higher quality healthcare services is likely to rise. A 1% rise in per capita income increases RN staffing intensity in doctors' offices by 0.33%.
- *Patient acuity levels.* A population with greater healthcare requires greater levels of services as measured by both the quantity of services provided and staffing intensity per unit of service provided. The NDM contains two measures that are proxies of population health status: (1) the mean age of the population, and (2) the average number of ADL limitations of nursing facility residents. (In addition, the Medicare and Medicaid).

Changes in staffing intensity will vary by state depending on the projected values for exogenous variables and changing demographics. Between 2000 and 2020 staffing intensity is projected to increase 34% in home health, from approximately 2.8 FTE RNs per 1,000 home health visits to approximately 3.8 FTE RNs per 1,000 visits. In ST hospital inpatient settings, FTE RNs per 1,000 inpatient days is projected to increase by 18% at the national level (from 6.5 up to 7.7). For nursing facilities and doctor's offices, we project a 13% increase in staffing intensity, while for ST hospital outpatient settings we project a 6% increase in staffing intensity. We project virtually no change in staffing intensity in ST hospital emergency settings and in LT hospitals. The staffing intensity measures for RNs in occupational health, school health, public health, nurse education, and "other" healthcare settings is assumed constant over time at their 1996 levels.

The overall impact of staffing intensity must be considered in conjunction with healthcare utilization projections to fully comprehend the magnitude of additional RN FTE's required.

3.3 Nursing Demand Projections

Baseline Projections

Under the baseline scenario, demand for FTE RNs is projected to increase 41% between 2000 and 2020 at the national level. In percentage terms, the fastest growth will occur in settings that predominantly serve the elderly (e.g., home health and nursing facilities) and in hospital outpatient settings (Table 2).

Alternative Scenarios

Future nurse demand will be determined, in part, by political decisions, changes in technology, changes in the healthcare operating environment and changes in other factors that are difficult to predict. In addition, projection models such as the NDM are relatively simplistic simulations of a complex healthcare system that try to capture the major trends affecting demand for nurses, so the RN demand projections are made with some level of imprecision. The degree of imprecision is difficult to determine. A sensitivity analysis shows how the projections change as we change key assumptions in the model. We present projections under four alternative scenarios (Figure 13):

- Scenario 1 assumes no changes in managed care enrollment rates (compared to the baseline that assumes an annual 0.5 percentage point increase). At the national level across all settings, this modest change in the growth rate of managed care enrollment has virtually no effect on demand for RNs. There are, however, substantial changes at the setting level. Managed care growth simply shifts care from inpatient to outpatient settings, and the decline in projected inpatient days is offset by a likely increase in staffing intensity as the average level of patient acuity increases.
- Scenario 2 assumes that RN wages increase 1% annually compared to LPN wages. (The baseline assumes that RN and LPN wages grow at the same rate.) Under this scenario, a rise in RN wages gives employers greater financial incentive to substitute lower-cost LPNs for higher-cost RNs, where possible. Between 2000 and 2020, the compounding effect of a 1% annual growth in relative wages for RNs results in a real increase of 22% relative to wages of LPNs. By 2020, demand for FTE RNs would be approximately 10% lower (or 285,000 FTE RNs) relative to the baseline.
- Scenario 3 assumes that the U.S. population grows 20% faster than projected by the Census Bureau. By 2020, this results in the demand for an additional 88,000 FTE RNs (or 3%) relative to the baseline.
- Scenario 4 assumes that the U.S. population grows 20% slower than projected by the Census Bureau. By 2020, this results in the demand for 85,000 fewer FTE RNs (or 3%) relative to the baseline.

4. Assessing the Adequacy of Future Supply

Comparing the baseline supply and demand projections suggests that the U.S. has a shortage of approximately 168,000 FTE RNs in 2003, implying

Table 2: Baseline Projections of FTE Demand for RNs

Setting	2000	2005	2010	2015	2020	% Increase 2000–2020
Hospitals[a]	1,239,500	1,324,800	1,427,900	1,555,600	1,698,900	37
ST hospitals, inpatient	874,700	930,200	999,100	1,086,800	1,187,000	36
ST hospitals, outpatient	83,500	95,900	110,400	126,400	142,000	70
ST hospitals, emergency	90,300	92,200	94,500	97,300	100,400	11
LT hospitals	191,000	206,500	223,900	245,100	269,400	41
Nursing facilities	172,800	197,200	224,500	253,600	287,300	66
Doctors' offices	155,000	166,400	178,800	191,600	204,700	32
Home health	132,000	157,300	187,500	226,200	275,600	109
Occupational health	20,200	21,000	22,000	23,100	23,900	18
School health	57,600	59,700	60,400	61,100	62,200	8
Public health	99,800	103,500	107,300	111,500	115,800	16
Nurse education	45,900	49,600	53,800	58,800	64,500	41
Other healthcare	78,500	81,700	84,900	88,400	92,000	17
Total[a]	2,001,500	2,161,300	2,347,100	2,569,800	2,824,900	41

[a] *Category totals might not equal the summation across component settings due to rounding.*

Figure 13: Projected Demand for FTE RNs Under Alternative Scenarios

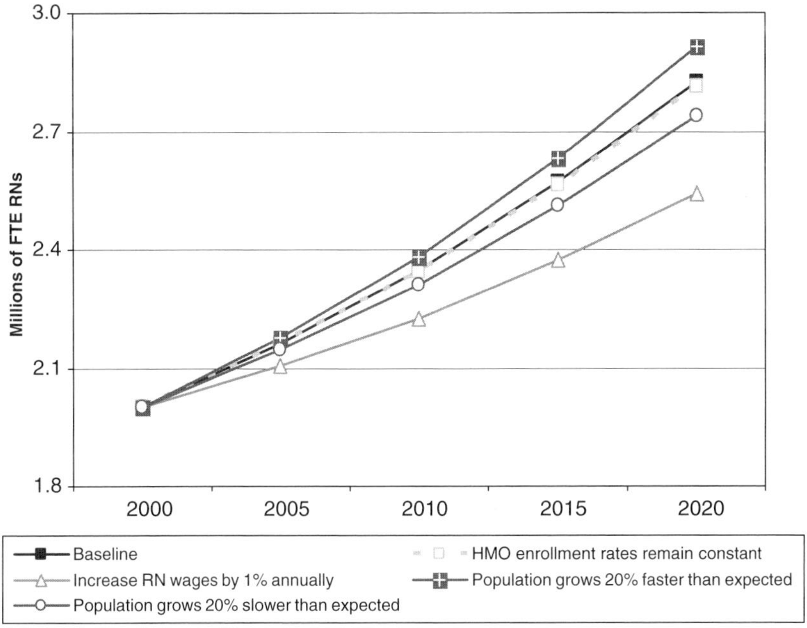

that the current supply would need to increase by 9% to meet estimated demand (Figure 14). By 2020 the national shortage is projected to increase to over one million FTE RNs, if current trends continue, suggesting that only 64% of projected demand will be met (Table 3).

The supply and demand projections most likely bound the range of the actual number of FTE RNs who will be employed over the projection horizon. As the nursing shortage becomes more severe, market and political forces will create pressures that either will increase supply, decrease demand, or both.

State-level shortages will vary substantially over time and across states. As the nurse shortage in any particular state becomes too severe, market forces will create financial incentives for nurses to migrate to states with more severe shortages.

5. Limitations of the Models and Areas for Future Research

The NSM and NDM are built on a theoretical foundation supported by empirical research. Still, efforts to update and enhance both models faced numerous challenges — many due to data limitations. Below we describe

Figure 14: Projected U.S. FTE RN Shortages: 2000 to 2020.

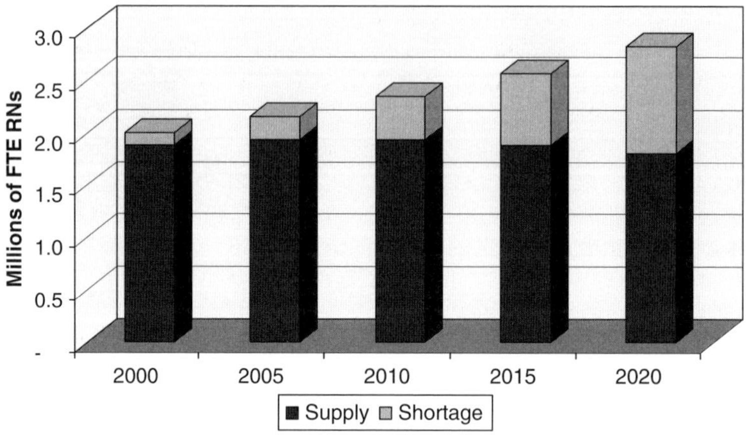

Table 3: Projected U.S. FTE RN Supply, Demand and Shortages

	2000	2005	2010	2015	2020
Supply	1,890,700	1,942,500	1,941,200	1,886,100	1,808,000
Demand	2,001,500	2,161,300	2,347,000	2,569,800	2,824,900
Shortage	(110,800)	(218,800)	(405,800)	(683,700)	(1,016,900)
Supply/Demand	94%	90%	83%	73%	64%
Demand Shortfall	6%	10%	17%	27%	36%

limitations of the two models and suggest areas for research that could address these limitations. Such research could improve the theoretical underpinnings of the models and improve the precision of key parameters in the model.

The NSM and the NDM are independent models. The demand model make projections without considering the potential supply of nurses, and vice versa. The future nurse workforce, in reality, will be influenced by the combination of supply and demand. A rising demand for nursing services at a time when supply is flat or falling will place upward pressures on nurse wages, which in turn will induce more supply. Rising nurse wages, on the other hand, will place downward pressures on demand for nurses. This phenomenon will occur at both the national and local level. A national shortage will tend to increase RN wages, both in real terms and relative to other occupations, across the nation. This rise in wages would increase the number of new graduates, increase employment participation rates, and delay retirement for some nurses — all actions that will increase supply.

Local shortages, on the other hand, could increase nurse wages locally contributing to local increases in the number of nurse graduates and an increase in the number of nurses migrating to that locality.

Both models use the NSSRN to estimate the number of RNs employed in the base year. The NSM uses the 2000 NSSRN to estimate the supply of RNs by age, education level and state. The NDM uses the 1996 NSSRN to estimate the number of FTE RNs by setting and state. Because the precision of estimates is proportional to sample size, the RN supply and employment estimates for the base year become less precise the smaller the unit of aggregation. Consequently, the base-year starting values and projections for future years are less precise the smaller the unit of analysis. For example, estimates of demand for RNs in a particular setting within a state likely will be less precise than the state-level estimates, which in turn likely will be less precise than the national-level estimates.

One criticism of many attempts to model nurse demand is the limited consideration of important determinants of nursing demand (see, for example, Dumpe et al., (1998); Prescott (2000)). Projections models such as the NDM and NSM are scaled-down versions of complex systems. Data and resource limitations prevented building models that include a wider array of determinants to better model the complexities of the supply of and demand for RN. Consequently, there are many determinants of RN supply and demand that are not included in these models. Still, these models attempt to account for the major trends affecting the supply of and demand for RNs and project future supply and demand under a set of assumptions that is an educated guess at whether current trends will continue in the future.

Regarding the NDM, we use state-level data to estimate the relationship between demand for RNs and its determinants. One consequence of using state-level data is that there are relatively few degrees of freedom for estimating the regression equations. Future efforts might investigate the use of alternative approaches or lower levels of data aggregation to estimate the relationship between healthcare use and its determinants, and between staffing intensity and its determinants.

Additional research could provide estimates of key parameters that improve the accuracy of the models and make the models more flexible policy tools. The NSM, for example, was built with the capacity to model the RN supply implications of changes in nurse wages, working conditions, tuition costs, and the number of nursing school faculty. The empirical research has yet to be conducted to estimate the parameters necessary to utilize these features.

The NSM models only the supply of RNs and, unlike the NDM, does not consider LPNs and nurse aides. The adequacy of the LPN supply has implications for both the supply of and demand for RNs. On the demand side, employers have some ability to substitute between RNs and LPNs — taking into consideration legal and practical constraints. On the supply side, some LPNs seek further training to become RNs. Using the 2000 NSSRN, we estimate that approximately 9.5% of the RN workforce, or 257,784 RNs, were employed as LPNs prior to starting their basic nurse education. The RN and LPN workforces are competing for the same candidates. Many of the people who are candidates for nurses could become either RNs or LPNs. Consequently, policies designed to recruit more RNs could have the unintended consequence of reducing the LPN supply.

Parts of both models are static. In the NSM, for example, the probability of cross-state migration is based on historical patterns that do not consider the current shortage of RNs in each state. The NDM has limited ability to model substitution between types of nurses and between nurses and other healthcare workers. The NDM does model substitution between RNs and LPNs if their relative wages change, but future research might look at other ways to incorporate substitution effects. Similarly, the NDM has limited ability to capture the interaction of healthcare settings. For example, some settings might be viable substitutes (e.g., home health vs. nursing facilities), while other settings might be complementary (e.g., increased use of outpatient services leading to the increased use of home health services).

Despite the limitations identified here, the value of the NSM and NDM remain unquestionable and provide two important benefits. First, the NSM and NDM serve as an early warning system capable of identifying shortages and describing their causes. In the current situation, the two models help quantify the growing shortage of RNs as the aging population increases demand for nursing services at the same time that an aging RN workforce and difficulties attracting new entrants to the nursing profession portent relatively little growth in the national supply of RNs. The second benefit of the NSM and NDM is that they provide policy makers with information that can lead to the development of various options for reducing demand or increasing supply and provide the ability to examine the relative value of these options. It is the ability to provide policy makers with tools for addressing shortages that make the NSM and NDM so valuable.

References

American Hospital Association. *Hospital Statistics*. Various years.

American Nurses Association. (2001). *Analysis of American Nurses Association Staffing Survey*. Presentation by Cornerstone Communications Group on February 6, 2001. Available from http://nursingworld.org/staffing/ana_pdf.pdf. Accessed November 2003.

Askildsen, J.E., Baltagi, B.H. and Holmas, T.H. (2002). Will Increased Wages Reduce Shortage of Nurses? A Panel Data Analysis of Nurses' Labor Supply. Unpublished manuscript. Available from http://www.eco.rug.nl/~espe2002/Askildsen.pdf. Accessed November 2006.

Buerhaus, P.I., Staiger, D.O. and Auerbach, D.I. (2000). Implications of an Aging Registered Nurse Workforce. *Journal of the American Medical Association*, 283(22), 2948–2954.

Bureau of Health Professions. (2001). *The Registered Nurse Population, March 2000: Findings from the National Sample Survey of Registered Nurses*.

Dumpe, M.L., Herman, J. and Young, S.W. (1998). Forecasting the Nursing Workforce in a Dynamic Healthcare Market. *Nursing Economics*, 16(4), 170–179.

Fritz, M.S. (1999). *The Nursing Demand-Based Requirements Forecasting Model*. 10th Federal Forecasters Conference, 1999: Papers and Proceedings.

Hogan, P.F., Dall, T.D., Smith, S.G., Mackin, P.C., Mackie, C.D., Darling, K.L., Harris, D.A., McCloy, R.A. and Statman, M.A. (1995). *Conceptual Framework for Analyzing and Developing a Compensation System*. Report prepared for the Eighth Quadrennial Review of Military Compensation Taskforce.

Lane, J. and Gohmann, S. (1995). Shortage or Surplus: Economic and Non-Economic Approaches to the Analysis of Nursing Labor Markets. *Southern Economic Journal*, 61, 644–654.

Minino, A.M., Arias, E., Kochanek, K.D., Murphy, S.L. and Smith, B.L. (2002). Deaths: Final Data for 2000. *National Vital Statistics Reports*, Vol. 50(15).

National Center for Health Workforce Analysis. (2002). *Projected Supply, Demand, and Shortages of Registered Nurses: 2000–2020*. ftp://ftp.hrsa.gov/bhpr/nationalcenter/rnproject.pdf. Accessed November 2003.

National Center for Health Workforce Analysis. (2004). *NDM User's Guide*. Report prepared by The Lewin Group for the National Center for Health Workforce Analysis.

National Center for Health Workforce Analysis. (2004). *NDM Development and Baseline Projections*. Report prepared by The Lewin Group for the National Center for Health Workforce Analysis.

National Center for Health Workforce Analysis. (2004). *Nursing Supply Model: Technical Report and User Guide*. Report prepared by The Lewin Group for the National Center for Health Workforce Analysis.

Prescott, P.A. (2000). The Enigmatic Nursing Workforce. *Journal of Nursing Administration*, 30(2), 59–65.

Robinson, E.S. and Mee, C.L. (2003). Nursing 2003 Salary Survey. *Nursing 2003*, Vol. 33(10), 50–53 http://www.nursingcenter.com/home/index.asp. Accessed November 2003.

Seago, J.A., Ash, M., Spetz, J., Coffman, J. and Grumbach, K. (2001). Hospital Registered Nurse Shortages: Environmental, Patient, and Institutional Predictors. *Health Services Research*, 36(5), 831–852.

Sloan, F.A. and Richupan, S. (1975). Short-run Supply Responses of Professional Nurses: A Microanalysis. *The Journal of Human Resources, X*,(2), 241–257.

Spetz, J. (1999). The Effects of Managed Care and Prospective Payment on the Demand for Hospital Nurses: Evidence from California. *Health Services Research*, 34(5), 993–1010.

Appendix A: National-Level Supply, Demand and Shortage Projections

TABLE A1: Baseline FTE RN Supply and Demand: 2000, 2005, 2010, 2015, 2020

Year	Supply	Demand	Supply–Demand	Supply/Demand (%)
2000	1,890,700	2,001,500	−110,800	94
2005	1,942,500	2,161,300	−218,800	90
2010	1,941,200	2,347,000	−405,800	83
2015	1,886,100	2,569,800	−683,700	73
2020	1,808,000	2,824,900	−1,016,900	64

Part V: Data Challenges

Chapter 17

Data Quality and Non-Response Effects when Using Logistical Regression in the Welsh Health Survey

Ruth Studley

National Assembly for Wales, Cardiff, Wales, UK

Abstract

The second Welsh Health Survey was conducted in 1998. The aim of the survey was to collect information from groups within the population representing those with a range of illnesses or disabilities and also representing healthy people — without using any medical records. The results provide a picture of health of the people of Wales, the way the National Health Service is used, and areas where service could be improved.

Self-completion questionnaires were sent to over 50,000 adults across Wales. A crude response rate of 60% was achieved. A follow-up non-response questionnaire was conducted and indicated that non-response was non-ignorable. Furthermore, the follow-up survey was conducted using interviewers who were present while the original non-responders completed the questionnaire. The response rate for the follow-up survey was 70%. This paper aims to discuss issues surrounding the data quality and the adjustments used for non-response bias.

A logistical model will be used to fit the weighted data and comparisons will be drawn between adjusting for the non-response and ignoring it. In particular, the model will consider the effect of age on the use of health services such as General Practitioners, hospitals, dentists and the level of patient satisfaction.

1. Introduction

The Welsh Health Survey was conducted in 1998. The objective was to survey a representative cross section of the population of Wales with a view to determining the range of illnesses and disabilities afflicting the Welsh

International Symposia in Economic Theory and Econometrics, Vol. 16

ISSN: 1571-0386 DOI: 10.1016/S1571-0386(06)16017-2

population, without using any medical records. A further outcome of the survey was to gain an understanding of how the National Health Service in Wales is used, and to provide an indication of how satisfied people were with the services supplied, (Welsh Health Survey 1998 (1999)).

This was the second Welsh Health Survey that had been conducted, with the first occurring in 1995. A further health survey is planned for 2003/2004. A substantial amount of the questionnaire used in 1995 was re-used in 1998.

Self-completion questionnaires were sent to just over 50,000 adults aged 18 and over in Wales in May 1998. No deadline for completion of the questionnaires was included, however, by the middle of June 1998 nearly 30,000 forms had been returned. This provided information on the respondents use of the National Health Service, the quality of the service provided, the general health and well-being of the respondents and data on their lifestyle. The questionnaire included the Short Form 36 (SF-36) which are standard questions that can be combined to give outcome measures of physical and mental well-being.

2. The Sample

The sampling frame used was the latest available electoral register, which had been compiled in Autumn 1997. The reason for using this sampling frame was to reduce the amount of non-response associated with frame errors, such as sampled units being non-contactable, e.g. where they had moved or died.

Within Wales there are (and were) 22 unitary authorities. These were grouped to make five health authorities and three regional office areas. To improve the chance for small area estimation, small unitary authorities were over sampled. The minimum target set for each area was 900 respondents, which would assume an overall response rate of 55%. This target was achieved. Over sampling occurred in 7 of the 22 unitary authority areas to achieve this response rate. The remaining sample was a probability proportional to size sample, with the balance of the sample distributed according to the share of the population of adults aged 18 and over.

The sampling fraction, f, was calculated as

$$f = \mathrm{TRUNC}\left(\frac{\sum_{\text{all } i} x_i}{x_i}\right) \tag{1}$$

where x is the total population of adults aged 18 and over in unitary authority area i.

The target sample was 50,000, however, using the above formula meant that the actual sample selected was 50,023. This is equivalent to one in every 45 adults in Wales being selected for the survey.

3. The Survey Questionnaire

A substantial amount of the questionnaire that was used in 1995 was re-used in 1998. This was to ease comparability between the two Welsh Health Surveys. However, areas that were not successful in the 1995 survey were removed or adjusted.

The questionnaire was piloted in two stages. First, a small postal survey was conducted, sampling 265 people from each of four unitary authorities within Wales, adding to 1,060 in all. A total of 605 questionnaires were returned. The unadjusted response rate is almost 60%, but once adjustments had been made for non-contacts, deaths and movers the response rate increased to 63%.

Simultaneously, a pilot survey was being conducted using a difference mode of data collection — face-to-face interviewing. The interviewers showed an amended covering letter and offered the selected respondents the opportunity to complete the questionnaire. Generally, the interviewers were present while the questionnaire was being completed. The data collection mode allowed the interviewers an opportunity to note any problem areas with the questionnaire. Following completion of the questionnaire the interviewers conducted an in-depth discussion to find out where any difficulties with the questionnaire may lay. These findings were then brought together.

Amendments resulting in findings from the pilot survey were made, mainly surrounding the layout of the questionnaire, but there were also some changes made to wording of the questions and coding of the responses.

A help-line was set up to be used during both the pilot survey and the survey proper. Information about non-contacts was kept to ensure that the response rate could be calculated accurately.

The questionnaire asked information on:

- the use and experiences of the National Health Service;
- the use and experiences of the doctor, hospital and Casualty departments;
- the use and experience of the dentist; the use of medicines;
- the views on the respondent's general health;
- the respondent's daily activities;
- the respondent's feelings over the previous four weeks;
- illnesses the respondent may have had;
- exercise the respondent may have taken;
- the use of alcohol and smoking; and
- demographic information about the respondent.

4. Data Collection and Validation

The survey was posted to the sampled units on 1st May 1998. Reminders were sent in the form of a postcard and then a repeat questionnaire on the 25th May 1998 and 18th June 1998, respectively. Different serial numbers were attributed to the questionnaires that were sent out as a reminder to enable analysts to identify the data associated with those responders.

All the questionnaires were treated with the strictest confidence. While there was a separate database which linked the unique identifier of the sampled unit with the questionnaire identifier, this was destroyed in a way that made it irretrievable once the survey proper had been closed. Furthermore, there was no place on the questionnaire to enable respondents to reveal their personal details. Therefore, there was no relationship between the names and addresses of personal replies and the data achieved.

A constraint of the survey was to obtain this information without using medical records. However, the survey questionnaire was copied to all General Practitioners in Wales via the, then, five health authorities. This was to enable General Practitioners to deal with any queries the survey may raise by respondents while in consultation with their family doctor. The survey questionnaire was accompanied by a covering letter from the Chief Medical Officer or Wales stating the purpose for conducting this research.

Of the 50,023 questionnaires that were posted, a response of 29,874 was achieved. There was an unadjusted response rate of just under 60%. Adjustments were made to account for those who had moved, died, were ill, refused to participate or were classed as address unknown. Further information was also made available to the help-line regarding the respondents who were too ill or too elderly, who refused, who had died or moved, who were too young or were on holiday. Those that contacted the help-line with this information totalled to 136, but unfortunately they did not leave details enabling the survey team to attribute them to particular areas. After accounting for those sampled units who had died or moved to the adjusted response rate was 61%.

The returned questionnaires were then coded for Government Social class using the 1991 (OPCS) Standard Occupational Classification. The nature of any complaints about the National Health Service and other services was also coded using the 1995 Welsh Health Survey coding frame.

Data were then validated to remove erroneous data items, for example, questionnaires completed by a 15-year old. The data quality was checked further using editing tools, this would automatically highlight implausible records where, say, a height was 3 ft or weight was 600 pounds. Where these sorts of records were found the data item was changed and classed as an item non-response. Most of the edits removed extraneous information, such as a complaint about a service, when that service had not been used for over 12 months.

The total amount of editing affected much less than 0.1% of the overall sample.

5. Non-Response Surveys

Self-completion postal questionnaires are renowned for having item non-response. Some of these items can be filled in on behalf of the respondent with a little bit of common sense. For example, if someone has not answered the question asking if they are pregnant, yet they have indicated they are male it is very easy to correct the form. However, it was accepted that higher levels of non-response would have to be accepted as a trade-off for using this cost-effective method of data collection.

As non-response was expected to be an aspect of the 1998 Welsh Health Survey a non-response survey was conducted. The survey was piloted after the pilot postal survey and conducted formally after the main postal survey.

For the pilot non-response survey, 100 people were sampled with a view to conducting a face-to-face interview. Where a response was achieved, the interviewers asked the respondent a small number of questions about receiving the questionnaire and returning it. They also asked some of the key questions regarding morbidity. A total of 45 responses were achieved.

The object of the pilot non-response survey was to establish how people would react to a non-response survey. An unfavourable reaction would probably have stopped the full non-response survey being conducted. This was not the case the non-response survey went ahead as planned.

Approximately 1,000 people were selected for the non-response survey in 22 unitary authorities. However, one area had particularly poor response to the main postal survey and therefore, this area was over sampled. About 100 people were selected in this area, leaving a total of 43 for each of the other 21 unitary authorities. The survey was conducted in October 1998, five months after the initial survey was posted.

The non-response survey suggested that people who did not complete the postal survey were put off by both its length and the fact that it looked complicated. There was a proportion that admitted they just could not be bothered. Others were either too ill or disabled.

About 91% of people sampled for the non-response survey were happy to answer a few questions about their general health and their use of the National Health Service, along with some questions about the main postal survey.

The results of the non-response survey suggested that non-respondents were generally in better health than respondents of the main postal survey.

This was particularly noticeable regarding heart disease. The results of the main postal survey suggested that 21% of respondents suffered from some type of heart disease, whereas only 6% of respondents to the non-response survey considered they were suffering from heart disease.

We should remember that the different modes of data collection will probably have an impact on the results given. Furthermore, the questions asked in the non-response survey were simpler than in the full postal survey.

6. Analysis

We know from the data collected that over 30% of the respondents have had an outpatient appointment in the last year. However, we also know that the non-responders tended to be more healthy than the responders. So is this an accurate representation of the population of Wales?

Is it possible to model how likely it is that someone would have had an outpatient appointment in the previous 12 months, using the demographic data that was collected, and that may even be available centrally? This includes data such as

- gender
- age
- marital status
- ethnicity
- home tenure
- employment status
- Government Social Class.

Using these variables we can conduct a logistic regression to model how many people would have had an outpatient appointment in the previous 12 months.

Using a backward stepwise method of choosing variables in SPSS we find that the fields that are significant in predicting whether someone would have had an outpatient appointment.

The model produced is below:

$$\log(y) = -1.221 + 0.078f + 0.174a - 0.169m + 0.260h + 0.900d - 0.241c + 0.478s + 0.441u + \varepsilon \quad (2)$$

where f denotes if the person is female, a if the person is aged over 65, m if they are single, h if their house is rented from a housing association or

Table 1: Confidence Intervals for Coefficients in the Model

	B	SE	95%CI
Constant	−1.22	0.03	(−1.27, −1.17)
f — if the person is female	0.08	0.03	(0.03, 0.13)
a — if the person is aged over 65	0.17	0.04	(0.09, 0.26)
m — if they are single	−0.17	0.04	(−0.25, −0.09)
h — if their house is rented from a housing association or similar	0.26	0.08	(0.10, 0.42)
d — if the person is disabled	0.90	0.06	(0.79, 1.01)
c — if the person is a carer	−0.24	0.07	(−0.37, −0.11)
s — if the person is a student	−0.48	0.08	(−0.64, −0.32)
u — if the person is unemployed	0.44	0.04	(0.36, 0.52)

similar, d if the person is disabled, c if the person is a carer, s if the person is a student and u if the person is unemployed.

Therefore, the probability of a person having an outpatient appointment in the previous 12 months is likely to be greater if the person is female, aged over 65, lives in a housing association residence, is disabled and/or is unemployed. The likelihood is reduced if the person is single, a carer and/or a full-time student.

The confidence intervals associated with the variables in the model are given in the Table 1.

Therefore, the odds of a person needing an outpatient appointment in Wales are

$$e^{-1.221+0.078f+0.174a-0.169m+0.260h+0.900d-0.241c+0.478s+0.441u+\varepsilon} \tag{3}$$

As an example, the odds of a single female disabled student aged 24 living in rented accommodation, and not caring for anyone are e^{α} where

$$\begin{aligned}\alpha = & -1.221 + 0.078(1) + 0.174(0) - 0.169(1) + 0.260(1) + 0.900(1) \\ & - 0.241(0) - 0.478(1) + 0.441(1) \\ = & -1.221 + 0.078 - 0.169 + 0.260 + 0.900 - 0.478 + 0.441 \\ = & -0.189\end{aligned}$$

Therefore, $e^{\alpha} = e^{-0.189} = 0.828$

So the odds of this particular type of patient needing an outpatient appointment are 0.828 and the probability of this person needing an outpatient appointment is

$$\frac{e^{\alpha}}{1+e^{\alpha}} = \frac{0.828}{1.828} = 0.453$$

For comparison purposes, if we consider exactly the similar person but without a disability the odds are e^{α} where

$$\begin{aligned}\alpha = & -1.221 + 0.078(1) + 0.174(0) - 0.169(1) + 0.260(1) + 0.900(0) \\ & -0.241(0) - 0.478(1) + 0.441(1) \\ = & -1.221 + 0.078 - 0.169 + 0.260 - 0.478 + 0.441 \\ = & -1.089\end{aligned}$$

Therefore, $e^{\alpha} = e^{-1.089} = 0.337$

So the odds of this particular type of patient needing an outpatient appointment are 0.337 and the probability of this person needing an outpatient appointment is

$$\frac{e^{\alpha}}{1+e^{\alpha}} = \frac{0.337}{1.337} = 0.252$$

This means the probability has nearly halved.

7. Conclusions

So what do these conclusions mean for Wales as a whole. Can we use this model to predict how many outpatient appointments we need to provide for the population of Wales?

If we assume that the sample is representative of the people of Wales, the model suggests that without knowing any information about the demography of Wales that the likelihood of a need for an outpatient appointment is $e^{-1.221}/(1+e^{-1.221}) = 0.228$. Therefore if the population of Wales is approximately 2.97 million, this equates to over 675,000 outpatient appointments every year. Over the past few years the number of outpatient appointments conducted in Wales has stood around 2.7 million. Of course, this can be broken down into the number of new outpatients and follow-up outpatients.

The non-response survey suggested that respondents to the Welsh Health Survey were sicker than non-respondents. However, there is very little data available to confirm this.

The model suggests that being female and/or aged over 65 increases the likelihood of needing an outpatient appointment. Furthermore disabled people, those living in housing association homes and the unemployed are all more likely to need to an outpatient appointment.

7.1 Next Steps

Ideally, it would be good to test this model further, to understand if the logit model was the most appropriate, or whether a probit or cloglog should have been used.

On a more pragmatic note, I would like to predict exactly how many outpatient appointments would be needed for Wales based upon the survey results and how this differs from the amount we are recording centrally. I would also like to see what other information we could use to produce a stronger model. I would then like to apply this methodology to other variables within the survey.

A more applied use for this would be to assist the Local Health Boards within Wales on their demand patterns, i.e. area-based analyses.

Reference

Welsh Health Survey 1998 (1999). *Government Statistical Service*, Her Majesty's Stationery Office, National Assembly for Wales, Wales.

Chapter 18

Confidentiality and Anonymised Survey Records: The UK Experience

Paul Williamson

University of Liverpool, UK

Abstract

A key input to any microsimulation model is a set of population microdata. However, supply of microdata is not unproblematic. Data supply agencies are becoming increasingly concerned about the protection of respondent confidentiality, leading to variable aggregation and suppression. In addition, there are significant problems relating to the issue of sample size. This paper reviews the UK experience in the context of the supply of samples of anonymised records from the UK census. Recent research into the problem of sample uniques is highlighted. The issue of sampling error is re-examined to show that it may be more pervasive than most researchers realise. The adoption of synthetic population microdata is offered as a possible solution to these problems. The paper concludes with the perhaps surprising conclusion that, in certain circumstances, synthetically generated microdata offer better accuracy than actual survey data, and provide better statistical estimates of multi-way distributions than those obtainable using iterative proportional fitting.

1. Overview

Without microdata, microsimulation models cannot function. Sources of microdata vary from country to country, but most commonly the core microdata in any model are supplied by the national statistical agency, and are based on respondents from national social surveys or samples of census returns. This paper addresses two aspects of data quality with respect to these core microdata. First, the trend for increasing levels of statistical disclosure control over time is reviewed. Some of the latest statistical developments in this area are outlined, and are shown to offer no hope of a reversal in this trend. Second, the analytical limitations imposed by sample

International Symposia in Economic Theory and Econometrics, Vol. 16

ISSN: 1571-0386 DOI: 10.1016/S1571-0386(06)16018-4

size are reviewed. The extent of these limitations is shown to be significantly greater than commonly acknowledged.

Having established the current and likely future shortcomings of current sources of microdata, this paper goes on to review the potential of synthetic microdata for overcoming some of these limitations. Synthetic microdata are shown to provide better estimates, over a defined range of control variables, than a 2 per cent sample of census records. They are also shown to offer better performance than statistical estimates derived using iterative proportional fitting. A final section reviews a number of issues yet to be resolved.

2. Statistical Disclosure Control

Unfortunately, at least from the modeller's point of view, national statistical agencies are imposing even greater restrictions on the availability of public use microdata. In part, these growing restrictions have risen in response to increases in the risk of disclosure over time. Increased disclosure risk is attributable to a dramatic growth in the availability of electronic data, coupled with commensurate improvements in both computing power and data-matching techniques. At the same time, there have been significant changes in societal attitudes to the risk of disclosure. In many countries, data protection laws have been introduced or strengthened. In response, statistical agencies have been forced to make protection of respondent confidentiality paramount. Trust in the discretion of data analysts has been replaced by anticipation of 'worst case' scenarios of 'data attack' by malign but statistically sophisticated and data-rich 'data intruders'.

Set against this backdrop, rapid advances have been made in minimising the risk of releasing public use microdata that inadvertently allow the identification of supposedly anonymised (confidentialised) survey respondents. These advances include both improved measures of disclosure risk (Samarati, 2001; Domingo-Ferrer and Torra, 2003) and more sophisticated methods of pre-release data modification and suppression (Bethlehem et al., 1990; Muralidhar and Sarathy, 2003). Two key developments in the UK have been the introduction of measures of file-level risk and of Relative Record-Level Risk (RRR) (Skinner and Elliot, 2002; Elliot et al., 2002). These new measures are outlined below, as they provide a clear insight into the changing nature of risk perception within statistical agencies.

File-level risk may be defined, for a given set of 'key' variables, as the probability of an apparent match between a unique sample record (sample unique) and an identical population record being a correct match. In other words, file-level risk may be defined as the probability of a correct match given a unique match; pr(cm|um). This may be measured as:

$$\Pr(\text{cm}|\text{um}) \cong \frac{Uf}{Uf + P(1-f)} \tag{1}$$

where U is the number of sample uniques (for given variable 'key'), P the number of matching sample record pairs and f the sampling fraction.

RRR may be measured using the concept of "a special unique is a record". In essence, a special unique is a record, which is not only sample unique, but also has a high likelihood of being population unique. Special uniques may be identified in a sample survey by first selecting a variable key (*a* set of k variables upon which to attempt record matching), and then calculating the number of combinations of key variables, m, that allow a record to be identified as sample unique (freqency (k)). The more combinations of key variables that identify a record as sample unique, the 'riskier' the record. Record-level risk also increases in inverse proportion to the number of key variables, m, required to identify a record as sample unique. For example, a record, which is sample unique simply by virtue of being a 16-year old widow, would have a high level of relative disclosure risk. On this basis,

$$\text{RRR} = \sum_{m=1}^{k} \frac{\text{frequency}(m)}{m} \tag{2}$$

for all frequency $(m) > 0$.

Of itself, RRR provides only a relative measure of risk. However, this risk score can be linked to pr(cm|um) to give an approximation to the level of Absolute Record-Level Risk (ARR) (Elliot and Manning, 2003). In crude terms, for a specific records, i,

$$\text{ARR}_i = pr(cm|um) \times \frac{\text{RRR}_i}{\Sigma\, \text{RRR}_i} \tag{3}$$

Given ARR, statistical agencies are in a position to identify potentially disclosive recos, and to undertake disclosure control measures appropriate to the level of identified record-level risk, ranging from suppression for high-risk records through data perturbation to minimal category collapsing for low-risk records. In the UK, this approach is currently being adopted by the Office for National Statistics in preparing for release samples of anonymised records from the 2001 Census. Given the frequent sharing of experience and expertise between statistical agencies, it would be unsurprising to see similar approaches adopted elsewhere. In the future, research suggests that it will also be possible to identify the relative contribution of each record attribute to its overall ARR, allowing the implementation of even more finely tailored record-specific disclosure control strategies (Manning et al., undated).

Irrespective of the measure of disclosure risk adopted, statistical agencies are likely to implement one or more of a number of core data modification techniques prior to data release. These include record and variable suppression, data perturbation, record swapping, top coding and category collapsing. More recently, interest has also been expressed in micro-aggregation (replacement of a variable value by a population sub-group average) (Domingo-Ferrer and Mateo-Sanz, 2002). Notably, especially for those interested in sub-national or sub-regional modelling, a key line of attack at the present time is the reduction of geographic detail. For example, the US Census Bureau is planning to raise the minimum population threshold for identified geographical units in the national public use microdata file (1 per cent sample) from 100,000 to 400,000. Geographical units in the state level 5 per cent samples will retain the 100,000 population threshold, but only at the expense of collapsing all variable categories with fewer than 10,000 representatives nationally (US Census Bureau, 2001). Similarly, in the UK, the current proposals for a 3 per cent Sample of Anonymised Records (SAR) from the 2001 Census include the replacement of a district-level geography (minimum population threshold, 120,000) with a regional geography (average population 4.8 million) (Office for National Statistics, 2003). Finally, the Australian Bureau of Census has taken a slightly different approach, but to the same effect. The basic Household Sample File (HSF) from the 2001 Census available as an input to microsimulation models has a coarser geography than the remotely accessible version of the HSF, as well as a reduced number of categories in many other variables (Australian Bureau of Statistics, 2001). Similar increases in statistical disclosure control have either been enacted, or are under active consideration, for the wider range of social surveys for which these statistical agencies are responsible.

In summary, increasingly aggressive disclosure control measures are degrading the informational content of released microdata. At the time of writing this trend appears more likely to accelerate than to slow down. The burgeoning availability of electronic data shows no signs of dissipating, whilst cultural attitudes to the protection of data confidentiality appear to be hardening rather than softening. As microdata provide a key input to microsimulation models, this reduction in microdata quality will pose an increasing challenge to microsimulation modellers in the future. However, this is to pre-suppose that currently available microdata actually meet modellers' needs. As the following section reveals, issues of sampling and rounding error seriously limit the utility of currently released microdata, even for relatively rudimentary analyses.

3. Inherent Problems with SAR-Based Analyses

Nearly all public use microdata are samples which have to be re-weighted to estimate 'true' population values (Section 3.3). These estimates are subject to sampling and rounding error (Sections 3.2 and 3.4), which add to the data quality problems caused by disclosure control that have already been touched upon in Section 2. For estimates based on large counts such errors are trivial and can be ignored for most purposes. However, for small counts the potential impact of estimation errors cannot be ignored. Unfortunately, as Section 3.1 shows, 'small' counts are hard to avoid when analysing public use microdata.

3.1 The Inevitability of Small Numbers

The cell counts in sample-based tabulations can become very small surprisingly rapidly, particularly when the focus is on an analysis of district-level variation in minority population sub-groups. For example, in the UK 2 per cent individual SAR, ~1.1 million individuals are drawn from ~430,000 households. Running a household-level analysis of car ownership (4 categories) by tenure (10 categories), and splitting by large Local Authority District (278 large LADs) produces a table with 11,120 cells, averaging 39 households per cell (far fewer in the less populous SAR LADs). As shown in Section 3.2, estimates based on these small cell counts are necessarily associated with wide confidence intervals.

The small numbers problem is not restricted to district-level analysis of the individual SAR. In the UK, 1 per cent household SAR, there are 215,761 households with full information for all residents (28 households with 12+ residents are suppressed). Of these households, 205,792 are 'white' (i.e., all persons in the household self-report their ethnicity as 'white'); leaving 2,354 'black', 4,022 'other unmixed' and 3,593 'mixed' households (a total of 9,969 households, with an average of 3,323 households in each minority ethnic split). Sub-dividing these groups by another variable with only *two* categories, and assuming an equal split across categories, gives an average of 1,662 households per cell. Further sub-dividing by SAR region (12 regions) gives an average of 139 households per cell.

Given the multivariate nature of many microsimulation-based analyses, and their common focus on minority population sub-groups, small counts are likely to be hard to avoid, especially when spatially disaggregated. The alternative would be data aggregation to the point at which users are left without any information of interest.

3.2 Sampling Error

The microdata used in microsimulation models are almost invariably *samples*, yielding only *estimates* of actual population counts. The degree of imprecision associated with each estimate may readily be calculated (Campbell et al., 1996; Dale et al., 2000). In essence, imprecision arises from a combination of sampling error, design effects and sample-size related under-enumeration. The smaller the size of the population sub-group being analysed, the wider the confidence interval. This is illustrated in Tables 1 and 2, which present the 95 per cent confidence intervals associated with the distribution of economic position, calculated using the UK 2 per cent individual SAR.

Table 1 concentrates on estimates of the joint distribution of economic position across the two SAR districts, Leeds and Babergh/Ipswich, with adult population totals of ca. 1,048,000 and 303,000, respectively. As can be seen from the table, the confidence intervals associated with estimates of the percentage of the adult population in each 'economic position' category vary widely. For the smallest category ('on a government scheme'), the associated 95 per cent confidence interval amounts to ± 42 per cent of the SAR estimate for the smaller district of Babergh/Ipswich. Although double that for Leeds (± 23 per cent), this value is by no means atypical. The Babergh/Ipswich district has a sample size almost identical to the SAR average, whereas the Leeds sample is the second largest district in the UK SAR (after Birmingham).

For most users, analyses will require far more than the type of simple univariate distribution presented in Table 1. Table 2 presents the confidence intervals associated with estimates of the proportion of adults within each economic position category who are female. For this analysis, the size of the associated design factors and under-enumeration corrections are unknown. But even on the basis of uncorrected standard error alone, the confidence intervals are, unsurprisingly, considerably widened.

Table 3 reproduces similar estimates of sampling error calculated by the Australian Bureau of Statistics for their 1 per cent HSF (Australian Bureau of Statistics, 2001). Where appropriate, these estimates take into account, additionally, the impact of the clustering of individuals within sample households. The figures quoted reinforce the degree of caution needed when undertaking analyses using 'small' sample counts.

3.3 Population Weights

The use of population weights further complicates the potential analysis of sample microdata. For example, the population weights supplied with the UK individual SAR rescale results not to published census counts, but to

Table 1: Confidence Intervals of Sample Survey Estimates: Joint Probabilities

Economic position	Total	% (SAR estimate)	SE p	Design factor (national)	Under enumeration correction	95% Confidence interval	95% Confidence interval as percentage of SAR estimate
SAR district: Leeds							
Employee full-time	4,146	39.5	±0.5	0.99	1.01	±0.9	2.4
Employee part-time	1,162	11.1	±0.3	0.98	1.01	±0.6	5.4
Self-Semployed w emps.	172	1.6	±0.1	1.00	1.01	±0.2	15.1
Self-employed no emps.	361	3.4	±0.2	0.99	1.01	±0.4	10.2
On a government scheme	77	0.7	±0.1	0.99	1.01	±0.2	22.5
Unemployed	573	5.5	±0.2	0.99	1.01	±0.4	8.0
Student	435	4.1	±0.2	1.01	1.01	±0.4	9.4
Permanently sick	414	3.9	±0.2	0.99	1.01	±0.4	9.5
Retired	2,116	20.2	±0.4	1.00	1.01	±0.8	3.9
Other inactive	1,029	9.8	±0.3	0.98	1.01	±0.6	5.8
Total	1,0485	100.0					
SAR district: Babergh/Ipswich							
Employee full-time	1,185	39.1	±0.9	0.99	1.04	±1.8	4.6
Employee part-time	367	12.1	±0.6	0.98	1.04	±1.2	9.8
Self-employed w emps.	69	2.3	±0.3	1.00	1.04	±0.6	24.4
Self-employed no emps.	152	5.0	±0.4	0.99	1.04	±0.8	16.1
On a government scheme	23	0.8	±0.2	0.99	1.04	±0.3	42.3
Unemployed	133	4.4	±0.4	0.99	1.04	±0.8	17.2
Student	79	2.6	±0.3	1.01	1.04	±0.6	22.9
Permanently sick	77	2.5	±0.3	0.99	1.04	±0.6	22.8
Retired	557	18.4	±0.7	1.00	1.04	±1.4	7.9
Other inactive	391	12.9	±0.6	0.98	1.04	±1.2	9.5
Total	3,033	100.0					

Note: *w emps. = with employees; no emps. = no employees.*

Table 2: Confidence Intervals of Survey Estimates: Conditional Probabilities

Economic position	SAR count			% Female (SAR estimate)	SE p	95% Confidence interval	95% Confidence interval as percentage of SAR estimate
	Male	Female	Total				
SAR district: Leeds							
Employee full-time	2,621	1,525	4,146	36.8	±0.7	±1.5	4.0
Employee part-time	117	1,045	1,162	89.9	±0.9	±1.7	1.9
Self-employed w emps.	130	42	172	24.4	±3.3	±6.4	26.3
Self-employed no emps.	280	81	361	22.4	±2.2	±4.3	19.2
On a government scheme	46	31	77	40.3	±5.6	±11.0	27.2
Unemployed	405	168	573	29.3	±1.9	±3.7	12.7
Student	222	213	435	49.0	±2.4	±4.7	9.6
Permanently sick	239	175	414	42.3	±2.4	±4.8	11.3
Retired	849	1,267	2,116	59.9	±1.1	±2.1	3.5
Other inactive	31	998	1029	97.0	±0.5	±1.0	1.1
Total	4,940	5,545	10,485	52.9	±0.5	±1.0	1.8
SAR district: Babergh/Ipswich							
Employee full-time	779	406	1185	34.3	±1.4	±2.7	7.9
Employee part-time	38	329	367	89.6	±1.6	±3.1	3.5
Self-employed w emps.	46	23	69	33.3	±5.7	±11.1	33.4
Self-employed no emps.	122	30	152	19.7	±3.2	±6.3	32.1
On a government scheme	17	6	23	26.1	±9.2	±17.9	68.8
Unemployed	100	33	133	24.8	±3.7	±7.3	29.6
Student	42	37	79	46.8	±5.6	±11.0	23.5
Permanently sick	39	38	77	49.4	±5.7	±11.2	22.6
Retired	239	318	557	57.1	±2.1	±4.1	7.2
Other inactive	5	386	391	98.7	±0.6	±1.1	1.1
Total	1,427	1,606	3,033	53.0	±0.9	±1.8	3.4

Note: No account taken of unknown under-enumeration and design factors. See Note in Table 1.

Table 3: Standard Error of Estimates for ABS 1% Household Sample File

Sample count	Size of estimate	Standard error	Relative standard error (%)
Dwelling/Family estimate			
5	500	225.0	45.0
10	1,000	310.0	31.0
50	5,000	650.0	13.0
100	10,000		
Clustered person estimate			
5	500	317.0	63.4
10	1,000	447.0	44.7
50	5,000	989.0	19.8
100	10,000	1,393.0	13.9

Source: Australian Bureau of Statistics (2001)

1991 mid-year estimates (adjusted to take account of Census under-enumeration). As the individual SAR is, in effect, a 2 per cent random sample of the underlying census data, inflation by the reciprocal of the sampling factor (1/0.02) should theoretically yield the target district counts. In practice, sampling error and design factors mean that there is not 100 per cent correspondence between census and inflated SAR counts. This discrepancy could be overcome by re-weighting the SAR to known district age–sex totals. Such an approach would ensure perfect agreement between SAR and census district totals, but could have an adverse impact on the relationships between variables not used in the weighting process. For this reason, throughout the remainder of this paper SAR counts have been inflated to 100 per cent through multiplication by the reciprocal of the sampling fraction, and most analyses are based upon proportional rather than absolute distributions.

3.4 Rounding Error

The calculation of standard error, design factors and under-enumeration corrections are all geared towards adjusting for variations in sample size away from the target fraction of 2 per cent. However, even if a sample represented a perfect, bias free sample of an underlying population, there would still be rounding error. For example, a SAR count of 50, once inflated, equals a count of between 475 and 524. This gives rise to a potential rounding error of ± 1 per cent. Smaller counts have commensurately higher levels of associated rounding error (see Table 4). Unfortunately, as Section 3.1 has already demonstrated, small counts are hard to avoid in district-level

Table 4: Inherent Limits to Sample Counts

Sample count	Sample count × 50[a]	Actual count		Possible rounding error (%)
		Minimum	Maximum	
1	50	25	74	±50.0
2	100	75	124	±25.0
3	150	125	174	±16.7
4	200	175	224	±12.5
5	250	225	274	±10.0
10	500	475	524	±5.0
20	1,000	975	1,024	±2.5
30	1,500	1,475	1,524	±1.7
40	2,000	1,975	2,024	±1.3
50	2,500	2,475	2,524	±1.0

[a] *Assumes sampling fraction = 2%.*

analyses of the 1991 individual SAR. This point is reinforced in the analyses that follow.

4. Using Synthetic Microdata in Place of Sample Microdata

A review of the variety of methods by which synthetic population microdata may be generated has been published elsewhere (Williamson, 2002a). One technique is to identify, for each (small) census output area, a set of sample records that, when aggregated, best fits published aggregate census statistics for that area (Voas and Williamson, 2000; Williamson, 2003). The remainder of this paper considers whether or not such synthetic microdata might help to address some of the shortcomings with sample-based microdata reviewed in Sections 2 and 3. All of the results presented are based upon analyses of synthetic microdata estimated for the 16 UK local authority districts comprising the 1991 counties of Cambridgeshire, Derbyshire, Norfolk and Suffolk, plus the metropolitan district of Leeds. The selection of these areas is entirely arbitrary: these were the areas for which synthetic microdata were available at the time of writing. However, unless there is a distinct and unanticipated problem associated with the estimation of microdata for the principal metropolitan area of London, there is no reason to think that the results presented would not apply more generally. Table 5 lists the constraints used in generating these synthetic microdata.

The following section focuses on the overall fit of synthetic microdata to the constraints used in the synthetic estimation process. Sections 4.2 and 4.3 examine the fit to one constraint, that of economic position by sex, in more

Table 5: Constraints Used During Creation of Synthetic Microdata

Constraint on synthetic microdata	SAS table	Tabulation constrained	Cells constrained per table
1	S35	Age/sex/marital status	84
2	S42	Household composition/ tenure	77
3	S01	Resident status/sex	6
4	S22	Household size/number of rooms/tenure	196
5	S12	Long-term illness/age/sex	14
6	S29	Dependants	7
7	S86	Socio-economic group of household head/tenure	100
8	S39	Age/sex/marital status of household head	28
9	S34	Sex/marital status/economic position	56
10	S08	Age/sex/economic position	180
11	S49	Ethnic group of household head/tenure	16
12	S09	Sex/economic position/ ethnic group	24
13	S42	Household composition/car ownership	33
14	S74	Occupation/age/sex	20
Total			817

detail. Section 4.4 summarises what light this examination sheds upon the adverse impact of sampling and rounding error on district-level SAR estimates.

4.1 Overall Fit of Synthetic Microdata to Census Estimation Constraints

The synthetic microdata evaluated in this paper were constrained to fit published constraints for the smallest level of 1991 UK Census geography output, the enumeration district (average population: ~120 households). The impact of spatial aggregation upon the quality of these synthetic microdata is assessed in Table 6. The table confirms a trend previously identified (Huang and Williamson, 2001). The greater the degree of spatial aggregation, the poorer the fit of synthetic microdata to known constraints. On this basis the district-level, the analyses that follow are likely to present synthetic

Table 6: Fit of Synthetic Microdata to Estimation Constraints

Area type	Number of areas	Average			
		NFT	NFT (%)	NFC	NFC (%)
ED	($n = 8{,}055$)	0	0	0.1	0
Ward	($n = 806$)	0	0	5.9	1
District	($n = 30$)	2.6	19	11.1	1
SAR district	($n = 17$)	4.4	32	15.2	2
County	($n = 4$)	7.8	55	40	5
SAR region	($n = 1$)	10	71	85	10

Notes: NFC = non-fitting cell: Z-score for constraining table cell exceeds Z-score critical value at 0.05 significance level.
NFT = non-fitting table: Sum of squared Z-scores for table exceeds chi-square critical value at 0.05 significance level.

microdata in a relatively unfavourable light. An obvious step for someone interested in district-level analysis would be to generate synthetic microdata constrained directly to district totals. In fact, to facilitate direct comparison of synthetic and SAR data, not districts but SAR districts are used in the analyses that follow. A SAR district comprises one or more census districts, combined to meet a specified minimum population threshold. In consequence, the results reported will be even less favourable than those that might have been expected if analyses had been undertaken using the smaller census districts normally of most interest to end users.

Out of the 17 SAR districts estimated to-date, the large metropolitan district of Leeds is the LAD with the greatest number of 'non-fitting tables' (7 out of 14). Comparison of synthetic and constraining counts for one table, for Leeds gives some idea of the stringency of the measures-of-fit used (see Table 7). A fuller comparison is presented in Huang and Williamson (2002). Even for non-fitting tables there is still a generally high degree of correspondence between the synthetic and constraining counts.

4.2 Fit to the Constraint of Economic Position by Sex

One of the constraints used in the synthetic microdata estimation process was Table 34 from the Census Small Area Statistics (SAS), which tabulates economic position by sex and marital status. In Table 8, comparisons are made between the 'true' census district counts and two alternative 'estimates': inflated SAR counts and synthetic estimation. Not shown are the alternative district counts derived by aggregation of ED-level census data. For presentation purposes, the marital status dimension of SAS Table 34 has been dropped. Results are presented for the two SAR districts of Leeds

Table 7: Fit of Synthetic Data to Constraining Census Counts for Leeds (SAS Table 39)

	Head of household							
Age	**Male**		**Female**		**Male**		**Female**	
	SWD	**M'rrd**	**SWD**	**M'rrd**	**SWD**	**M'rrd**	**SWD**	**M'rrd**
	Census count (target)				*Synthetic count (estimate)*			
16–39	13,550	11,925	13,920	3,121	13,563	11,895	13,844	3,109
30–44	12,131	45,681	12,801	5,871	12,106	45,833	12,827	5,825
45–59	8,212	41,729	10,605	2,968	8,192	4,1849	10,571	2,970
60–64	2,875	12,733	5,315	654	2,819	12,660	5,288	653
65–74	5,431	20,302	14,607	950	5,412	20,354	14,650	945
75–84	4,140	8,328	15,502	598	4,094	8,369	15,589	593
85+	1,008	925	4,739	182	984	897	4,723	176
	Cell-level error				*Cell-level Z-score*			
16–39	13	−30	−76	−12	0.12	−0.28	−0.66	−0.21
30–44	−25	152	26	−46	−0.23	0.79	0.24	−0.60
45–59	−20	120	−34	2	−0.22	0.65	−0.33	0.04
60–64	−56	−73	−27	−1	−1.05	−0.66	−0.37	−0.04
65–74	−19	52	43	−5	−0.26	0.39	0.37	−0.16
75–84	−46	41	87	−5	−0.72	0.46	0.72	−0.20
85+	−24	−28	−16	−6	−0.76	−0.92	−0.23	−0.44

Notes: Total non-fitting cells ($|Z|>1.96$): 0.
Table sum of Z^2: 7.25 (< Table critical value of 41.3; $p<0.05$).
M'rrd = Married; SWD = Single/Widowed/Divorced.

and Babergh/Ipswich. These two districts were chosen for illustration purposes as representing SAR districts with average (Babergh/Ipswich) and worst fit (Leeds) to estimation constraints.

Given the known mismatches between synthetic estimates and their constraints (Section 4.1), it is no surprise that the synthetic and census district counts differ. The discrepancy between synthetic and census district totals amounts to 0.4 per cent of the population of Leeds and 0.2 per cent of the population of Babergh/Ipswich. This discrepancy is attributable to a combination of modelling and ED SAS aggregation error. Aggregation error is readily calculable, being the difference between census district counts and their aggregated ED equivalents. Modelling error is equal to the overall synthetic data error less the aggregation error. For Leeds, aggregation error (−0.09 per cent) is one-third that of the modelling error (−0.28 per cent). For Babergh/Ipswich, aggregation error (0.15 per cent) is two-fifths the size of modelling error (−0.37 per cent).

Table 8: Example of Fit to Census Data for Selected SAR Districts

Economic position	District SAS		2% SAR count × 50		Synthetic	
	Male	**Female**	**Male**	**Female**	**Male**	**Female**
SAR district:leeds						
Employee full-time	132,641	75,384	131,050	76,250	132,365	74,338
Employee part-time	5,821	52,445	5,850	52,250	6,255	52,994
Self-employed w emps.	8,424	2,680	6,500	2,100	8,126	2,490
Self-employed no emps.	16,216	4,512	14,000	4,050	15,787	4,342
On a government scheme	2,443	1,589	2,300	1,550	2,271	1,502
Unemployed	21,455	8,918	20,250	8,400	21,268	8,667
Student	11,012	10,411	11,100	10,650	10,730	10,174
Permanently sick	12,339	8,460	11,950	8,750	12,363	8,365
Retired	43,323	64,115	42,450	63,350	43,199	64,454
Other inactive	1,693	52,597	1,550	49,900	1,561	53,237
Total population	536,478		524,250		534,488	
Percentage difference from SAS district total			−2.28		−0.37	
Goodness of fit to district SAS counts						
Total absolute error			15,252		5,962	
Goodness of fit to district SAS proportions						
Total absolute error			2.78			

SAR district: Babergh/Ipswich						
Employee full-time	39,902	19,342	38,950	20,300	40,092	19,401
Employee part-time	1,886	16,415	1,900	16,450	1,789	16,347
Self-employed w emps.	2,567	771	2,300	1,150	2,496	716
Self-employed no emps.	6,437	1,526	6,100	1,500	6,379	1,420
On a government scheme	547	345	850	300	537	297
Unemployed	4,855	1,936	5,000	1,650	4,827	1,896
Student	2,303	2,361	2,100	1,850	2,356	2,331
Permanently sick	2,295	1,541	1,950	1,900	2,249	1,491
Retired	13,321	15,663	11,950	15,900	13,330	15,688
Other inactive	412	19,918	250	19,300	400	19,956
Total population	154,343		151,650		153,998	
Percentage difference from SAS district total						
			−1.74		−0.22	
Goodness of fit to district SAS counts						
Total absolute error			7,553		1,093	
Goodness of fit to district SAS proportions						
Total absolute error			4.61		0.81	

Note: See Note in Table 1.

Table 8 also contains SAR-based estimates of the collapsed SAS Table 34 counts. To produce these estimates all SAR counts have been inflated by the reciprocal of the overall sampling fraction (1/0.02) (see Section 4.3). The discrepancies between the district SAS and inflated SAR-based totals are more than five times as large as the observed discrepancies between synthetic and district SAS counts (2.3 and 1.7 per cent respectively for Leeds and Babergh/Ipswich). These discrepancies help to give some indication of the scale of sampling error to be encountered when using the SAR.

But a focus on counts disadvantages both synthetic and SAR-based estimates. District-specific weights could be added to the SAR, and district-level constraints could be introduced to the synthetic estimation process. In any case, accuracy of proportional distribution is often of more importance to users. For this reason, for each estimate of the 'true' district SAS, Table 8 also presents a measure of the difference in proportional distributions (total absolute error, TAE). The size of the TAE echoes the findings relating to differences in overall district totals. First, for synthetic data, aggregation errors are smaller than model errors. Second, the combined impact of modelling and aggregation error on synthetic estimates remains smaller than that of sampling and rounding error on SAR-based estimates. Considering the small count size in some cells (e.g., only six females in the SAR Babergh/Ipswich sample are on a government scheme), the adverse impact of sampling and rounding error on SAR-based estimates is perhaps unsurprising.

4.3 Fit to the Constraint of Sex Given Economic Position

Table 9 presents a set of analyses based on the distribution of the conditional probability of being female given economic position. This might at first appear to be a slightly idiosyncratic choice, but reflects a common user interest in identifying proportions (or probabilities) *within* population subgroups. It is perhaps no coincidence that the largest distributional discrepancy between the district SAS and its SAR-based equivalent (proportion of persons on a government scheme in Babergh/Ipswich) is associated with the smallest underlying SAR count.

Given a sample of only two districts, some caution in generalising these findings might be appropriate. However, they are confirmed by an analysis based on all 17 SAR districts for which synthetic microdata are currently available. The average difference from census district conditional probabilities (as measured by TAE) is 33.4 for SAR-based estimates, but only 3.8 for the equivalent synthetic estimates. A similar ranking of differences exists whether comparing probabilities, odds or log-odds. There is a clear relationship between SAR district sample size and the extent to which SAR and SAS district distributions differ ($r = -0.75$ for difference as measured by TAE).

Table 9: Example of Fit to Census Data for Selected SAR Districts: Joint Distribution

Economic position	District SAS	Individual SAR	Synthetic
		Female (%)	
SAR district: Leeds			
Employee full-time	36.2	36.8	36.0
Employee part-time	90.0	89.9	89.4
Self-employed w emps.	24.1	24.4	23.5
Self-employed no emps.	21.8	22.4	21.6
On a government scheme	39.4	40.3	39.8
Unemployed	29.4	29.3	29.0
Student	48.6	49.0	48.7
Permanently sick	40.7	42.3	40.4
Retired	59.7	59.9	59.9
Other inactive	96.9	97.0	97.2
Goodness-of-fit to district SAS proportions			
Total absolute error		4.7	3.4
SAR district: Babergh/Ipswich			
Employee full-time	32.6	34.3	32.6
Employee part-time	89.7	89.6	90.1
Self-employed w emps.	23.1	33.3	22.3
Self-employed no emps.	19.2	19.7	18.2
On a government scheme	38.7	26.1	35.6
Unemployed	28.5	24.8	28.2
Student	50.6	46.8	49.7
Permanently sick	40.2	49.4	39.9
Retired	54.0	57.1	54.1
Other inactive	98.0	98.7	98.0
Goodness-of-fit to District SAS proportions			
Total absolute error		45.5	6.9

Note: See Note in Table 1.

4.4 The Impact Of Sampling Error

The conclusion to be drawn from Tables 8 and 9 is that, despite not being optimised for use at district level, synthetic microdata provide a better fit to the 'true' census district distribution than the (unweighted) SAR. This performance advantage would appear to be attributable to sampling and rounding error in the SAR. It is possible that re-weighting to known district age–sex profiles might improve SAR fit to census counts. On the other hand, re-weighting by age and sex is likely to have an adverse impact on the distributional fit of other variables. In either case, as discussed in Section

3.4, the SAR would remain at a disadvantage due to the problem of rounding error, which is significant for counts of less than 50. As Table 8 shows, even for a SAR district of average size, such as Babergh/Ipswich, many counts in a simple two-way distribution fall below 50.

5. Comparison of Synthetic Microdata to SAR and IPF-Based Estimates

Section 4 evaluated the fit of synthetic microdata to tables and cell counts used as constraints in the synthetic microdata estimation process. These types of synthetic estimates might be described as 'fully constrained'. In contrast, 'margin-constrained' estimates comprise constrained marginal cells, but unconstrained interior table counts. In principle, it should be possible to identify published equivalents to these 'margin-constrained' distributions, allowing assessment of the fit of margin-constrained synthetic to actual census distributions. Unfortunately, the set of published tables used as direct constraints on synthetic estimation (Table 5) is sufficiently exhaustive as to leave only one published table of interest for comparison purposes, Local Base Statistics Table 45. This four-way table cross-tabulates household head's age and sex by economic position and household tenure. The success of synthetic microdata in capturing this unknown multi-way relationship, relative to other estimation strategies, is assessed below.

Two main alternatives exist for estimating unknown multi-way relationships. One is estimation via sample survey. In the UK, the most spatially detailed sample survey currently available is the 2 per cent SAR from the 1991 Census. The released data have a spatial resolution of large LAD (ca. 80,000 households). The other is the use of a technique known as Iterative Proportional Fitting (IPF) or 'entropy maximizing' (Wong, 1992; Johnston and Pattie, 1993). Two variants of the IPF approach are considered. One uses a uniform distribution as a starting position, the other the national distribution (as recorded in the 2 per cent SAR). Both use, as marginal constraints, distributions that were also used during synthetic estimation (head's age by sex; head's tenure by economic position). The marginal constraint on economic position lacks a sub-category for the unemployed. Consequently, to avoid disadvantaging the IPF approach, the initial target for estimation is a version of LBS Table 45 in which the sub-category of 'unemployed' has been collapsed into the 'economically active'.

Table 10 summarises the relative performance of synthetic microdata, IPF and SAR-based estimates in capturing the district-level distribution of household head's age and sex and head's tenure by economic position. The results are based on an assessment of 17 districts: the city of Leeds and the 16 districts forming the counties of Derbyshire, Norfolk and Suffolk.

Table 10: Relative Performance of Alternative Estimates of LBS Table 45

Measure of difference from LBS (error)	Method of estimation				No. of Districts where error for (1) < (2) ($n = 17$)	Ratio of error (1):(2)
	Synthetic microdata (1)	2% Individual SAR	IPF (National Distribution as seed) (2)	IPF (Uniform Distribution as seed)		
LBS Table 45 (no sub-category for the unemployed)						
	Goodness-of-fit to SAS district counts					
TAE	2,961	8,882	4,598	60,967	14	0.64
TAE^2	381,781	3,897,949	1,122,860	259,403,014	17	0.34
	Goodness-of-fit to SAS district proportions					
TAE	3.60	11.00	5.49	70.84	17	0.66
TAE^2	0.50	5.38	1.44	276.44	17	0.35
$Z\text{-score}^2$	441	2,995	1,033	353,198	16	0.43
NFC (%)	18	32	22	37	14	0.81
LBS Table 45 (with sub-category for unemployed)						
	Goodness-of-fit to SAS district counts					
TAE	3,258	10,088	5,952	89,118	16	0.55
TAE^2	352,379	3,995,754	1,528,355	429,446,801	16	0.23
	Goodness-of-fit to SAS district proportions					
TAE	3.92	12.48	7.13	104.30	16	0.55
TAE^2	0.44	5.47	2.05	473.49	16	0.22
$Z\text{-score}^2$	539	4,249	1,906	5,723,336	17	0.28
NFC (%)	33	68	48	84	15	0.70

(Continued)

Table 10. *Continued.*

Measure of difference from LBS (error)	Method of estimation				No. of Districts where error for (1) < (2) ($n = 17$)	Ratio of error (1):(2)
	Synthetic microdata (1)	2% Individual SAR	IPF			
			(National Distribution as seed) (2)	(Uniform Distribution as seed)		
Percentage of overall TAE due to the unemployed sub-category	16.5	11.3	20.6	24.9		

Notes: TAE = Total Absolute Error.
NFC = Non-fitting cells: Cells in table with an associated Z-score > ±1.96.

The clear message is that, on average, IPF and SAR-based estimates are out-performed by those derived from synthetic microdata, irrespective of whether absolute counts or proportional distributions are considered. This statistical hegemony is disputed only in a few districts, and even then not across all measures of fit. In all cases, the closest challengers are estimates derived from a nationally seeded IPF (IPF_N). At the other end of the spectrum, the outcome of IPF seeded with a uniform distribution (IPF_U) clearly represents a worst case 'minimum information' scenario.

It is perhaps surprising that SAR-based estimates are out-performed by those derived from both synthetic microdata and IPF_N. Brief reflection reveals the cause. A 2 per cent national sample yields an average of only 1,544 households per district. Further sub-division across the 64-cell target distribution under consideration leaves an average sample per cell of 24. Such small counts greatly amplify the effects of both sampling and rounding error. For example, a 2 per cent-sample count of 24 yields an estimated district-level count of 1,200. Allowing for potential random sampling error, this estimate has a 95 per cent confidence interval of ± 243 (± 20 per cent). The estimated count is also subject to a potential rounding error of ± 25 (± 2.1 per cent). Further allowance should be made for systematic biases (design factors) introduced via the sampling process used in extracting the SAR. Even though the sampling frame for the SAR is identical to that on which the LBS are based (all census records), these biases can inflate the standard errors of estimates by ± 0–15 per cent, depending upon the variable(s) of interest (Campbell et al., 1996). These problems are avoidable only by substantially increasing the sampling fraction, decreasing the spatial resolution or collapsing table dimensions and variable categories to the point that they are of little use to end users.

The performance advantage of synthetic microdata over IPF_N can also be explained. Both are directly constrained by the marginal distribution of head's age, sex, tenure and economic position. However, during the creation of synthetic microdata a wide range of additional 'indirect' constraints are also used (Table 5). Three types of indirect marginal constraint may be identified. First, there are constraints involving a combination of attributes that include at least one drawn from the target distribution. Second, there are constraints that include one or more attributes from the target distribution, but cover a different sub-population. Third, there are constraints that involve no attribute from the target distribution. In all three cases, correlations between the indirect constraints and the target distribution, however slight, will help to improve the estimate of the target distribution.

The benefit derived from indirect constraints may be illustrated by estimating counts for the full version of LBS Table 45, in which a sub-category is included for the unemployed. As previously mentioned, the number of unemployed *household heads* is not a direct constraint on either synthetic microdata or IPF-based estimates. However, the number of unemployed *residents* present in the synthetic microdata is directly constrained, providing an indirect marginal constraint on the number of unemployed household heads. Target and estimated counts are presented in Table 11. Summary measures of estimate accuracy are presented in the lower half of Table 10. Not surprisingly, the addition of an 'unemployed' sub-category leads to a general decrease in levels of fit. Yet, at the same time, the average performance advantage of synthetic microdata over IPF_N increases across all measures of fit. This reflects the competitive advantage enjoyed by synthetic microdata as a result of its additional indirect marginal constraints.

Repetition of this analysis for another margin-constrained distribution is precluded by lack of suitable LBS tables. However, synthetic microdata may be compared directly to margin-constrained tabulations derived from the SAR although, as already noted, these 'targets' are subject to both sampling and rounding error. SAR-based analyses of this type are reported elsewhere (Williamson, 2002b). The results indicate broad agreement between a range of SAR distributions and their margin-constrained synthetic microdata equivalents.

6. Conclusions

There is clear evidence to suggest that the margin-constrained distributions captured by synthetic microdata approximate to reality better than estimates derived from either IPF or a sample survey with a sampling fraction $\leq$2 per cent. An additional benefit of synthetic microdata is that, once generated, they contain best estimates of all possible multi-way margin-constrained distributions (32,752 in a dataset with 15 variable constraints, ignoring the potential for combining categories within variables). In contrast, IPF has to be undertaken separately for each multi-way distribution to be estimated.

This above conclusion is based on an assessment of a handful of selected SAR tabulations and one LBS tabulation, and therefore should be treated with some caution. A fully exhaustive assessment of the full range of ca. 32,000 multi-way margin-constrained tabulations is precluded by both lack of time and by lack of appropriate target data against which to evaluate estimates. Nor has a rigorous mathematical proof of the superiority of one approach over another been offered. However, in many other ways the conclusion offered appears robust. The SAR provides a 2 per cent sample, drawn directly from the census records on which each target distribution was based. Other surveys are likely to have smaller sample sizes and less reliable sampling frames. IPF marginals were similarly taken directly from the target distribution. In contrast, the particular set of synthetic microdata

Table 11: Target and Estimated Counts for the District of Suffolk Coastal and Waveney

Tenure	Economic position	Male household heads				
		Age				
		16–29	30–44	45–<p.a.	p.a.+	Total[a]
Target: census distribution (LBS Table 45)						
Owner-occupied	Active	4,247	13,643	14,277	1,074	33,241
	Unemployed	143	414	799	2	1,358
	Inactive	27	180	2556	11,174	13,937
Privately rented	Active	1,950	2,432	1,437	150	5,969
	Unemployed	225	184	189	2	600
	Inactive	36	65	228	1,086	1,415
Housing association	Active	64	158	177	27	426
	Unemployed	19	26	17	2	64
	Inactive	4	17	61	559	641
Council rented	Active	308	898	1,157	122	2,485
	Unemployed	130	179	218	2	529
	Inactive	21	127	459	2,369	2,976
Total		7,174	18,323	21,575	16,569	63,641
Estimate: synthetic microdata						
Owner- occupied	Active	4,164	13,612	14,605	1,050	33,431
	Unemployed	130	442	878	3	1,453
	Inactive	28	158	2,535	11,053	13,774
Privately rented	Active	2,020	2,529	1324	152	6,025
	Unemployed	218	150	129	1	498
	Inactive	53	70	146	1,227	1,496
Housing association	Active	65	113	102	9	289
	Unemployed	5	15	22	0	42
	Inactive	0	20	44	604	668
Council rented	Active	332	889	1,144	123	2,488
	Unemployed	118	179	179	0	476
	Inactive	29	132	487	2,381	3,029
Total		7,162	18,309	21,595	16,603	63,669
Estimate: 2% individual sample of anonymised records (× 50)						
Owner- occupied	Active	4,550	13,950	14,750	900	34,150
	Unemployed	100	550	1100	0	1,750
	Inactive	0	150	2,400	11,150	13,700
Privately rented	Active	17,50	2,800	2,150	200	6,900
	Unemployed	300	250	150	0	700
	Inactive	150	100	250	950	1,450
Housing association	Active	50	150	150	50	400
	Unemployed	50	0	50	0	100
	Inactive	0	0	150	900	1,050

(*Continued*)

Table 11. *Continued.*

Tenure	Economic position	Male household heads				
		Age				
		16–29	30–44	45– <p.a.	p.a. +	Total[a]
Council rented	Active	450	1,000	1,000	0	2,450
	Unemployed	100	250	250	0	600
	Inactive	100	50	400	2,900	3,450
Total		7,600	19,250	22,800	17,050	66,700
Estimate: iterative proportional fitting (seeded with national distribution)						
Owner- occupied	Active	4,114	13,761	13,861	1,026	32,763
	Unemployed	196	597	950	12	1,755
	Inactive	52	220	2,693	11,144	14,109
Privately rented	Active	1,719	1,976	1,629	229	5,553
	Unemployed	291	281	247	8	828
	Inactive	123	80	200	1,203	1,606
Housing association	Active	67	134	124	19	344
	Unemployed	30	46	41	2	118
	Inactive	12	28	85	488	614
Council rented	Active	345	778	892	105	2,120
	Unemployed	190	300	328	5	824
	Inactive	34	122	523	2,329	3,008
Total		7,174	18,323	21,575	16,569	63,641
Estimate: iterative proportional fitting (seeded with uniform distribution)						
Owner- occupied	Active	1,633	4,170	4,910	3,771	14,483
	Unemployed	1,633	4,170	4,910	3,771	14,483
	Inactive	1,919	4,901	5,771	4,432	17,023
Privately rented	Active	335	855	1,007	773	2,970
	Unemployed	335	855	1,007	773	2,970
	Inactive	267	683	804	618	2,372
Housing association	Active	28	71	83	64	245
	Unemployed	28	71	83	64	245
	Inactive	131	334	393	302	1,159
Council rented	Active	161	411	484	372	1,429
	Unemployed	161	411	484	372	1,429
	Inactive	545	1,391	1,638	1,258	4,832
Total		7,174	18,323	21,575	16,569	63,641

[a] *For IPF estimates, row marginal totals sum to the published univariate census distribution when the 'active' and 'unemployed' categories within each tenure category are combined.*

under evaluation were estimated using small-area (ED) constraints. As a result of disclosure control measures, it is known that these constraints do not add up precisely to the target district distribution totals. Future versions of the synthetic estimation algorithm could readily be adapted to include these district-level constraints. In addition, plausible theoretical explanations, if not mathematical proofs, have been advanced for the relative performance (dis)advantage of each estimation approach. IPF-based estimates lack the indirect constraints involved in the estimation of synthetic microdata, while district-level survey-based estimates suffer from severe rounding and random sampling errors that can be eliminated only by substantially increasing sample size, or substantially reducing distributional detail.

Even so, some areas of doubt remain, which could usefully provide a focus for future research.

(1) Evaluation of fit at ward level (average population ~10,000), reported elsewhere (Voas and Williamson, 2000), suggests that the fit of margin-constrained synthetic microdata distributions is lower when a combination of household- and individual-level marginals are involved. The impact of such cross-hierarchy marginals on the fit of IPF-based estimates has not been considered. It is possible that in such situations synthetic microdata might be out-performed by IPF.
(2) In the assessment undertaken of IPF, two marginal constraints were used. It is, of course, possible to use three or more constraints. These additional constraints can either overlap, thereby serving to reinforce existing constraints, or extend the constraints into further dimensions (Johnston and Pattie, 1993). In such circumstances, synthetic microdata might lose their performance advantage over IPF (although not their ease-of-use advantage).
(3) It has been claimed that indirect constraints serve to improve the accuracy of synthetic microdata-based estimates. At present, this claim is supported by only one empirical assessment. Further assessments would help to quantify the impact of additional constraints on synthetic microdata accuracy. It is hypothesised that a U-shaped relationship may exist. If there are too many indirect constraints, their simultaneous satisfaction may actually lead to a decrease in the accuracy of margin-constrained tabulations.

References

Australian Bureau of Statistics. (2001). *Census of Population and Housing Household Sample File.* Technical Paper 2037.0, Australian Bureau of Statistics, Australia.

Bethlehem, J.G., Wouter, J.K. and Pannekoek, J. (1990). Disclosure Control of Microdata. *Journal of the American Statistical Association*, 85(409), 38–45.

Campbell, M., Holdsworth, C., Payne, T. and Dale, A. (1996). *Sampling Variance and Design Factors in the Samples of Anonymised Records*. CCSR Occasional Paper No. 6, University of Manchester, UK.

Dale, A., Fieldhouse, E. and Holdsworth, C. (2000). *Analyzing Census Microdata*. Arnold, London.

Domingo-Ferrer, J. and Mateo-Sanz, J.M. (2002). Practical Data-Oriented Microaggregation for Statistical Disclosure Control. *IEEE Transactions on Knowledge and Data Engineering*, 14(1), 189–201.

Domingo-Ferrer, J. and Torra, V. (2003). Disclosure Risk Assessment in Statistical Microdata Protection via Advanced Data Linkage. *Statistics and Computing*, 13, 343–354.

Elliot, M.J., Manning, A.M. and Ford, R.W. (2002). A Computational Algorithm for Handling the Special Uniques Problem. *International Journal of Uncertainty, Fuziness and Knowledge-Based Systems*, 10(5), 493–509.

Elliot, M. and Manning, A. (2003). *Using DIS to Modify the Classification of Special Uniques*. Working Paper 22, Proceedings of Joint Economic Commission for Europe and EuroStat Work Session on Statistical Data Confidentiality, Luxembourg, 7–9 April. www.unece.org/stats/documents/2003/ 04/confidentiality/ wp.22.e.pdf, accessed date 4/11/2003.

Huang, Z. and Williamson, P. (2001). *Comparison of Synthetic Reconstruction and Combinatorial Optimisation Approaches to the Creation of Small-Area Microdata*. Working Paper 2001/2, Population Microdata Unit, Department of Geography, University of Liverpool, Liverpool. http://pcwww.liv.ac.uk/~william/microdata/ Methodology/WorkingPapers.html, accessed date 4/11/2003.

Johnston, R.J. and Pattie, C (1993). Entropy-Maximising and the Iterative Proportional Fitting Procedure. *Professional Geographer*, 45(3), 317–322.

Manning, A., Elliot, M. and Ma, B. (undated). *Automated Statistical Disclosure Risk Assessment*. Unpublished manuscript, Department of Computer Science, University of Manchester, Manchester.

Muralidhar, K. and Sarathy, R. (2003). A Theoretical Basis for Perturbation Methods. *Statistics and Computing*, 13, 329–335.

Office for National Statistics (2003). *SARS Consultation*. http://www.statistics.gov.uk/census2001/sar_consultation.asp, accessed date 4/11/2003.

Samarati, P. (2001). Protecting Respondents' Identities in Microdata Release. *IEEE Transactions on Knowledge and Data Engineering*, 13(6), 1010–1027.

Skinner, C. and Elliot, M.J. (2002). A Measure of Disclosure Risk for Microdata. *Journal of the Royal Statistical Society Series B*, 64(4), 855–867.

US Census Bureau. (2001). The US Census Bureau's Plans for the Census 2000 Public Use Microdata Sample Files. http://www.census.gov/population/www/ cen2000/pums.html, accessed date 31/10/2003.

Voas, D. and Williamson, P. (2000). An Evaluation of the Combinatorial Optimisation Approach to the Creation of Synthetic Microdata. *International Journal of Population Geography*, 6, 349–366.

Williamson, P. (2002a). Synthetic microdata, in Rees, P.H., Martin, D.J. and Williamson, P. (eds), *The Census Data System*, Wiley, Chichester, pp. 231–241.

Williamson, P. (2002b). *The Aggregation of Small-Area Synthetic Microdata to Higher-Level Geographies: An Assessment of Fit*. Working Paper 2002/1, Population Microdata Unit, Department of Geography, University of Liverpool, UK. http://pcwww.liv.ac.uk/~william/microdata/Methodology/WorkingPapers.html, accessed date 4/11/2003.

Williamson, P. (2003). *Synthetic Small-Area Microdata: An Evaluation*. Paper Presented at Technical Workshop, International Microsimulation Conference on Population Ageing and Health, Canberra, 7–12 December.

Wong, D.W.S. (1992). The Reliability of Using the Iterative Proportional Fitting Procedure. *Professional Geographer*, 44(3), 340–348.

Part VI: Overview of Existing Microsimulation and Health Human Resources Models

Chapter 19

The Search for Ideas among Existing Microsimulation Models

Mike McCracken and Anil Gupta

Informetrica Limited, Ottawa and Applied Research and Analysis Directorate, Health Canada, Canada

Abstract

Modelling activity has rapidly grown in the recent past. The use of microsimulation modelling is expanding and so are the number and types of microsimulation models. Modellers would love to have access to the latest advances in modelling techniques on the one hand and innovative ways of data gathering and data synthesis on the other. This chapter attempts to answer this need by bringing together some of the leading edge microsimulation (and some hybrid) models presently actively in use in real policy processes around the world. In particular, some key learnings from each of the models are highlighted.

1. Introduction

Readers of a collection of articles like this book are not usually planning to use the specific models. If so, they should go to the model developers and obtain the current documentation. Nor are they reading these articles for the sheer pleasure, as exciting as some might be. Rather they seek ideas for their own models, an appreciation of the possible applications of the models, and an assessment of the current state of the art of microsimulation.

The balance of this overview assumes that the reader is interested in building a model for purposes of shedding some light on issues dealing with health, ageing, or other social policies. He or she will look at the model descriptions and the applications discussed elsewhere in this and the companion volume (Harding and Gupta, 2006), with a number of different categories or dimensions in mind. A tabular summary of the models in this volume appears as an appendix to this chapter. We now turn to what these categories might be.

International Symposia in Economic Theory and Econometrics, Vol. 16

ISSN: 1571-0386 DOI: 10.1016/S1571-0386(06)16019-6

2. Categories for Description and Comparison

2.1 Naming of Models

If you are going to build a model, then a simple acronym or name will be helpful in identifying the product. Start with anything, but early on have a naming contest among the builders. Inspiration will show up, usually quite quickly. Some of the better ones described here: *SAGE, DESTINIE*, and *LOTTE.*

2.2 Survivability of Models

Some of the models were first built in the 1970s (*LOTTE*), while the bulk of them started in the 1990s. In this study we see the "survivors". Many other micro and macro models have been built and subsequently disappeared. Success factors include being developed by a statistical agency or a government department. In Australia, NATSEM has a long history of developing microsimulation models and applying them to policy issues. The dedication and leadership of Ann Harding has much to do with this success.

If policy departments use the model or their outputs, then this too ensures on-going support and continual improvement. As a rule-of-thumb maintenance of a model requires an outlay of about 30% of the initial construction costs per year. Having the assistance of a Finance department in support of your budget can be very helpful.

2.3 Users of Models

Many of the models have multiple users, either directly as with *STINMOD* in Australia or through custom runs for a client as with *LOTTE* in Norway. The evolution of software, computers, and devices for handling data securely are leading to increased direct use of microsimulation models. The ideal combination is to provide for both custom runs and direct use, reflecting the needs of the users.

2.4 Microsimulation Unit

One of the first choices that a new modeller must make is the basic unit for the microsimulation. Will it be a person, a household, or a special person (e.g., client, beneficiary of a program, employed worker[s])? Too narrow a focus here can limit the types of policies that can be simulated. For example, focusing on current customers or beneficiaries only, precludes possible expansion of the "universe" through changes in age, income, or other attributes. It is also useful to compare the population of beneficiaries to non-beneficiaries.

Many programs are specified at the individual level. However, family income tests may apply and policy analysts may want to consider the effects of changes on the family or household unit. The most flexible approach would include all people in the family in the sample along with their linkages to each other. Then simulations can be done with an individual focus, a family focus, or on people with particular roles in the family. A second approach is to keep the person as the basic record, with its status in a family indicated. This allows some analysis to be done along types of family roles, but does not define the family unit. If a policy affects multiple people in a family, then that change will not be visible in an individual file.

The models examined here sometimes use only people, others households only, and some a mixture of both. There are also other "units" that are part of some of the models as well. One model, *NSW Hospital*, includes hospitals as part of the microsimulation model, with people being associated with the various hospitals in their area. Another model, *CuSP*, uses data on customers and channels of service, with a matching of customers to channels as part of the model.

People live in a family context. In turn, families usually live in a Community, Neighbourhood, or special area (e.g., First Nations reserve). It will probably be useful to at least note that context in the individual or family records. Going further may require defining the membership in particular clusters, called neighbourhoods, and allowing the data to be aggregated by cluster. Another approach is also possible, and is discussed below in the section on spatial information.

The universe of people should also be defined with some care. Usually models use the "normal" population as the universe. However, there are a significant number of people who are institutionalized in hospitals, prisons, nursing homes, military barracks, and university dormitories. Are they a population of interest? For some social programs they may be major users. The Australian model, *STINMOD*, has added this population group to some versions of its database to allow broader analysis.

For some microsimulation models the units might be business units such as establishments and enterprises, or housing units. Such units might be additional units or the basic units, depending on the nature of the model.

2.5 Matching Processes

Should your model have specific matching processes or "markets" embedded? Do you want to form families through matching males and females through a marriage or partnering algorithm? How should children be generated (in the model)? See the *SAGE* and *SVERIGE* models for details.

Should people be matched with vacancies by occupation? This is done in *SVERIGE*, along with geographic constraints.

One could also imagine matching households and houses in the same geographic area. In turn, the houses and communities could be linked. At this point, serious thought should be given to the incorporation of spatial information more formally.

2.6 Spatial Information

At a minimum, distinction should be made between major entities, like Provinces or States, particularly if taxes and transfers vary across these jurisdictions. It may also be the case that these jurisdictions could be customers for your model, another good reason for having this breakdown in the data. The problem is that larger samples may be necessary to obtain decent estimates by jurisdiction. Fortunately, increases in computer speeds have reduced the computational problems. However, statistical agencies still must collect the data and privacy issues can occur with smaller regions.

The distinction in the data between urban and rural can also be helpful, particularly since the housing types and occupational mixes can be quite different. (Definitions of rural abound as well.)

Sub-provincial areas can also be defined. Some models have chosen the "labour market" as the unit for analysis (see *SVERIGE*-2). If survey data are available to support this level of geography then it might be useful to consider for new models.

NATSEM has developed a new and innovative approach for small-area microsimulation. In essence, they use information from a Census with small-area measures for key variables such as age, sex, effective family income, housing type, and other socio-economic characteristics. These variables are in turn used to create population weights within the small area. Records with more extensive information from a *national* survey are then selected as the records for the small area. Tests of this approach are promising (see the summary of *spatialMSM* for further details or go to the NATSEM website).

Spatial information can also be based on a more extensive approach with multi-country models (see *OECD Tax-Benefit* and *EUROMOD*). The major advantage of such models is the ability to simulate the effects of a policy change in different countries and to explore the reasons for the differences. Is it the population composition, elasticities of labour supply, income types, interaction with other tax systems? Are their lessons to be learned about subpopulations in your country?

2.7 Time Dimension

Microsimulation models usually start with data on units of one year, from a census or a survey. The supporting surveys are usually not annual, but a longer interval of every five or 10 years. This creates an inevitable lag in data. Generally the data lags by 2 3 years and the policies are intended, e.g. budgets, for the next year. It is not surprising that policy makers want the "latest data", even if the only choice is to forecast it. This desire is driven by trying to avoid a common criticism of any empirical work — it is not current and therefore is irrelevant.

Static models are used for a given year, with individual outcomes determined by the characteristics of the person in that year (the *variables*), the *parameters* of the tax system and transfer programs or other propensities for that year, and the population *weights* used to inflate the records to represent the total population in that year.

To create a static model for another year involves updating the population weights (if population is not modelled) to reflect changes in birth rates, death rates, net immigration, and movements between regions, if there is a spatial dimension.

The updating of the population weights is sometimes referred to as population ageing. It does scale the results for population changes, but is not the same as incorporating demographic processes into the microsimulation model, through a dynamic population component in the model.

Parameters of tax and transfer systems need to be updated as well to reflect budget changes. This may include CPI price indexes for indexed programs and unemployment rates for certain transfer programs triggered by labour market conditions.

What makes a model "dynamic"? If equations or "rules" depend on variables for an earlier time period as well as the current period, then the model is "dynamic". If a "stock" (accumulation of past flows) appears in a rule, then again the model is dynamic. Of course, if the model is being calculated for only one year, then these lagged variables can be stored as regular variables and the model remains comparable to a static model. If, however, the model calculates outcomes in subsequent years, then the results in a later year depend on the outcomes in earlier years. And if a policy change, for example, has altered the outcomes of an individual in an earlier year, then the results in a later year will also change. This "path dependency" indicates that the model is "dynamic".

The effects of stocks (e.g., wealth levels, accumulated capital losses) are to create persistent differences into the future. Equations defining these lagged variables need to be incorporated into the model to update their values from period to period (see Table 1).

2.8 Behavioural Elements

Some models are pure calculators, applying a set of parameters to variables of an individual and calculating various tax liabilities and transfer entitlements. Take-up rates on programs can be incorporated into the model by

Table 1: Two Important Characteristics

Time dimension	Behaviour?
Static	No
Dynamic	Rules
Stock-flow	Optimization
Unknown	Stochastic

using a random number generator and selecting whether the individual selects the program or not, based on the value of the random number. This is a stochastic element in the model.

It is also possible to go further and to have behavioural equations, reacting to current or past variables of the individual, Behavioural responses may determine labour market participation, take-up rates on a program, or decisions about retirement. Since the estimated equations often have an error term, a stochastic element can also be combined with the behavioural equation.

3. Links with Other Models

Several microsimulation models are linked to macroeconomic models. It is common for models to use population forecasts from other models to age their populations (*IPDSM, NSM, NDM, Medisim, and NSW Hospital*). The Norwegian models (*MOSART* and *LOTTE*) also use macro model linkages, with information about populations, pensions, and labour supply driving a GE model in the case of MOSART. For LOTTE, macroeconomic forecasts help update the microsimulation into the future, and details from the tax, transfer, and consumer blocks can feed back to the macro model forecasts or econometric model, through a process of "manual simultaneity".

Links are also evident between microsimulation models. The Australian group at NATSEM often uses *STINMOD* to drive other microsimulation models (e.g., *CUsP* and *spatialMSM*). *PHARMASIM* in Canada feeds off of a general-purpose microsimulation model (CHTSIM) for income and demographic information. *PHARMASIM* also links to a typical pharmacare use model (TPU) for development of policy parameters through impact analysis on typical households.

4. User Dimensions

Only a few microsimulation models are publicly available or even accessible by researchers. The reason often given is that privacy laws prevent the disclosure of information about persons, particularly if they can be identified by some of the information. Much progress has been made in creating anonymous records, where information is not identifiable yet the statistical properties of the records are maintained. The imputation of data values into records adds further to this creation of "fictitious" people, but with enhanced value to the records.

Another barrier in the past has been the sheer size of the microsimulation files, with hundreds of thousands of records. Advances in computing storage and processing speeds have reduced this problem substantially.

Committing to make a model available requires careful documentation, full disclosure of equations and rules, databases, and output routines. Is it worthwhile? The benefit comes in the feedback from users, the studies that can build on your work, and the potential improvements that can occur over time. It also creates more confidence in the results, if people can look inside the "black box".

An even more pro-active approach is also possible. Some organizations are working to make microsimulation models available on-line through the Internet, with no restrictions on access. This is seen as a form of E-democracy (e.g., *GLADHISPANIA, OECD Tax and Benefit Model*).

4.1 Model Size

There is no single indicator of model size that conveys all of the dimensionality of a model. For macroeconomic models, the number of equations (behavioural and identities), the number of exogenous variables, and the size of the underlying database in years would give some sense of the model size. In the case of microsimulation models, the number of records (people) in the file, the number of variables about them, and the number of parameters describing the tax and transfer system would be a good starting point for sizing the model. Unfortunately these measures were not available to us in the short summaries received. The numbers of records (where available) vary from 6,000 households (*GLADHISPANIA*) to about 9,000 households with *STINMOD*, to hundreds of thousands with the statistical-agency or government-based models. The largest database is the total population of the country, with longitudinal histories. This base serves as a sampling frame for small-area studies as well (*SVERIGE*).

4.2 Software

Many models have started to use standard packages such as SAS, STATA, Excel, and Access for the analysis of results and the management of databases. Others have written their models in a programming language such as C, C++, C#, Pascal, and Visual Basic. On-line systems are using Java.

5. Why Microsimulation?

The studies in these volumes serve as examples of the rich texture that can be developed when policy is analysed for different groups in the society. Similar and different groups become evident. This can be further developed into a winners/losers analysis by subgroup within the population.

Description of the details of government tax systems and transfer programs through specific parameters and the application of equations or rules can be quite close to the actual administration of the programs. This ensures an accurate portrayal of policy, and allows for changing policy through the specific parameters of a program.

As a general rule, disaggregation helps clarify the response of each element to a policy change and often requires a simpler equation to describe behavioural response. With the detailed records, then re-aggregation can be done in a number of ways — by region, by age, by gender — each shedding light on the policy effects.

6. Challenges

Updating databases with new information and linking different databases together remains a challenge. Nevertheless, techniques are becoming standard and success breeds further application.

Imputation of variables onto records also offers a way of linking databases using regression models. By cloning the records and assigning values from a distribution of a variable, variance can be maintained in the database.

Specifying dynamic effects requires some care and substantially richer databases. The best predictor of a person's state in the next year is the state in the current year. This inertia model requires the longitudinal information to support it. As well, events need to be triggered in the model to "wake up" the individual represented by the record and provoke a change — marriage, becoming a parent, losing a job, retiring, becoming disabled, etc. Economists also like to calculate permanent income, wealth effects, and learning by doing. All of these concepts require histories of the income flows, the education and experience records, and accumulated saving flows.

The idea of simulating the matches of people into family formation and parenting offers an opportunity for a deeper understanding of the processes of family formation. Matching of households to available housing offers an opportunity to exploit the information about the housing stock as well as the information about the households. Employment positions of firms in an area being matched to employees in the area should provide additional insights into the processes of firm growth, the effects of layoffs, and the independent role of the demographic base in sustaining businesses in an area.

Usually variables about an individual record pertain only to that person or family. However, the response of an individual may reflect its response to neighbourhood effects, provincial or national variables. This is in addition to parameters that may affect the rules of the tax or transfer system, such as the CPI inflation factor.

In the past, computational limitations have been a challenge to many researchers. However, the introduction of high-speed PCs, large storage devices, and standard statistical software is making microsimulation modeling much easier than in the past. As always, gains are used to further complicate the models, to introduce large datasets, more spatial detail, and more sectors into the models.

There is more complementary use of microsimulation models with other models, taking advantage of the relative strengths of the models. It is now possible to link models together on the same computer, allowing simultaneous modelling of policies on macro and micro fronts.

Computer systems are also allowing better communication of the results of models to users. This occurs through better graphics, better tables, a variety of comparisons, and even the possible direct interaction of the user with a model. More efforts to extend the results of microsimulation to the media, researchers, and citizens are to be encouraged.

Reference

Harding, A. and Gupta, A. (eds). (2006). *Modelling Our Future: Population Ageing, Social Security and taxation.* International Symposia in Economic Theory and Econometrics, North-Holland, Amsterdam.

Appendix

	1	2	3	4	5
Model Name	**MOSART**	**DYNAMOD**	**SAGE**	**SESIM**	**DYNACAN**
Country	**Norway**	**Australia**	**Britain**	**Sweden**	**Canada**
Started in?	1988	1992	1999	1999	1994
Developer	Statistics Norway	NATSEM	Centre for Research on Ageing, Southampton & LSE	Swedish Department of Finance	Canada Pension Plan
Main User(s)	Ministry of Finance, Ministry of Labour and Social Inclusion				HRSDC, Office of the Chief Actuary, Finance
Model Type	microsimulation	microsimulation	microsimulation	microsimulation	microsimulation
Unit(s) modelled	People	People	People	People, households	People
Matching Processes	NO	NO	Marriage, parenting	NO	NO
Spatial Information				characteristic of people	
Time Dimension	**Dynamic**	**Dynamic**	**Dynamic**	**Dynamic**	**Dynamic**
Behavior?	Transitional Probabilities, survival functions	Transitional Probabilities, survival functions	Transitional probabilities		Equations estimating probabilities
Time Frame?	20-30 years ahead	to 2050	1991-2031		1971-2100
Unit Records	1 % Census sample	1 % Census sample, 150,000 persons	0.1% Census sample, 54,000 records	3.5% population sample, admin data, 350,000 households, 786,000 people	1 % Census sample, 200,000
Reference Year(s)	1993	1986	1991		1971
Links to Other Models	Input to GE model	macro model			no
Software	Simula/SAS	Windows/C	C++, STATA, Excel	Visual Basic, SAS & Excel	C/SAS
Policy Areas?	Reforms of the Norwegian National Insurance Scheme	Taxes & Transfers	Pensions, health care, long-term care, social policy	Pensions, health care, long-term care, population ageing, intergenerational wealth transfers	Canada Pension Plan, disability outlays
Features		One-month stepping and event-driven. Alignment processes key to successful applications over time	Incorporates labour market & pensions as well as healthcare and disability. Annual steps	Geographic distances between elderly and caregivers	Working on education module and tax module
Available to Others?	Custom Runs		SAGE researchers	Model code on website	Internal - government
Contact Point			Jane Falkingham, School of Social Sciences, University of Southampton		Rick Morrison
Frequency of Update	current				current

Appendix (*Continued*)

	6	7	8	9	10
Model Name	**DESTINIE**	**GLADHISPANIA**	**STINMOD**	**EUROMOD**	**PSSRU Long-term Care Finance**
Country	**France**	**Spain**	**Australia**	**EUROMOD**	**United Kingdom**
Started in?	1993	2000	1994	1996	1996
Developer	INSEE	University of Balearic Islands-Spain	NATSEM	Academic consortium	PSSRU, LSE
Main User(s)	Département des Etudes Economiques d'Ensemble, Conseil d'Orientation des Retraites	Teaching tool, Media, researchers	Commonwealth Government departments	Academics	Department of Health, Royal Commissions, EC
Model Type	microsimulation	microsimulation	microsimulation	microsimulation	subaggregate model + microsim link
Unit(s) modelled	People	Households	People, Households	Households, People	Groups of People
Matching Processes	NO	NO	NO	NO	NO
Spatial Information		NO		15 European countries	England, UK
Time Dimension	**Dynamic, stochastic**	**Static**	**Static**	**Static**	**Static-Macro Dynamic-Micro**
Behavior?	Endogenous retirement	Labour supply	no	NO	YES
Time Frame?	1998-2050	1998-2005	2010-11		to 2051
Unit Records	Financial Asset Survey	EC Household Panel (Spain), 6,420	Synthetic database	EC Household Panel	Group of people, by age, gender, household type, household tenure
Reference Year(s)	1998	1995	2003-2005	2001	
Links to Other Models		no	no		CARESIM
Software	Turbo Pascal, SAS & Excel	Excel, Java	SAS, Excel	C++, Excel, Access	Excel, SAS
Policy Areas?	Pension, health care system	Tax policy, basic income	General-purpose, training tool	comparative tax-benefit analysis; effects of inflation by country; child tax credits	Long-term care expenditure; balance between public and private care
Features	Incentive effects on retirement decision	Accessible by anyone on Internet; e-democracy application	Institutionalized population included in some versions	Comparative changes across countries; being expanded to 25 countries	Link between micro and macro models to determine distribution of users and financing
Available to Others?		Publicly available, on Internet	Publicly available	Students, policy researchers	
Contact Point		www.gladhispania.es	NATSEM	University of Essex (I-CUE)	
Frequency of Update		on-going	on-going	Periodic	on-going

Appendix (*Continued*)

	11	12	13	14	15
Model Name	**OECD Tax-Benefit Model**	**PHARMASIM (CHTSIM)**	**LOTTE**	**IPDSM**	**NSM/NDM**
Country	**OECD**	**Canada**	**Norway**	**Canada**	**USA**
Started in?	1995	2000	1970s	2003	1999
Developer	OECD and EU	Health Canada	Statistics Norway	Health Canada	Health Resources and Services Administration (HRSA), USA
Main User(s)	OECD, EU	Health Canada	Finance	Health Canada, provinces	HRSA
Model Type	Typical household	microsimulation	microsimulation	subaggregate model	subaggregate model
Unit(s) modelled	Households (5 typical HH)	People	People, households	Groups of People (supply), FTEs (demand)	Groups of People (supply), FTEs (demand)
Matching Processes	NO	NO	NO	NO	NO
Spatial Information	OECD- 29 countries	By province		By province (supply & demand);	State (supply and demand)
Time Dimension	**Static**	**Static**	**Static**	Stock-Flow, lags	Stock-Flow, lags
Behavior?	NO	NO	YES (under development)	NO	NO
Time Frame?	Recent years	2006	Macro forecasts used	1975-2020	
Unit Records		Synthetic database, 80,000 people	Merged database, 17,000 households		
Reference Year(s)		2000	2003		1996-2000
Links to Other Models	**NO**	Typical Pharmacare Use Model (TPU)	macro models	Population forecasts	Population forecasts
Software	STATA			Visual Basic, Excel, Access	
Policy Areas?	Analyses of work incentives, income poverty and adequacy of benefit entitlements	Evaluation of catastrophic drug plans, tax assistance for pharmaceuticals	Tax-benefit analysis; budget analysis	Health human resource planning, gap analysis, supply planning	Supply & demand for nurse resources
Features	Comparative analyses across countries. On-line version for 2006	Extends multi-purpose microsimulation model (CHTSIM)	expenditure taxes and real income measures; labour supply functions	Interprovincial movement of physicians; provincial differences for most reasonable diagnosis (MRD)	Regression equations pooling State data with short time series used for healthcare utilization and nursing intensity
Available to Others?	Online access		custom runs provided to Parliamentarians	NO	
Contact Point	www.oecd.org/els/social/workincentives	Anil Gupta, Health Canada		Anil Gupta, Health Canada	Steve Tise and Marilyn Bivian
Frequency of Update	on-going	on-going	on-going	on-going	

Appendix (*Continued*)

	16	17	18	19	20
Model Name	**Medisim**	**SVERIGE (1,2,3)**	**NSW Hospital**	**CuSP**	**spatialMSM**
Country	**Australia**	**Sweden**	**Australia**	**Australia**	**Australia**
Started in?	1998	1998	2003	2000	2003
Developer	NATSEM with funding of Medicines Australia	Spatial Modelling Centre in Kiruna	NATSEM	NATSEM	NATSEM
Main User(s)	Commonwealth Department of Health and Family Services	Umeå University, Sweden	NSW Health department	CentreLink (Australia)	Australian Research Council, ABS, State departments
Model Type	microsimulation	microsimulation	microsimulation	microsimulation	microsimulation
Unit(s) modelled	people, HH, drugs	people, HH	patients, hospitals	customers and channels of use	people, households
Matching Processes	Drugs to people	Marriages, jobs to vacancies	YES	YES	NO
Spatial Information		counties, towns, 100 meter squares	hospital catchment areas	Small area data	Small area data, SLA
Time Dimension	**Static**	**Dynamic, Annual and Event-driven**	**Static**	**Annual usage**	**Static**
Behavior?	NO	YES	NO	NO	NO
Time Frame?	5 year forecast		1996-2000	2005-2009, 2014	
Unit Records		100% population "sample", sampling as needed for spatial detail	1.9 million records for patient separation (1.2 million patients)		9,000 households in pool; used to populate each small area
Reference Year(s)	2001	longitudinal, 1968 - 2003	1996-2000	1998	2001
Links to Other Models	Population forecasts		Population forecasts	STINMOD	STINMOD
Software	SAS, Excel	Turbo, C++, C#	SAS	SAS	SAS
Policy Areas?	Drug pricing, listing, prescribing practices, copayment schemes, etc.		Effects of private health insurance incentives, roles of public and private hospitals	Decision support tool, analyze social security policy changes, and socio-economic developments	Regional policies for poverty reduction, housing affordability, tax benefit analysis for small areas
Features	Linking of health and drug utilization information to individuals	Variable rate of sampling, reflecting needs; power of longitudinal database in predicting income sources, etc.	Equivalent family income (EFI) used for SES imputation to people in small areas; use of administrative records by hospital	concepts of customers, areas, and channels of service linked together	Concept of reweighting of national results to portray small area is innovative
Available to Others?		NO	NO	NO	YES
Contact Point	NATSEM		NATSEM	NATSEM	NATSEM
Frequency of Update	on-going	on-going			on-going

Dynamic Microsimulation Models

Model 1

MOSART (Dynamic Cross-Sectional Microsimulation Model)

Dennis F. Fredriksen and Nils M. Stølen

Statistics Norway, Research Department, P.O. Box 8131 Dep., N-0033 Oslo, Norway

Introduction

Statistics Norway has since the 1970s projected population, education, labour force and public pension benefits both for improving the basis for policy making and own research. Until 1988, when the development of the dynamic cross-sectional microsimulation model MOSART started, these subjects were analysed by different transition matrix models. The first version of MOSART was completed in 1990 and included demographic events, education and labour force. The second version of the model was completed in 1993, and the model was extended with public pension benefits and labour market earnings. A more matured variant of this version is later on documented in Fredriksen (1998). The work on the third and current version started in 1995 by extending the model with household formation and a simple representation of other sources of income, taxation, savings and wealth. This version has not been properly documented yet. In addition to the use of the model in research projects in Statistics Norway, The Ministry of Finance and The Ministry of Labour and Social Inclusion are the main users. Specifically, MOSART has been, and is, extensively used in the process of reforming the Norwegian public pension system.

Overview

MOSART is a dynamic microsimulation model with a cross-section of the Norwegian population and a comprehensive set of characteristics. The model starts with a representative sample of the population in a base year and simulates the further life course for each individual in this initial population. The transition probabilities depend on individual characteristics

International Symposia in Economic Theory and Econometrics, Vol. 16

ISSN: 1571-0386 DOI: 10.1016/S1571-0386(06)16020-2

and are estimated from observed transitions in a recent period. Events included in the simulation are migration, deaths, births, household formation, educational activities, retirement, labour force participation and income and wealth. Public pension benefits are calculated from the simulated labour market earnings and other characteristics included in the simulation according to an accurate description of the public pension system. The pensions covered by the model include old age pensions, disability pensions, survival pensions and early retirement benefits.

MOSART projects the Norwegian population and its characteristics for the coming decades. The modelling of demographic events and the underlying demographic assumptions of the model are to a large degree based on the public population projections from Statistics Norway. New-borns and new immigrants are added to the initial population each year, and mortality depends on gender and age. The result of the simulation is a model population with the life course of each individual.

Before running the model, the model user must make assumptions on how the behaviour underlying each event will develop in the future. The usual approach is to define a base line scenario based on the conditions in the most recent year with available statistics, and with a few exceptions let the transition probabilities stay at this level. One interpretation is that the base line scenario shows the development ahead if "everything continues as today". Policies or other circumstances leading to shifts in the underlying assumptions can be analysed by comparing two or more projections. The MOSART model may also be used to analyse income distribution in a life course context.

Data Sources

The current version of MOSART starts with a 1 per cent random sample of the population in Norway from 1993. Together 12 disjoint 1 per cent samples are available as initial population for the model. Each 1 per cent sample comprises 40,000 persons with actual information on marriage, birth histories, educational level and activities, pension status and pension entitlements in the National Insurance Scheme. Most of the information is represented as annual data back to 1985, and pension entitlements are represented as annual labour market earnings back to 1967. The information is gathered from administrative registers in the Directorate of Taxes, the National Insurance Administration and Statistics Norway. The sample is stratified by gender, age, birth histories and household status, and the sample includes both spouses from all married couples and from cohabitating couples with children.

In addition to be the starting point of the simulation, the initial population is also used to estimate the transition probabilities. The probabilities may be adjusted to make the expected number of simulated events equal to some external constraints, for example, the historical number of events in the same year. The underlying assumptions are generally kept up to date by using adjustment factors from the last year with historical data at an aggregate level. This is the case for aggregate observations regarding net immigration, periodic life expectancy at birth by gender, number of births, number of pupils and students by gender and age groups, number of early retirees, retirement age, number of persons in the labour force and person-years by gender, total labour market earnings by gender and the basic pension unit, and rules for calculating pension entitlements and benefits. At present the model is calibrated to annual data from 2001. When calibrating new annual data we assume that the effects from different explanatory variables (gender, age, education, etc.) on the transition probabilities are the same as estimated from the initial population, and that the adjustment factors capture the interesting part of time variation.

A second level of maintenance is to keep the initial population up to date, but a frequent updating of the initial population seems to be less important for the use of the model. However, updating the initial population and reestimation of the transition probabilities will be given priority in the near future.

Technical Details

The MOSART model is run from a UNIX platform, and the simulation part of the model is written in Simula, an object-oriented language developed in Norway in the 1960s. An object-orientation both seems to ease a flexible handling of the model population and the division of the simulation programme into separate pieces that are small enough to be handled in a proper manner with respect to readability, etc. A standard simulation with 1 per cent of the population requires approximately 60 MB RAM, since computing the National Insurance Scheme benefits require access to annual labour market earnings from the entire working career. The need for hard-disk depends on to which extent the model population is written to a file, and that is seldom necessary at all to create standard tables. As Simula is not further developed and is thus not compatible with Statistics Norway's digital computers, we still run MOSART on old Sun Sparc servers. These computers use from 3 to 6 h to complete a standard simulation with 1 per cent of the population until 2100. With an ordinary up-to-date server, it would probably be possible to run the model well below 1 hour. We therefore intend to reprogram the model into a modern object-oriented language compatible with Statistics Norway's modern servers in the near future.

The outputs from a simulation consist of extensive self-documentation (making the user able to find errors in the results afterwards), a set of standard tables produced by the simulation programme with aggregated figures covering most frequently asked questions, and at last an option to produce a model population consisting of an ASCII-file with one record per selected person per selected year with selected variables. Special tables may be produced from this file with a suitable table production programme, usually SAS.

The user interface of the MOSART model is very simple and consists of a few shell scripts handling the set up of new simulations and the execution of necessary computer programs. Every new simulation is given a separate directory with the directory name also being the identification (the name) of the simulation. Each simulation directory includes six small text-files with names of input files and values for other external parameters, and all simulation results are stored in this directory. Operating the system requires some training, but the simplicity of the user interface means that there is no obstacle against developing the model in any direction.

Usage and Usability

MOSART is operated at Statistics Norway only, both due to technical obstacles, restrictions from the Data Authorities regarding the merged administrative registers, and because understanding the full meaning of changing any parameter requires detailed knowledge of the model. Besides our own analyses, the main users are the Ministry of Finance and the Ministry of Labour and Social Inclusion. The users in these ministries are either former model developers themselves or economists with a realistic sense of how economic models work. They are therefore critical and capable users of the simulation results, and this has proved beneficial to the development and validation of the model. For this reason we can also transfer the results with a low degree of preparation, often as tables supported by some verbal explanations. Other public institutions, private organisations and media use the results from the MOSART model occasionally. In these cases the results are handed over with a higher degree of preparation.

Development and maintenance of the model is partly financed through general funding from Statistics Norway, partly through a contract with the Ministry of Finance and the Ministry of Labour and Social Inclusion renegotiated annually, and occasionally through special research projects financed by the Norwegian Research Council or the Norwegian government. If private organisations or other public institutions than the two ministries want to use the model, they usually have to pay for the use of resources, unless the results are already available.

In the last couple of years the MOSART model has been intensively used in analysing effects from reforms of the Norwegian National Insurance Scheme. As in many other countries the pension system in Norway is rather complicated, including non-linearities regarding the accumulation of pension entitlements. A microsimulation model including demographic characteristics, labour supply and an accurate description of the pension system therefore seems to be the most appropriate tool to obtain accurate estimates of the direct effects on individual benefits, government expenditures and the future pension burden. Distributional effects may also be included in a consistent way. The results from the analyses are heavily used and documented in two reports from the Norwegian Pension Commission (who finished their work in the beginning of 2004) and a White Paper from the Government in the spring 2005. An overview of some of the questions analysed may be found in Fredriksen and Stølen (2005). New simulations are presently in progress for the preparation of a new White Paper in summer 2006.

Results from the MOSART-model have also been incorporated in a general equilibrium model to analyse macroeconomic effects of pension reforms. Projections of the demographic development and effects from different pension reforms on public expenditures and labour supply, including retirement behaviour, are made by MOSART and used as input in the general equilibrium model. These analyses are documented in Fredriksen, Heide, Holmøy and Solli (2005). In general, the Ministry of Finance uses the results from Statistics Norway's official population projections and from MOSART regarding supply of labour and pension expenditures as input in their macroeconomic analyses when discussing challenges in the long run for the Norwegian economy in their white papers.

References

Fredriksen, D. (1998). Projections of Population, Education, Labour Supply and Public Pension Benefits. *Social and Economic Studies 101*, Statistics Norway.

Fredriksen, D., Heide, K., Holmøy, E. and Solli, I. (2005). *Macroeconomic Effects of Proposed Pension Reforms in Norway*. Discussion Paper no. 417, Statistics Norway.

Fredriksen, D. and Stølen, M. (2005). *Effects of Demographic Development, Labour Supply and Pension Reforms on the Future Pension Burden*. Discussion Paper no. 418, Statistics Norway.

Model 2

DYNAMOD

Simon Kelly

NATSEM, University of Canberra, Australia

Introduction

DYNAMOD is a dynamic microsimulation model of the Australian population developed at the National Centre for Social and Economic Modelling (NATSEM). It is similar to other international microsimulation models in that it has a base population representative of the population; uses functions to model change; and has a set of alignment modules that ensure the output match external reference data. However, the methods used to model probability and align the data are unique.

In the early (1992) stages of the development of DYNAMOD the decision was taken to move away from the traditional approach to dynamic microsimulation and to include some innovative, albeit untested, new methodologies. Noteworthy aspects of the design for DYNAMOD included the use of survival functions; the division of the model into simulation and analysis modules; and the inclusion of an integrated macroeconomic model.

An overambitious development schedule resulted in faltering progress and culminated in a major break in the project when in late 1994/early 1995 the entire DYNAMOD team of four researchers resigned. An internal review began in March 1995 and three major changes were identified for implementation — the internal macroeconomic model was to be abandoned in favour of a simpler and more controlled micro–macro link; the use of survival functions were to be restricted and more reliance was put on the more traditional transition probability approach; and a more flexible model structure was to be implemented.

Following the review, development recommenced and DYNAMOD-2 was delivered at the end of 1997 to the Department of Employment, Education and Training.

The current DYNAMOD is version 3. A number of major changes have occurred between versions 2 and 3. The model was redeveloped and

International Symposia in Economic Theory and Econometrics, Vol. 16

ISSN: 1571-0386 DOI: 10.1016/S1571-0386(06)16021-4

transported from the Unix to the Windows/DOS environment. This reduced processing times and provided access to a vastly improved development environment. Alignment of demographics and labour force transitions were improved in version 3 and household wealth, superannuation, taxation and government transfer modules were added. Finally, better accounting of labour force participation and earnings were implemented.

The model is now being used operationally, a number of papers based on simulated outcomes from DYNAMOD are contributing to debate on social policy in Australia (e.g. Kelly, 2001, 2002; Kelly et al., 2002).

Technical Details

The latest version of the model is DYNAMOD-3. This version runs on a PC, contains around 40,000 lines of code and is written in the programming language C. It is able to project the characteristics of the Australian population up to the year 2050. It starts with a base population of 150,000 people (a 1 per cent sample from the 1986 Census), who are representative of the Australian population and then simulates events that will occur in their lives — births, deaths, migration, education, leaving home, forming couples, divorcing, being employed, earning money, accumulating and drawing down household assets, paying taxes, receiving government benefits, becoming disabled and recovering from a disability.

How the Simulation Works

The simulation model has the same structure as other microsimulation models — an initial base population, a simulation cycle and an output. Within the simulation cycle is a set of functions for calculating the probability of events occurring.

The Initial Base Population

At the start of the simulation the initial population of 150,000 records are read in. A 1 per cent sample file from the 1986 Australian Census is the source of these data. Other characteristics are imputed for each person to be simulated, links to other family members are created, and the births of children are scheduled. At the time of reading in this base data, labour force details are also initialised, status lists are created and dates of disability and death for each person are calculated. These events are added to the 'crystal ball'.

The Simulation Cycle

The simulation uses two methods to replicate events that happen during people's lives. The first — transition probabilities — is the one normally used and makes use of the simulation clock. This clock steps through time (in DYNAMOD the steps can be as small as one month). At the start of each increment, the chance of a person transitioning from one state to another is considered (e.g. changing from the state of 'employed' to the state of 'unemployed'). The chance that a person makes the transition varies with their circumstances at that time.

The calculation of transition probabilities are done through the use of regression equations that apply weightings to each of the influences based on historical data. This method is used extensively by DYNAMOD to simulate changes in relation to the labour force.

The second method used to simulate an event in a person's life is through survival functions. With this method, rather than do a calculation for every person every month, the calculation is only done when trigger events take place. When a trigger event occurs, a calculation is made of when a subsequent event will occur. For example, when a birth occurs (a trigger event), the date of death of the baby is decided (the subsequent event). The advantage of this method is that calculations only have to be made a few times rather than every month (as an example, date of death is only calculated once or twice in a person's life — at birth, if a person becomes disabled, or if a person recovers from a disability — rather than 12 times per year). The disadvantage of the survival function method is that estimated durations of being in a given state are required and only limited amounts of data are available in this form. DYNAMOD uses survival functions to model most demographic occurrences.

At the simulation steps through time, DYNAMOD uses a diary called the 'crystal ball' to keep track of the various events that are due to occur. The crystal ball contains details of dates, events and people.

Output

The method used to record what happens during a simulation is to write the details of every person and any change in their circumstances to a series of 'history files'. The files can then be analysed after the simulation.

The items stored relate to each person, relatives, parents, residences, qualifications, education types, educational institutions, education levels, the labour force, industries, occupations, sectors, income and employment status (full-time, part-time, unemployed, not in the labour force, marital statuses, pregnancies, migration, disabilities, deaths and wealth).

These history files enable comparisons at various points in time to be undertaken or allow the circumstances of an individual to be analysed over time.

Alignment

The output obtained from the original DYNAMOD model design was not in harmony with expected answers and a number of papers questioned whether DYNAMOD could become a credible and useful model in its then form. The key element missing was identified to be alignment processes — a point supported by the experiences of the successful CORSIM and DYNACAN dynamic microsimulation models. Importance of alignment as an essential element for a useful model has subsequently been emphasised during development of the recent versions of DYNAMOD. The various versions of alignment and its increasing sophistication are described in detail in Kelly and King (2001).

Conclusions

Despite a number of early setbacks, DYNAMOD-3 is now an operational dynamic microsimulation model that is providing a significant input into the Australian policy debate.

References

Kelly, S. (2001). *Trends in Australian Wealth — New Estimates for the 1990s*. Paper Presented to the 30th Annual Conference of Economists, University of Western Australia, September.

Kelly, S. (2002). *Simulating Future Trends in Wealth Inequality*. Paper Presented to the 2002 Annual Conference of Economists, Adelaide, South Australia, October.

Kelly, S. and King, A. (2001). Australians Over the Coming 50 Years: Providing Useful Projections. *Brazilian Electronic Journal of Economics*, 4(2), 1–23.

Kelly, S., Percival, R. and Harding, A. (2002). Women and Superannuation in the 21st Century: Poverty or Plenty? *Competing Visions: Proceedings of the National Social Policy Conference*, SPRC Report 1/02 University of New South Wales, pp. 223–249.

Model 3

The SAGE Model: A Dynamic Microsimulation Population Model for Britain

Maria Evandrou[a], Jane Falkingham[a], Paul Johnson[b], Anne Scott[b] and Asghar Zaidi[c]

[a]*Centre for Research on Ageing, University of Southampton, UK*
[b]*London School of Economics, UK*
[c]*European Centre for Social Welfare Policy and Research, Vienna, Austria*

Introduction

The ESRC Research Group 'Simulating Social Policy for an Ageing Society' (SAGE) was established in November 1999 with funding from the UK Economic and Social Research Council. The aim of the SAGE Research Group has been to carry out high quality academic research on the future of social policy within an ageing society that is of direct relevance to policy makers and the broader user community. One of the core activities of the Group has been the construction and use of a dynamic microsimulation model to provide projections to inform the development of social policy in Britain for the twenty-first century, focussing on the implications of population ageing for pensions and issues regarding health and long-term care needs. The model generates projections of the likely future socio-economic characteristics of the older population, including their financial resources, health and dependency, and family circumstances. This provides important information for policy makers regarding the likely demand for health and social care, the supply of informal carers and the degree to which older people will be able to resource their own retirement.

Overview

The SAGE model is a partially closed, discrete time, time-based dynamic microsimulation model. It is a full population model, and covers demographic processes, education, labour market participation, earnings, pension accumulation, and health and disability. The SAGE model takes a cross-section of

International Symposia in Economic Theory and Econometrics, Vol. 16

ISSN: 1571-0386 DOI: 10.1016/S1571-0386(06)16022-6

the British population drawn from the 1991 census and projects them forward through time to 2031, with each individual experiencing the risk of dying, forming a partnership, having children, obtaining educational qualifications, working, contributing to a pension (both state and private), experiencing ill health and disability and providing informal care. Using simulation techniques, the model builds a complete picture of the life histories of the model individuals, providing a picture of the likely pension entitlements, health and health care needs of the older population in 2031. The model can then be used to assess the impact of different policy options within the fields of pension provision and long-term care.

Data Issues

The choice of base data was an early and important decision in the model building process. No single sample dataset can be expected to provide all information required for the base population, so trade-offs had to be made between different requirements. The representativeness of the base sample and its size have been SAGE's principal concerns, and for these reasons it was decided to use a sample from the Samples of Anonymised Records (SARs) from the 1991 Census of Great Britain as the base dataset for the SAGE model, representing 0.1% of the British population (see SAGE Technical Note 1). Clearly, in this choice, greater importance is assigned to the sample representativeness of the base survey than its contents, mainly because an initial bias in representativeness is likely to be magnified during the simulation period. The disadvantage is that various matching and imputing techniques are required to compensate for the shortage of variables of interest. The base data have been supplemented with additional information taken from a variety of sources. In particular, summary information on work and caring histories and pension accumulation was matched on the base data from the 1994 Family and Working Lives Survey. This means that the base population starts with some history rather than being a pure cross-section (see SAGE Technical Note 8).

Data are also required to determine the probabilities of transitions between different states within the model. Where possible, transition probabilities have been estimated using longitudinal data, including the British Household Panel Survey, the Quarterly Labour Force Survey, and the ONS Longitudinal Study. However, panel data are not available to cover all the model requirements and cross-sectional surveys such as the General Household Survey have also been used.

Projection Component

Transitions within the SAGE model are based on 'rules' specified by the model designer. These may take the form of look-up tables of probabilities, or regression equations, or other functional transformations, and may be deterministic or stochastic. For the latter case, pseudo-random numbers are supplied by a random number generator built into the simulation program. The population is closed with respect to partnership and parenthood, and a partnership market is implemented for marital and cohabiting relationships. However, for extra-family members open relationships are possible, with a limited number of characteristics of secondary individuals being modelled as attributes of the primary individual.

Data Ageing

The SAGE model uses time-based processing with a discrete time frame. The entire population is processed simultaneously, allowing matching between sample individuals, and state changes are computed at fixed time intervals using transition probabilities. The different model processes take place in a fixed order within an annual cycle, and each transition may depend only on the outcomes of transitions in the previous cycle, or transitions that have occurred earlier in the same cycle. This means that the ordering of the transitions in the cycle needs to be carefully considered. As the model population is based on a nationally representative sample of the national population, no re-weighting of cases is required.

Technical Particulars

Language

The SAGE model program has been developed using the Borland C++ compiler, command-line version 5, for Windows 32 operating systems. The program utilises Object-Oriented Programming to produce a very flexible implementation that maximises separation between content and implementation. An important feature is a simple scripting language that enables transition rules to be declared and modified without the need for specialist programming skills. Further details are available in SAGE Technical Note 3. A variety of other software, particularly Excel and STATA, contribute to the extraction and presentation of the model's results.

System Requirements/Type of Computer

The model is currently being run under Windows 2000 on a desktop computer with a 1.7 GHz processor and 1GB of RAM. The executable file is under 600 K in size, and the data, principally the population database with just under 54,000 individual records, fit easily into available core memory, avoiding the need for swapping into virtual memory on disk, which would significantly degrade performance.

Data Storage

The base population data and output data are stored in tab-delimited files. They may be viewed using a text editor, but are best prepared and analysed using a statistical or spreadsheet package, such as STATA or Excel The script and rules files, and the log file, are in text (ASCII) format and can be viewed and edited using any text editor or word processor.

Typical Run Time

The running time depends on the number and complexity of included events, the frequency of output, and the speed of the output media. Currently, the most time-consuming event is the Labour Market, which takes under 2 s per simulation year. Events that are 'hard-coded', which include all the demographic events, run much faster than scripted events, such as the Labour Market. A full simulation of all events from 1991 to 2031, with output of results on an annual basis, takes under 420 s.

Interactivity

Currently a simple user interface allows the user to set the start and end year of the simulation, the population size and the output interval. There is no interactivity in the actual simulation itself, which is run in batch mode and relies upon thousands of parameters. However, the script and rules files are easily accessible and it is possible to change key parameters such as the rate of earnings growth or the real interest rate without specialised programming skills.

Usage and Usability

The main aim in developing the model was to provide projections of the future characteristics of older people in Britain and to inform the development of alternative policy options within pensions and long-term care. To date, the model has been used to examine the labour market trajectories and pension accumulation patterns of different birth cohorts among the British population. It has also been used to investigate the distributional impact of changes in the operation of the British pension system.

This has involved:

1. simulation of demographic and labour market histories for the current (base) and reform (option) pension systems;

2. calculation of pension contributions (state, occupational and private) and entitlements in the base system;
3. calculation of pension contributions (state, occupational and private) and entitlements in the option system; and
4. comparison of the base and option outputs and analysis of the distributional impact of policy reform, particularly the characteristics of winners and losers.

A unique feature of the SAGE model is that it also incorporates health and disability status. Thus an additional application of the model is the investigation of the likely future demand for long-term care and how this is related to the ability to pay for such care.

Most Recent Use

The SAGE dynamic microsimulation model is in active use and undergoing further development and enhancement.

Availability

Use of the SAGE model is currently restricted to members of the ESRC SAGE Research Group. The SAGE Research Group is jointly based in the Centre for Research on Ageing within the School of Social Science at the University of Southampton and at the London School of Economics. The model is located within the Centre for Research on Ageing.

Contact: Jane Falkingham, School of Social Sciences, University of Southampton, Highfield, Southampton SO17 1BJ, Great Britain:E-mail: j.c.falkingham@soton.ac.uk

Educational Value

The model is primarily a research tool. However it does have educational value in that results from the model may be used within teaching. Moreover enhancements to the model may form the basis of PhD study.

Macro–Micro Links

There are no explicit links to a macro model. However the model is aligned to macro data with regard to the population age and sex structure and the SAGE model uses the same assumptions regarding future mortality and fertility as the Government Actuary.

The SAGE Technical Notes are available free of charge at www.lse.ac.uk/depts/sage

Model 4

LifePaths Model

Geoff Rowe and Steve Gribble

Statistics Canada, Canada

Introduction

The LifePaths simulation model is the latest in a series of longitudinal microsimulation models produced at Statistics Canada. It is in turn the basis for a number of more specialized longitudinal microsimulation models used in the areas of health policy, time use analysis, and intergenerational equity.

Overview

The model is a dynamic overlapping cohort model. The unit of simulation consists of a "core" individual whose complete lifetime is simulated from birth to death. Additional individuals related to the core individual through marriage or childbirth are also simulated. Thus the model simulates both individuals and families. The dates of birth of the core individuals are chosen in such a way as to allow cross-sectional and longitudinal tabulation over the periods and cohorts of interest.

The model operates in continuous time, implementing state changes of individuals through competing events, which move the individual through their life trajectory.

The population simulated is that of Canada (with provinces represented). The model is able to reproduce the cross-sectional distribution of the living population from 1976 to the present. The first version of LifePaths was constructed in 1994, based largely on earlier work on a cohort microsimulation model named Demogen. The model has evolved greatly since that time. LifePaths contains detailed modules of birth, death, migration, marriage, education progression, labor force, and earnings.

The LifePaths model has been used for various studies, including intergenerational equity, pension privatization, lifetime time use accounting, and rates of return to education. It has also supported the policy development

International Symposia in Economic Theory and Econometrics, Vol. 16

ISSN: 1571-0386 DOI: 10.1016/S1571-0386(06)16023-8

process in other government departments, in particular with respect to Canada's post-secondary student loans program. A public release version of LifePaths is available on the Statistics Canada web site together with other supporting software.

LifePaths has been designed to facilitate the development and evaluation of government policies that have an essentially longitudinal dimension at the individual level. It can also be used to evaluate other programs and issues in a longitudinal context, for example the redistributive effect of the tax system across complete lifetimes.

Database

In order to ensure continuity and consistency across the simulated lifetime, LifePaths uses a synthetic approach, as discussed elsewhere in this book. Multiple data sources are used, sometimes simultaneously, in equation estimation, and in some cases the distributional properties of micro data sources are represented in a non-parametric form and are then used during simulation to re-create the longitudinal patterns found in the original source data. In some cases, particularly when reproducing history, data sources are lacking for equation estimation. In such cases, a process of calibration is used to find parameter values that will reproduce historical aggregates (which typically come from past censuses). This calibration process is automated, and uses numerical algorithms that run the model in an iterative fashion.

Analytical Facilities

Modgen includes a longitudinal tabulation facility with built-in Monte Carlo variance estimation, as well as various non-procedural language constructs that simplify the model development process. Modgen fully supports multiple foreign languages in the generated models. A companion application, BioBrowse, allows generated histories to be examined in detail in a visual environment.

Mode of Use

The model has a complete graphical user interface that allows the user to examine and change input parameters, perform the simulation, and examine result tables. It also incorporates facilities for scenario management.

Technical Details

LifePaths is implemented using the Modgen language developed at Statistics Canada. Modgen is an object-oriented extension of C++, and provides the model developer with an integrated environment for creating microsimulation models. Generated models run on Windows 32-bit platforms. Microsoft's C++ compiler is required to author or modify models, but is not needed to run them. Modgen has been designed to maximize the efficiency of CPU use, and to this end performs no file operations when in its simulation phase. Simulation runs make use of multiple processors, if present, and can also be distributed across a network of machines.

Modgen models can be distributed to end users with no additional commercial software. They contain a complete self-contained environment for simulation, including model-specific on-line help, scenario management, parameter input, and result viewing. Untrained users can modify parameters, run the model, and examine results, and can use on-line help to examine a model's structure in detail without needing to access the source code.

Typical Run Time

The model's run time varies depending on how many cases the user has requested. The run time scales linearly with the number of cases. The user sets the number of cases to a value that reduces Monte Carlo variance to acceptable levels for the result tables of interest. The current version of LifePaths simulates 200,000 cases per hour, where a case consists of complete lifetimes of the "core" person as well as those of the core individual's spouse and children. To reduce Monte Carlo variance to acceptable limits for narrowly defined table cells it is sometimes necessary to perform runs consisting of millions of cases.

Educational Use

The public version of LifePaths is available for educational use, but is likely too complex to use as an introductory microsimulation course. The Modgen language is also available, and includes a very simple longitudinal microsimulation model together with source (about 100 lines of Modgen code) that could form a useful starting point for developing more complex models in a course.

Availability

The public release version of the LifePaths model can be freely downloaded from the Statistics Canada web site, as can the underlying simulation language, Modgen and associatedincluding the BioBrowse data visualization application (http://www.statcan.ca/english/spsd/LifePaths.htm).

Macro–micro links

The model contains no macro–micro links, although it has been calibrated to replicate the last several decades of Canada's economic history insofar as this is reflected in the attributes of individuals and families.

Model 5

SESIM (Longitudinal Dynamic Microsimulation Model)

Olle Sundberg

Ministry of Finance, Sweden

Introduction

The SESIM dynamic microsimulation model is developed at the Swedish Ministry of Finance, in close cooperation with researchers at Swedish universities. The work started in 1997 as a tool to evaluate the Swedish education financing system. Since year 2000 the focus has shifted from education to forecasts and analysis of the new Swedish old-age pension system and the effects of the ageing population on the public finances. This new focus has also implied that SESIM has been developed into a general microsimulation model that can be used for a broad set of analyses. However, the most important purpose remains to analyse the financial sustainability of the pension system. SESIM has later been extended for other purposes, e.g. for analyses of health among the elderly. More detailed documentation can be found in Flood et al. (2005) or at www.sesim.org.

Overview

SESIM can be characterized as a mainstream dynamic microsimulation model in the sense that the variables (events) are updated in a sequence, and the period between the updating processes is a year. The starting year is 1999 and the initial sample of the Swedish population is ~110,000 individuals.[1] All individuals are then subjected to a large number of possible events,

[1] If necessary the sample can be extended

International Symposia in Economic Theory and Econometrics, Vol. 16

ISSN: 1571-0386 DOI: 10.1016/S1571-0386(06)16024-X

Figure 1: Structure of SESIM

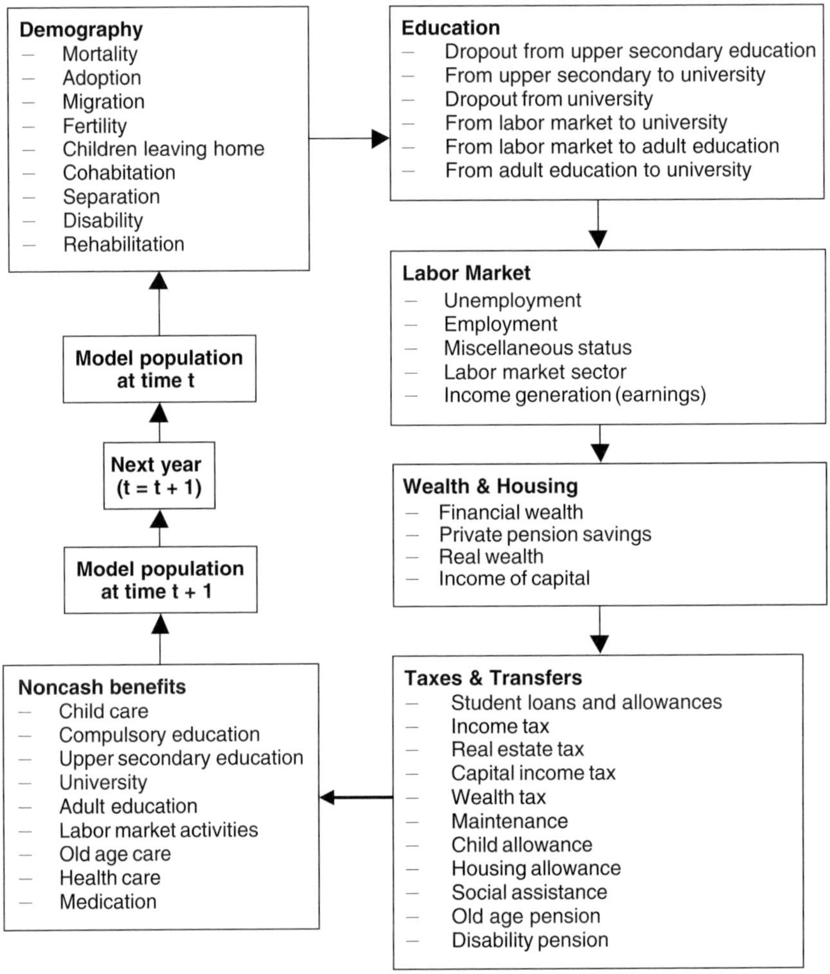

reflecting real-life phenomena, e.g., education, marriage, have children, work or retirement.

SESIM has a recursive structure consisting of a set of modules executed in a predetermined order (see Figure 1). The unit of simulation is the individual but the household also plays a significant role. Many of the simulated processes refer to household as well as individual properties. The simulation sequence starts with a set of demographic modules (mortality, adoption, migration, household formation and dissolution, disability pension, rehabilitation and regional mobility). After that follows a module for education.

Next module deals with the labour market, unemployment, employment, sick absence and employment sector.[2]

Every year the individuals are assigned a status. Each individual can only have one out of nine different statuses during a specific year.[3] Every status is related to a source of income; working results in earnings, retirement brings pensions, etc. For employed an earnings equation is used to determine the income. For other kind of statuses, e.g. unemployment, different rules are applied to obtain the income. After the calculation of income, a module for wealth capital income and housing is entered. Four separate assets are considered in the household portfolio: financial wealth, owned home, other real wealth and private pension savings.[4]

After the wealth/housing calculations a large module describes all relevant tax, transfer and pension rules. The rules for public and occupational old-age pensions have been implemented in all relevant details. Given the information above the household disposable income can be defined.

SESIM allows for an extensive definition of income since the value of various non-cash benefits can be included, e.g. education, childcare and health care. The value of the subsidy is assumed to equal production costs net of fees. Only benefits that can be attributed to a specific individual are included.

An important update in the latest model version is the health module, where the need for care is imputed. To evaluate the importance of informal care the geographical distance to relatives is imputed. The health status is calculated and the number of days with inpatient care followed by severe disability and finally assistance for elderly is imputed.

Data Issues

The primary database for SESIM, concerning estimation of statistical models as well as construction of the base population, is the Statistics Sweden longitudinal database Linda. This database is created from administrative registers and covers ~3.5 per cent of the Swedish population. In 1999 the primary sample was 308,000 households. Including their household members the total sample size was 786,000 individuals. The selected individuals

[2] The sector is required, e.g. for calculations of second pillar occupational pensions. There is also a module for endogenous old-age retirement decisions.

[3] The different statuses are: Child (0–15-years old), Old-age pension, Student, Disability pension, Parental leave, Unemployed, Employed, Miscellaneous, Emigrated (individuals living abroad with Swedish pensions rights).

[4] See also Flood (2003b).

are followed backward and forward and all relevant information is collected. Some information, for instance pension rights, can be traced back as long as to 1960. Thus this is a panel data since the same individuals are followed overtime. Selected individuals, who disappear from the data by death or emigration, are replaced by new individuals in such a way that the statistical representativity is maintained. More details about LINDA can be found in Edin and Fredriksson, 2000.

As Linda is completely created from administrative registers, no interviews are needed and therefore a major advantage is that there are no problems of attrition bias. The database is created by merging a large number of registers, and includes data about income and wealth, earnings, pension rights, sickness and unemployment benefit, schooling, etc. The base population used in SESIM is formed by a random draw of individuals from LINDA. Considerable work has been done with the initial dataset to make it consistent with macro outcome data, e.g., when assigning the individuals initial statuses.

In the construction of the base population in SESIM two main adjustments have been done:

- *Adjustment of the household definition.* The households in LINDA are not defined in an economically optimal sense. First, individuals are assumed to live in the municipality where they are recorded according to the national tax registry, second, adults living together without being married or having common children are considered as separate households. Also the number of young people, aged 18–29 years, who still live in their parent's household, are over-reported. Therefore other data sources are used to impute a more realistic family structure.
- *Adding emigrants with pension rights.* Individuals with Swedish pension rights will keep these entitlements even if they have emigrated. As LINDA does not include individuals living outside Sweden, information from the National Social Insurance Board about this has been added.

Apart from the sources mentioned above, some additional data are used for estimation or imputation. The Statistics Sweden income distribution survey, HEK, which is based on interviews merged with register information is, apart from being used in the correction of the household composition, also used in the estimation of public consumption and housing variables. Regional mobility and tenure choice is based on a database named GEOSWEDE.[5] The Statistics Sweden household expenditure survey is used for

[5] A database constructed from Louise, RTB, geography database and tax-assessed values.

calculation of indirect taxation. The health and care modules are based on some other surveys.[6]

Technical Details

Programming. The model is programmed in Visual Basic 6.0.[7] Microsoft Excel and Access is used for handling of macroeconomic and demographic assumptions and parameters. All programming has been made by statisticians and economists and no dedicated programmers have been used.

System requirements. To run the model a computer with at least 256 MB of RAM memory is recommended. To edit the model Visual Basic version 6.0 SP5 is required. The system requirements increase with the sample size and the simulation period.

Data storage. The initial population data is stored in binary form. The Linda database is in SAS format, and the start data is thus generated with a combination of SAS and Visual Basic.

Typical run time. A 100,000 individual's sample and 50-year long simulation takes ~30 min to execute on a modern standard PC.

Interactivity. The program can be controlled in three ways: from the "user interface", from the "Excel report generator" or in batch mode. Normally the "user interface" is used in the early stage of development, and the "Excel report generator" is used to produce standard outputs as graphs and tables. More extensive analysis of the results is performed in standard statistical packages like SAS or R. It is easy to implement different macroeconomic assumptions in SESIM, but more time-consuming to change population scenarios. If the files with demographic and macroeconomic assumptions are in place and relevant reports available, it is easy to make several model simulations in batch mode. When the model is run repeatedly, e.g., to assess the sampling variance, it is also appropriate to use the batch mode.

Usage and Usability

Usage of the model. An overview of the use and plans for SESIM is presented in Table 1 below. SESIM is regularly used for calculations and analysis of pensions and other public age-related expenditures within the Swedish Ministry of Finance. The model has also been used by the Ministry

[6] The Kungsholmen study by Mårten Lagergren and Statistics Sweden, Level of Living Survey, ULF.

[7] Also some Fortran subroutines are used for, e.g. sorting and random number generation.

Table 1: Overview of the Use of SESIM in 1999–2006

Year	Activity	Publication or principle
1999	Modelling budget estimates of student grants and loans	Studiebidraget i det långa loppet (Swedish only)
2000	Modelling budget estimates of student grants and loans	Distributional effects of student grants in Sweden
2003–2004	Long-run forecasts of pension expenditures	Long-term survey
2003 onwards	Periodical long-run forecasts of pension expenditures	Ministry of Finance
2003	Calculation of replacement ratios in the new Swedish pension system	The Accumulation of Wealth and Early Retirement
2004	Calculation of replacement ratios in the new Swedish pension system	Can we afford the future? An evaluation of the new Swedish pension system (Flood, 2003a)
2004	Life-cycle analysis	Lifetime redistribution through taxes, transfers and non-cash benefits (Pettersson and Pettersson, 2003)
2004	Analysis of the financial stability of the new Swedish pension system	Ministry of Finance
2004	Analysis of the ageing population, health care, housing, etc.	"Baby boom"-project, Anders Klevmarken, Uppsala university
2004 onwards	Pension projections for EU AWG	EU, EPC
2005	Analysis of financing of elderly care	National board of health and welfare
2006	Generational analysis	Ministry of Finance
2006	Analysis of tax-deductible private pension savings	Pensions tax commission

for long-run calculations of pensions for the EU Ageing Working Group (AWG).

An interesting ongoing application of SESIM is a research project under the leadership of Professor Anders Klevmarken at Uppsala University. In this project different economic aspects of the ageing population, "the ageing baby-boomers", are studied. The focus is health and care issues among the elderly, but also housing, labour market activities, etc. are studied. The researchers use SESIM as a tool to integrate their work into a common framework. Results are planned to be published in mid-2006. In another interesting project within the Ministry of Finance, SESIM is used in a project about intergenerational redistribution. Also the results from this project are planned to be published in mid-2006. During 2006 the model will also be used for analysis of private tax-deductible pension savings.

The first calculations with SESIM were carried out in 1997. The model was used to evaluate different reforms of the Swedish education financing system. Part of that work has been documented in Ericson and Hussénius (2000). Later the model was developed further and given a focus on pension calculations. The primary aim was to analyse the financial stability of the new Swedish old-age pension system. Today SESIM has been developed into a general microsimulation model that can be used for a broad set of analyses.

Availability of model. The model is in principle open source. The code is freely available on www.sesim.org. Because of the official data secrets legislation no individual start data are provided, though.

Educational value. SESIM's primary design focus on conducting policy analyses and forecasts for the Swedish economy and public finances. Most of its major applications so far have been in this area, but the model has also been used within the university sphere. Thus, at least in principle, the model could be used for educational purposes. For example, it should be possible for students in econometrics to use the model framework for making simulations and analyses of estimated partial models.

Macro–micro links. To make SESIM useful within the Ministry of Finance environment it is necessary to make it simple to implement exogenous assumptions and forecasts. The model has therefore been designed to make it easy to use different exogenous demographic and macroeconomic assumptions, e.g. from the Ministry of Finance or Statistics of Sweden. For implementation of demographic and labour market assumptions aligning techniques are used.

References

Edin, P. A. and Fredriksson, P. (2000). *LINDA — Longitudinal Individual Data for Sweden.* Working Paper 2000:19, Uppsala Universitet, Economics Department.

Ericson, P. and Hussénius, J. (2000). Studiebidragen i det långa loppet, Rapport till Expertgruppen för studier i offentlig ekonomi (ESO). Ds 2000:19.

Flood, L. (2003a). *Can We Afford the Future? An Evaluation of the New Swedish Pension System.* Paper presented at the International Microsimulation Conference on Population Ageing and Health: Modelling Our Future, Canberra.

Flood, L. (2003b). *Formation of Wealth, Income of Capital and Cost of Housing in SESIM.* SESIM Working Paper, www.sesim.org.

Flood, L., Jansson, F., Pettersson, T., Pettersson, T., Sundberg, O. and Westerberg, A. (2005). *The Handbook of SESIM — A Swedish Dynamic Micro Simulation Model*, www.sesim.org.

Pettersson, T. and Pettersson, T. (2003). *Lifetime Redistribution Through Taxes, Transfers and Non-cash Benefits*. Paper presented at International Microsimulation Conference on Population Ageing and Health, Canberra.

Model 6

DYNACAN (Longitudinal Dynamic Microsimulation Model)

Richard J. Morrison

Human Resources and Social Development Canada, Canada

Introduction

Following four years of preliminary feasibility investigations, formal DYNACAN development began in 1994, using Steven Caldwell's CORSIM model as a template. After some very limited policy application in 1996 and 1997, DYNACAN became part of the formal process for assessing the impacts of prospective changes to the Canada Pension Plan (CPP), Canada's contributory, earnings-based public pension plan. Challenges in adapting CORSIM's logic included differences in variable definitions between Canadian and U.S. surveys, the higher levels of immigration in Canada, re-estimating the equations for the model's operating characteristics using Canadian data, implementing the desired degree of consistency between the results from DYNACAN and counterpart results from the Chief Actuary's CPP actuarial valuation model, and ensuring the realism of the synthetic individuals' lifetime earnings histories relative to Canadian administrative data.

Overview

DYNACAN is a closed, stochastic, longitudinal, dynamic microsimulation policy model, simulating the longitudinal evolution of individuals and many of their characteristics within family contexts. DYNACAN's primary objective lies with ascertaining the detailed, distributional policy impacts of prospective changes to the CPP, presented within the context of the broader retirement income system. The model simulates, on an annual basis, the evolution of the Canadian population from 1971 as far into the future as the year 2100. However, it concentrates on the roughly three-quarters of the population participating in the CPP. (The province of Quebec administers its own, very similar, plan for the other quarter of the population.) The synthetic individuals are

International Symposia in Economic Theory and Econometrics, Vol. 16

ISSN: 1571-0386 DOI: 10.1016/S1571-0386(06)16025-1

born, age, immigrate or emigrate, leave home, work, marry, divorce, become disabled or recover, retire and eventually die. DYNACAN simulates a variety of characteristics for these individuals, concentrating on annual CPP contributions and benefits, and the variables, particularly earnings, necessary to calculate them. The Office of the Chief Actuary initially developed DYNACAN at the request of the government department that then administered the CPP. In early 1999, the DYNACAN project was formally transferred to the department that was the primary user of DYNACAN's results. It is currently housed in Human Resources Social Development Canada (HRS-DC), the department that has the primary responsibility for CPP policy.

Data Sources

DYNACAN uses, as its starting point, a heavily modified version of the public use microdata file for the 1971 Canadian Census, roughly a 1% sample of the Canadian population. Publicly available DYNACAN documentation describes the nature of these modifications. The several modifications, and the derivation of DYNACAN's equations and its alignment data, depend heavily on a variety of surveys and other statistics publicly available from Statistics Canada, e.g. the Canadian Survey of Consumer Finances series, subsequent censuses, vital statistics data, and educational surveys. Aggregate administrative data from the CPP are also used, along with a sample of earnings histories that has been rigorously screened to respect Canadian privacy and confidentiality requirements. Case weights are equal for all individuals in the initial sample. They remain constant throughout the run, and are identical to the case weights assigned to individuals on birth or immigration.

Projection Component: DYNACAN's individuals evolve through time primarily via annual events whose probabilities are governed by equations, constrained by alignment to yield desired (historical or assumed future) collective rates. The alignment targets include rates for mortality, fertility, migration, marriage and divorce propensities, etc. The equations and alignment data are derived using the data sources described above. An aggressive program of model validation tracks the extent to which, over the historical period, DYNACAN's synthetic individuals and families resemble, distributionally, their real world counterparts. The validation effort extends, in a cross-model validation sense, to comparing various DYNACAN projections for the future with their counterparts from other models, particularly the Chief Actuary's ACTUCAN model.

Data ageing: Because DYNACAN is an explicitly longitudinal model, it ages the population, and the characteristics of the component individuals, simulation period by annual simulation period, via the simulated events as driven by the various equations. Because the population is a scale model of the national population, at the same scale throughout each run, no re-weighting of cases is necessary. Links to other models are indirect and non-interactive, implemented via the parameters used in a run of the model.

However, the preparation of the initial 1971 database, roughly 200,000 individuals, uses a number of techniques that are fairly standard for micro-simulation models and analyses. For example, that development uses imputation, to assign specific ages to children whose ages are known only as far as falling in a particular age range. It adjusts for under-reporting or mis-reporting of earnings by alignment to distributions drawn from exhaustive administrative data. The preparation merges data from the family and unattached versions of the public-use microdata, adjusting for definitional differences, to provide a population representative of Canada as a whole. Other adjustment techniques are also relevant, e.g., adjusting the ages of individuals to counteract age heaping on five year multiples.

Technical Details

Language: The DYNACAN modules' source code is all ANSI standard C. However, a variety of other software (Perl, SAS, Java, Excel, etc.) contributes to the extraction and presentation of the model's results.

System requirements/Type of computer: The primary production machines are dual-processor Athlon MP 1900+ PCs with 4 GB RAM, and large, fast hard disks. DVDs and a purpose-built results-browser play a central role in the dissemination of model results. The operating system is Linux, chosen for its capacity for memory management and the maximization of computational throughput. The production machines operate in a networked environment in conjunction with other machines that are used for the extraction and presentation of results, and for project administration.

Data storage: The initial population data are stored in ASCII format, and then compiled into a more useable binary form. The large numbers of parameters are stored and manipulated in ASCII format, but are converted to a more computationally efficient binary form during the course of a run.

Typical run time: The demographic projection portion of a run requires roughly half an hour for a 90-year projection, with a non-trivial portion of this resulting from the internal validation checks. The simulation of CPP contributions and benefits requires less than half an hour for either the base system or an option system. The extraction of results requires about 45 min for simple summary results, and about an hour for the generation of a complex slate of more than 800 SAS tables and graphics that form the standard outputs for the analysis of a policy option.

Interactivity: DYNACAN's basic calculations run in a batch mode that is very heavily informed by tens of thousands of parameters. Many of the results extractions involve standard SAS scripts run in a batch mode. However, custom analyses involving SAS and/or custom scripts may be done interactively on the outputs from a model run.

Usage and Usability

Process: An important design requirement for DYNACAN is that its structure permit behavioural feedback, and the differential evolution of the base and option systems, e.g., because of differential mortality conditioned on the levels of CPP benefits. However, in practice, the demographic evolution for the base and option systems is typically held constant between the two systems in order to permit the identification of winner and loser individuals and their characteristics. In this typical mode, DYNACAN's use consists of the following four major steps:

- Simulation of the common demographics and earnings to be used for the base and option systems.
- Calculation of CPP contributions and benefits in the base system.
- Calculation of CPP contributions and benefits in the option system.
- Comparisons of the base and option outputs to ascertain policy impacts in the form of aggregates, distributions, and winners/losers analyses.

The only direct, hands-on, users of DYNACAN itself are the members of the DYNACAN team. Results from the model go primarily to its principal clients, policy analysts within HRSDC. Results may also be shared with the Office of the Chief Actuary and the Department of Finance.

Most recent use: DYNACAN is in current, active use. The most recent impact projections have involved a variety of assessments of possible changes to CPP contribution and benefit rules, e.g., for survivors' benefits and child-rearing dropouts, conducted on behalf of the federal government and the provinces.

Availability: Rights to the DYNACAN model software rest with the Government of Canada. The licensing agreement with respect to its CORSIM foundation does not permit secondary distribution of this software. The 1971 census public use microdata file that serves as the primary starting point for the simulations is available from Statistics Canada. However, as noted, considerable modification was required to achieve a starting data base suitable for longitudinal microsimulation.

Educational value: DYNACAN's primary design focus lies with conducting policy impact analyses for possible changes to the CPP. All of

DYNACAN's major applications to date have been in this area. However, the developers believe that there is, at least in principle, an educational value to the model. For example, even in its present form, it provides a powerful test bed framework for examining the evolution of Canada's demography. On the educational research front, it could provide a comparable test bed for exploring behavioural feedback, or the impacts of alternative demographic assumptions.

Macro-micro links: A major design consideration for DYNACAN requires consistency with the Chief Actuary's ACTUCAN model. ACTUCAN is a traditional actuarial valuation model with cell-based (semi-aggregate) longitudinal projections of Canada's demographics, earnings, and of CPP contributions and benefits. DYNACAN typically runs using the same assumptions/parameters that the Chief Actuary has chosen for ACTUCAN. Those assumptions in turn employ, as inputs, the results from several macro models, at both the intermediate and longer-run horizons. To date, there has been substantial consistency for the key CPP aggregates and distributions that both ACTUCAN and DYNACAN project.

Development priorities: Although DYNACAN is fully operational, and already an established part of the CPP policy development process, it is not finished. Current priorities include revising the education module, with implications for several of the other modules that use educational attainment as an explanatory variable, more effective presentations of the model's results, and a more ambitious set of validation studies. However, the single highest priority remains implementing an approximation for the after-tax impacts of prospective policy options, rather than the pre-tax impacts that DYNACAN currently projects.

Model 7

DESTINIE ("Modèle Démographique Economique et Social de Trajectoires Individuelles Simulées, i.e. Demographic, Economic and Social Model of Simulated Individual Trajectories")

Cédric Afsa and Sophie Buffeteau

INSEE, France

Introduction

The dynamic microsimulation model DESTINIE has been built to analyse the long-run situation of pensioners, accounting for the heterogeneity of careers and preferences and for changes in the labour market, as well as for the demographic structure and retirement rules. In this respect it has been used to simulate the impact of the 2003 French Pension Reform on, for example, the age of retirement, the replacement rate as well as the long-term number of retirees or financial equilibrium of the pension system.

The scope of the model is national: it is based on a representative sample of the whole French population.

Overview

DESTINIE is a stochastic, dynamic microsimulation model built by the French National Statistical Institute (INSEE). Its construction began in 1993 for simulating the distribution of pensioners' incomes up to the year 2050. In the first version of the model the age of retirement was deterministic: the individual was supposed to take up her pension at the age of eligibility to the "full rate". The model has been then improved by implementing a module where the age of retirement is endogenously determined according to a labour-leisure trade-off in the line of Stock and Wise (1990). The parameters of the utility function were first estimated on the

International Symposia in Economic Theory and Econometrics, Vol. 16

ISSN: 1571-0386 DOI: 10.1016/S1571-0386(06)16026-3

"Echantillon Inter-Régimes des retraités" (inter-scheme sample of pensioners) which is an administrative data source collected by the Ministry of Social Affairs. However, the parameters had to be calibrated because of the extreme concentration of observed retirement ages which makes very difficult any structural estimation. More recently, a new unit was added to the model, which simulates transitions between various states of old age disability for individuals aged 60 and above.

Data Issues

DESTINIE is based on individual data derived from the 1998 Financial Assets Survey collected by INSEE. The original sample has been reweighted to account for the demographic structure of the whole French population as known from the 1999 French Census. Thus, the initial sample of DESTINIE contains about 20,000 households and 50,000 individuals. In order to study intergenerational relationships individuals from the sample are connected to each other through the artificial imputation of kinship ties. Some other individual information has been imputed, for example, the school leaving age for children of the initial sample who have not yet completed their studies. This variable is of primary importance for the model as it sums up the social class and the qualification. The other data sources used by DESTINIE are the INSEE prospective mortality and activity tables by sex and age.

Data Ageing

Owing to its longitudinal nature DESTINIE ages each individual of the sample via the simulated events driven by various equations. More precisely, the model simulates both demographic and economic trajectories from the initial year (1998) up to 2050, using a mix of deterministic rules, behavioural hypotheses and random transitions. The demographic events are union, breaking-up, birth of a child, death and migration. The parameters of the equations are adjusted so that the probabilities predicted by the model fit the long-term demographic projections made by the INSEE and the French Demographic Institute (INED).

The economic events are mainly the transitions on the labour market. These transitions are treated as a first-order Markovian process. The parameters of the transition equations are adjusted to account for the increasing labour force participation and to allow for changes in the macroeconomic environment (rate of unemployment in the long run). Conditional on the labour market status annual wages are then imputed as a sum of a deterministic component (depending on sex, school leaving age, tenure and economic sector) and a stochastic one (including an individual fixed effect and an autocorrelated residual). Lastly, as noted above, the age of retirement is endogenous: it depends on a trade-off between the utility the individual can expect if she retires now and the one she can get if she defers her withdrawal.

Technical Particulars

Language

The source code of the core of DESTINIE is Turbo Pascal (about 10,000 lines of program). The initial sample is created using SAS. The data are then coded in ASCII format. The results of the simulations are in ASCII format too. They are then manipulated with SAS or Excel.

System Requirements

The execution of the simulations requires PCs with 512 MB RAM. The operating system is Windows NT. Data (initial sample, programs and simulated data) are all stored in a networked environment. A 10 GB storage capacity is sufficient for a standard use of DESTINIE. All things considered, simulations as well as analyses of the results can be done interactively.

Typical Run Time

The simulations up to 2050 require about 90 min. As the results of the simulations (i.e. the individual trajectories up to 2050) are stored at the end of the program execution, any manipulation of the simulated data does not take very long.

Conclusions

The main use of DESTINIE is to analyse the effect of alternative pension rules on the participation rate and the amount of pension of successive cohorts. A great advantage of the model and its retirement module lies in that it can simulate the impact of changes in retirement incentives such as the ones introduced by the recent 2003 reform. In this respect DESTINIE has been used intensively during the preparation of this reform.

The most recent uses of the model consist in studying the *ex post* effects of this reform of the French pension system and the earlier one that has occurred in 1993. The main focus is on the intra- and intergenerational redistribution induced by these reforms.

Although, DESTINIE's primary focus is the simulation of pension the model can cope with distributional aspects of other public policies especially if one is interested in a life-cycle approach. In this regard one of the future developments of the model is to implement individual health expenditures in order to analyse the redistributive properties of the French health care system.

The direct users of the model are the members of the division "Redistribution et Politiques Sociales" which is a subunit of the "Département des Etudes Economiques d'Ensemble" (department of global economic studies) within INSEE. The model is maintained and developed by these members. Second-hand users are, for example, economists of the "Département des Etudes Economiques d'Ensemble" who have used outputs from DESTINIE as inputs for medium and long-term macroeconomic projections, and also the "Conseil d'Orientation des Retraites" (Pensions Advisory Committee), an organism aimed at evaluating the French pension system.

Reference

Stock, J.H. and Wise, D.A. (1990). Pensions, the Option Value of Work, and Retirement. *Econometrica*, 38(5), 1151–1180.

Static Microsimulation and Macro/Micro Approaches

Model 8

GLADHISPANIA (A Spanish Tax-Benefits Microsimulation Model)

Xisco Oliver[a] and Amedeo Spadaro[b]

[a] *Universitat de les Illes Balears, Palma de Mallorca, Spain*
[b] *PSE -Paris-Jourdan Sciences Economiques, France, FEDEA, Madrid and Universitat de les IIles Balears, Palma de Mallorca, Spain*

Introduction

GLADHISPANIA is an interactive web-based static and partial equilibrium microsimulation model that allows the user to simulate the effects of Spanish Income Tax legislation and several reform proposals. It is built on the Spanish database from the European Community Household Panel (ECHP) that provides a representative sample of the Spanish population with detailed information on socio-demographic characteristics and income sources for each member of the household.

Overview[1]

The relevance of the debate about the costs and benefits of the recent reforms of the Spanish income tax motivated the construction of a microsimulation model that can be used freely, easily and in an independent way by economists, politicians, journalists and analysts. GLADHISPANIA covers this necessity. The model provides several predefined scenarios that allow the user to simulate the existing redistributive system from 1998 until today. It gives also the possibility to simulate the effects of several reforms. The main characteristics of GLADHISPANIA are the flexibility in the implementation of the scenarios to be analysed and the facility of the use given by its user-friendly interface. The model allows the user to have a clear

[1] See Oliver and Spadaro (2004a) for further details about the microsimulation model.

International Symposia in Economic Theory and Econometrics, Vol. 16

ISSN: 1571-0386 DOI: 10.1016/S1571-0386(06)16027-5

picture of the effects of the fiscal instruments on the aggregate figures and at the individual level. The microsimulation research group at the University of Balearic Islands has built it with the financial support of several public and private institutions.

GLADHISPANIA uses the household as unit of the analysis and it simulates changes in the budget set due to changes in the direct taxation (personal income taxes and social security contributions).

Currently, there exist two versions of GLADHISPANIA. The first one (available on the web at www.gladhispania.es) does not consider behavioural reactions. The second one takes into account changes in labour supply of the individuals. Using a discrete choice model of labour supply (Van Soest, 1995) it computes a utility function to measure changes in labour supply and in participation of the members of the household.

Data Issues

GLADHISPANIA uses the Spanish database from the ECHP, designed by the Statistical Office of the European Community (Eurostat) and collected by the Spanish National Statistics Institute (INE). The information available in the database is representative of the Spanish population. The ECHP contains detailed information on the income sources, housing and other demographic, social and economic characteristics of the respondents.

All individuals in the household who are aged 16 or more are interviewed. The information available for individuals below that age is restricted to basic demographic characteristics such as age, gender and relationship with the other household members. The last Spanish wave available (when the microsimulation has been developed) was the 1995. The updating procedure takes into account only the nominal growth rate (inflation plus real growth). Gross figures are computed by a fixed-point algorithm, iterating several times until reaching the withholdings, the income tax and the social insurance contribution patterns fitting the net income observed in the reference years. The calibration procedure has been performed very carefully in order to ensure the reliability of the microsimulation model. The number of households in the model database is 6,420, representative of the 12,068,375 households in the Spanish population (in 1995, source INE).

Technical Details

Language: Following the experience developed in the microsimulation model EUR3 for France, Italy and United Kingdom (see Bourguignon et al., 1998), the calculations are carried out in spreadsheets. Three spreadsheets are used. The first contains the dataset (the input file). Each line represents one household and contains all the socio-demographic and economic variables of each member. The second represents the true budget constraint of each household. Cell references are used to compute all the intermediate and final steps to obtain individual and household disposable income, income taxes and social contributions. Finally, the results are stored in a third spreadsheet (the output file). Visual Basic programs are used to run the model and to compute the results (tax collection, redistribution, inequality, poverty measures).

To implement the microsimulation model in the web, the programs have been rewritten in JAVA. The user accesses the model through any navigator with an installed virtual JAVA machine. She introduces the values of the parameters of the simulated scenario and runs the simulation. The microsimulation model, the data and the routines needed to perform the simulation are downloaded in the RAM of the user's PC. In this way the web does not collapse. Finally, after the numerical computation, the results are stored in the RAM and shown in HTML pages. There is no way for the user to keep the routine and the data in her PC.

System requirements/type of computer: A minimum of 128 MB of RAM and a high-speed Internet connection with a navigator including a virtual JAVA machine.

Typical run time: It depends on the Internet connection speed, the processor and the RAM of the PC. Using a Pentium IV 2.66 GHz processor with 1 GB of RAM memory and high-speed Internet connexion, each simulation takes around 1 min.

Interactivity: GLADHISPANIA is extremely interactive and user-friendly. It allows the user to modify the parameters defining the tax-benefit system and to customise the results (i.e., the user must choose the equivalence scale used in the calculation of the inequality measures and the poverty line).

Usage and Usability

Most recent use: GLADHISPANIA is a model in permanent evolution. It tries to replicate any potential reform that is object of debate in the academic or political environment. Several articles used it. Oliver and Spadaro (2004b) use the model to reveal the social planner preferences implicit in the tax-benefit system (assuming that the tax-benefit system is optimal). Oliver and Spadaro (2003) explore the effects on redistribution and inequality when the 1999 system is replaced by a flat tax combined with a vital minimum (i.e., an amount of income that is not taxed) or a basic income (i.e., an amount of money that is given to everyone, independently of the economic status). Labeaga et al. (2005) use the behavioural version of GLAD-HISPANIA in order to analyze the impact of several reforms on the labour supply, the individual utility and social welfare.

The model has been used also by several newspapers' political analysts (El País, Cinco Días, Expansión, El Mundo, La Vanguardia, etc.) for comments about several proposals of reform of the Spanish income tax. It has been cited as an example of *e-democracy*.

Availability: As previously commented, there exist two versions of the model. The arithmetical version is freely available in the web (www.gladhispania.es), while the behavioural version is available upon request.

Educational value: GLADHISPANIA is a good tool to introduce students to the world of policy evaluation with microsimulation models. The user-friendly appearance and the flexibility of the model helps promote the use of microsimulation models and their direct application to policy analysis. Just a small knowledge of the Spanish fiscal system and of inequality and poverty measures is required. The model is used in Policy Evaluation and Public Economics courses both at undergraduate and graduate level.

References

Bourguignon, F., O'Donoghue, C., Sastre, J., Spadaro, A. and Utili, F. (1998). *Technical Description of Eur3: A Prototype European Tax-Benefits Model.* DAE Research Note N.9801 Micro-simulation Unit, Cambridge University.

Labeaga, J.M., Oliver, X. and Spadaro, A. (2005). *Discrete Choice Models of Labour Supply, Behavioural Microsimulation and the Spanish Tax Reform.* PSE Working Paper 13. Available at http://www.pse.ens.fr/document/doc2005.html.

Oliver, X. and Spadaro, A. (2007). Basic Income or Vital Minimum? A Note on the Distributive Effects of Possible Reforms of the Spanish Income Tax in Harding, A and Gupta, A. (Coord.). *Modelling Our Future: Population Ageing, Social Security and Taxation.* International Symposia in Economic Theory and Econometrics, Vol. 15; 2006, North Holland, Amsterdam.

Oliver, X. and Spadaro, A. (2004a). *A Technical Description of GLADHISPANIA: A Spanish Micro-Simulation Tax-Benefit Model.* DEA Working Paper 7, Universitat de les Illes Balears. Available at http://www.uib.es/depart/deaweb/deawp/.

Oliver, X. and Spadaro, A. (2004b). Are Spanish Governments Really Averse to Inequality? A Normative Analysis using the 1999 Spanish Tax Reform. *Investigaciones Económicas*, 28(3), 551–566.

Van Soest, A. (1995). Structural Models of Family Labour Supply: A Discrete Choice Approach. *Journal of Human Resources*, 30(1), 63–88.

Model 9

STINMOD (Static Incomes Model)

Richard Percival, Annie Abello and Quoc N. Vu

NATSEM, Australia

Introduction

STINMOD is NATSEM's static microsimulation model of Australia's tax and transfer system. The first version of STINMOD was released in 1994 and since then, two versions of the model are normally released each year. The model is used to analyse the distributional impact of current tax-transfer policy and to estimate the fiscal and distributional impacts of policy reform.[1] It is used by several Australian Commonwealth departments as well as a small number of research and welfare institutions and some individual researchers.

Overview

There are two major components to STINMOD. The first is the model's base population, which is a database of income units representing the Australian population. The second major component of STINMOD is the suite of entitlement modules that simulate the policy rules of the major federal tax and transfer programs, including eligibility, entitlement and interaction. The model is built using SAS software.

Each year, the model is updated to incorporate legislated changes in personal income tax or income support policies and to ensure the currency of the model's base population and program parameters. This involves keeping the government programs up-to-date, keeping the microdata up-to-date, making enhancements, correcting errors, ensuring that the documentation

[1] For more information on STINMOD, see Lambert et al. (1994) and Bremner et al. (2002).

International Symposia in Economic Theory and Econometrics, Vol. 16

ISSN: 1571-0386 DOI: 10.1016/S1571-0386(06)16028-7

reflects the current model and, archiving old versions of the model and its documentation to enable historical comparisons to be made.

There are two main versions of STINMOD available to users — a source code version and an interface version. There is also an 'outyears' version, that is basically the source code version with a projection component. The interface has been designed in a PC Windows environment, but it is portable — with minor modifications — to other operating systems. It allows users to simply 'point and click' on a number of menus and option windows to run a simulation that they have specified. The user can then analyse and print the simulation outcomes of interest to them. Users can run their simulation against the entire base population or for one or more synthetically generated hypothetical (i.e. 'typical') families. The public release of STINMOD with a user interface has made distributional analysis of government policy at the micro-unit level available to a wide range of users who previously would not have had access to this type of model. Nevertheless, while the interface version of STINMOD contains an easy to use 'point and click' interface, the policy changes able to be made through the interface are somewhat restricted. For any structural changes, such as the implementation of a new program or a change in the eligibility criteria for an existing payment, the source code that underlies the interface model needs to be amended.

Data Sources

For each version of STINMOD released to date, Table 1 shows the microdata from the Australian Bureau of Statistics (ABS) used to construct the basefile, and the type of STINMOD model produced. The basefile for the most current version of STINMOD (05B) was constructed using the following data sources:[2]

1. 2000–01 and 2002–03 ABS Surveys of Income and Housing Costs, for information on the Australian population members and their socio-economic characteristics.
2. May 2005 ABS Labour Force Survey, for demographic reweighting.
3. Various administrative datasets from FACS, DEWR and DEST, for calibration of entitlement numbers for government programs.
4. Various parameter datasets on federal government pensions, allowances and other types of assistance, the taxation system, consumer price index and other indexation parameters, for costing and uprating income components.

[2] For more details on the steps involved in creating the basefile, see Percival (1994) and Bremner et al. (2002).

Table 1: Microdata Used for STINMOD Model Versions

Version of STINMOD	Survey(s) for basefile	Type of STINMOD model		
		Source code	Outyears	Interface
94A	1990 ABS Survey of Income and Housing Costs and Amenities (SIHCA)	√		√
94B	1990 ABS SIHCA	√		√
95	1990 ABS SIHCA	√		√
96A	1993–94 ABS Household Expenditure Survey	√		√
98A	1994–95 and 1995–96 ABS Surveys of Income and Housing Costs (SIHC)	√		√
99A	1994–95 and 1995–96 ABS SIHC	√		√
99B	1995–96 and 1996–97 ABS SIHC	√		
00A	1995–96 and 1996–97 ABS SIHC	√	√	√
00B	1996–97 and 1997–98 ABS SIHC	√	√	
01A	1998–99 ABS Household Expenditure Survey	√	√	
01B	1996–97 and 1997–98 ABS SIHC	√	√	√
02A	1996–97 and 1997–98 ABS SIHC	√	√	
02B	1996–97 and 1997–98 ABS SIHC	√	√	√
03A	1996–97 and 1997–98 ABS SIHC	√	√	
03B	1996–97 and 1997–98 ABS SIHC	√	√	
04A	1999–00 and 2000–01 ABS SIHC	√	√	√
04B	1999–00 and 2000–01 ABS SIHC	√	√	
05A	1999–00 and 2000–01 ABS SIHC	√	√	
05B	2000–01 and 2002–03 ABS SIHC	√	√	√

The institutionalised population, or persons living in non-private dwellings, was first added to the basefile that underlies STINMOD in version 99B. This subset of the population is of interest because of the high incidence of cash transfers to this group. The institutionalised dataset that was included in all versions of STINMOD from 99B to 03B, excluding the HES-based STINMOD/01A. Owing to lack of currency, this institutionalised dataset is not present in current versions but it is intended to once again incorporate them using more current ABS microdata in future versions.

Projection Component

Prior to the 00A version of STINMOD, the basefile was current at a single point in time. In response to requests from users in federal government departments who needed to provide 'outyear' costings as part of the budget process, STINMOD is now an outyears model, with users able to choose the financial year they wish to analyse.[3] The most recent version of STINMOD — STINMOD/05B — has basefiles for the December and June quarters of each financial year from 2005–2006 to 2010–2011.

The inclusion of outyear basefiles required the development of a projection methodology. Private incomes are updated based on expected changes to average earnings and the consumer price index. The projected basefiles are reweighted against projected population characteristics and customer numbers. In addition to the base datasets, STINMOD also generates a set of parameter files that contain values for the parameters of the tax and transfer programs modelled in STINMOD. The user has the option to use average parameter values for each financial year, or to use point-in-time parameter values for one of the four indexation periods in each financial year. The parameters are projected in line with projections in the consumer price index and male total average weekly earnings. The way in which the outyears functionality has been developed has made it easier for users to include their own assumptions about future labour force, economic and demographic outcomes. This is done by editing a spreadsheet containing those assumptions and then using custom menu options to create new STINMOD basefiles and parameter files that reflect those assumptions.

Imputation

Owing to the unavailability of some variables required in STINMOD in the ABS surveys, a number of variables have been imputed. For the most

[3] The development of the outyears capacity in STINMOD stemmed from an outyears version of the model created by the federal treasury.

current version, the imputed variables include family links between away-from home dependants and parental records; workforce independence for single income units still living with their parents; disability level for Department of Veteran's Affairs pension recipients; take-up of private health insurance; number of children aged under one year; number of children in age ranges; and more detailed marital status for 15–24 year olds.

Technical Details

Language: The source code, outyears and interface versions are all SAS-based.

System requirements/type of computer: IBM compatible PCs — Pentium III minimum although we recommend a faster computer if possible; minimum 256 MB of RAM; 2 GB hard disk space minimum.

Data storage: basefiles and parameter datasets are stored in SAS and Excel.

Typical run time: A one-year simulation would take no more than a few minutes to run.

Interactivity: Simulations using the source code and outyears version of STINMOD are generally run from within an interactive SAS session, as are simulations using the STINMOD interface.

Conclusions

STINMOD is a publicly available and easy-to-use model for quantifying the immediate distributional and revenue implications of a wide range of government programs, and is now the standard model used by several Australian federal government departments for their analyses of possible budget policy options. STINMOD provides reliable estimates of the first-round distributional impact of changes in tax and transfer policy. It provides estimates of the number of winners and losers, the net impact on government outlays or taxation revenue, and the magnitude of the gains or losses for families of different composition and at different income levels.

NATSEM continues to enhance and develop STINMOD in response to requests from client departments and users, to meet internal needs and to improve the quality of the model. It has been used for a wide range of policy input — including analysing the major changes to the tax and transfer system introduced in Australia in July 2000, effective tax rates, and most recently, as input to the safety net wage case and the distributional impact of the recently enacted Welfare to Work legislation. STINMOD has been used as an educational tool in a training course entitled *Microsimulation techniques for social and economic analysis*, run by NATSEM as part of the University of Canberra's Professional Management Program. STINMOD has also been used as the starting point for modelling research across a wide range of other areas, including housing, legal aid, pharmaceutical benefits and child support payments.

References

Bremner, K., Beer, G., Lloyd, R. and Lambert, S. (2002). *Creating a Basefile for STINMOD.* Technical Paper no. 27, National Centre for Social and Economic Modelling, University of Canberra.

Lambert, S., Percival, R., Schofield, D. and Paul, S. (1994). *An Introduction to STINMOD: A Static Microsimulation Model.* STINMOD Technical Paper no. 1, National Centre for Social and Economic Modelling, University of Canberra.

Percival, R. (1994). *Building STINMOD's Base Population.* STINMOD Technical Paper no. 2, National Centre for Social and Economic Modelling, University of Canberra.

Model 10

EUROMOD — The Tax-Benefit Microsimulation Model for the European Union

Holly Sutherland

Institute for Social and Economic Research, University of Essex, UK

Overview

EUROMOD is a microsimulation model that calculates static effects of tax and benefit policy on household incomes; it also can be used as a platform for other more sophisticated modelling exercises and can, in principle be linked to other types of economic or statistical models. Its distinguishing feature is that it covers many countries within one framework: currently the 15 countries that made up the European Union (EU) prior to the 2004 enlargement. As such it can simulate the rules behind all 15 tax-benefit systems, which are very diverse, as well as including databases broadly representative of 15 household populations (Immervoll et al., 1999; Sutherland, 2000).

EUROMOD provides estimates of the distributional impact of changes to personal tax and transfer policy, with (a) the specification of policy changes, (b) the application of revenue constraints and (c) the evaluation of results, each taking place at either the national or the European Level. Thus, EUROMOD is of value both in terms of assessing the consequences of consolidated social policies and in understanding how different policies in different countries may contribute to common objectives. It can be used to evaluate national policies within a European perspective, as well as policies at the level of the EU.

History and Organisation

The idea of EUROMOD first originated among a group of academics from several countries working together on social policy and taxation comparisons. It was constructed specifically to maximise comparability across

International Symposia in Economic Theory and Econometrics, Vol. 16

ISSN: 1571-0386 DOI: 10.1016/S1571-0386(06)16029-9

countries, recognising that national models tend to run with national assumptions and conventions "hardwired" in, and that access to many models at once may be difficult to negotiate. Its initial construction (starting in 1996) and subsequent development and use have been mainly funded by a succession of European Commission research grants. These have the particular advantage of funding many institutions in different countries at once. This is important because EUROMOD development needed to draw on national expertise at each stage. The large consortium has developed the model: a total of 60 or so individuals, with 35 at any one time in 18 institutions across the 15 countries. This has required a significant amount of management and scientific coordination, a task carried out by a team based originally at the University of Cambridge, and now at the University of Essex. A particular focus for this coordination has been on the comparability of model results across countries. This team also designed the structure of the model and continues to coordinate its development, with national modelling teams contributing their particular expertise.

Examples of Use

The model construction consortium also worked together on a project which explored the impacts of national social and fiscal policies, and reforms to these policies, on poverty reduction in the EU-15. The developing Social Agenda of the EU and the Social Inclusion process in particular, provided the policy context and shaped many of the project's activities. Highlights include:

Which policies make a difference? We have demonstrated that an assessment of the relative redistributive and poverty-reducing effects of national tax-benefit systems depends on which components are included in the system. Including the effect of taxes can be important, through the counting of tax concessions as quasi benefits or through accounting for the taxation of benefits. Whether public pensions are included as part of the transfer system, and contributions as part of the tax system can have a large impact on conclusions from cross-country comparisons.

Policy learning across countries. Much can be learned from cross-country comparisons of the effects of common policies. Examination of *pension reform* scenarios under budgetary constraints in four countries shows that the variations in fiscal and distributive effects of a given reform can be very significant. The different starting points in terms of inequality among the elderly, the proportion of them below the national poverty lines, and existing pension arrangements, result in differential effects of some illustrative reform packages designed to protect the most vulnerable pensioners through a period of reform. Different paths for reform are necessary to achieve common objectives across countries.

Taking account of changes in labour supply following the adoption of systems from other countries — in this case, *Making Work Pay* policies shows that labour market conditions in one country may make the design of a policy from a country with different conditions quite inappropriate or indeed damaging. For example, in France or Germany, the application of the British Working Families Tax Credit would have a net negative impact on employment since the strong decrease in the participation of married women (with working partners) would not be offset by a positive effect on single parents.

Replacing the minimal *child-targeted social transfer systems* of the countries of Southern Europe with child benefits borrowed from Northern European systems reduces child poverty significantly. While expensive if introduced on a universal basis, there is scope for designing non-means-tested benefits for example those targeted on young children or large families that can be cost effective in terms of child poverty reduction.

Macro changes and micro outcomes. Even when the rate is low, inflation can have a significant effect on both the equalising and revenue-generating properties of income tax and social contribution systems. More broadly, changes such as the level of unemployment, the extent of earnings inequality and the rate of real income growth can change the operation of tax-benefit systems and their effectiveness in reducing the risk of poverty. The size of the effect of such changes on relative poverty rates, and sometimes the direction of the effect varies across the 15 countries. If relative poverty rates are to be used as generally accepted indicators of the outcomes of policy, then it is important that these differential sensitivities are fully understood.

Inequality and policy at the regional level. National tax-benefit systems appear particularly efficient at inequality reduction in the poorer regions in a country but much less so in the richer regions. Since some of the new forms of poverty are associated with richer and more urban regions, this calls for further intervention at the level of the regional governments. At the same time, similar regions in Europe in terms of economic performance and levels of original income inequality achieve quite different degrees of income inequality once the redistributive role of the national tax-benefit system is accounted for. This may provide an argument on equity grounds for EU intervention in the design of tax-benefit policies.[1]

[1] For more information see www.iser.essex.ac.uk/msu/emod/micresa-final.php

Relationships with National Models

EUROMOD can also be used for national tax-benefit modelling exercises and has provided the impetus for the construction of associated national models in four countries where they did not exist before (Austria, Greece, Luxembourg and Portugal). Many of those in the original EUROMOD consortium run their own national models in parallel with their involvement in EUROMOD.[2] Generally national models cover the tax-benefit system in more detail or less selectively than EUROMOD and are more up-to-date.[3] On the other hand, EUROMOD is much more flexible than a national model and this flexibility is essential if comparability (or results) and transferability (of system components) are to be achieved. So, typically, national models are used for national (single country) analysis and EUROMOD for comparative and comparable multi-country analysis.

Current Developments

The model is being expanded to cover the 10 new Member States of the EU and is being re-designed and upgraded in the light of enlargement and also of the lessons learned from operating and using the first version. EUROMOD is entirely unique in being a multi-country microsimulation model and much of its architecture was originally developed without prior or parallel experience to draw on.

This new project, known as I-CUE ("Improving the Capacity and Usability of EUROMOD") is laying the technical basis for a 25-country comparative research infrastructure by up-grading the design of the model, and providing greater clarity in presenting the knowledge base embodied in it. It is also beginning to involve researchers, data providers and institutions from the 10 new Member States in the long-standing EUROMOD collaboration.

A second project is involving a large network of researchers across Europe in a programme of research called "Accurate Income Measurement for the Assessment of Public Policies" (AIM-AP). This is designed to improve the comparability, scope and applicability of tools, methods and data for the

[2] For example, ESPASIM for Spain (Levy et al., 2001), SWITCH for Ireland (Callan et al., 1996), POLIMOD for the UK (Redmond et al., 1998) and TUJA for Finland (Viitamäki, 1998).

[3] For example, at the time of writing in 2006 a typical national model would be running 2006 or 2007 policies. At this time, EUROMOD is running 2001 policies for all countries, 2003 for the majority and 2005 for a few. Making EUROMOD easier to update and maintain is one of the goals of the I-CUE project, described below.

measurement of income and the analysis of the effects of policies on inequality, poverty and social inclusion. It includes three linked projects on:

- The distributional effects of non-cash incomes (such as education and health services) and the implementation of a more comprehensive income definition,
- The implications of (and methods to account for) errors in targeting social benefits, tax evasion and measurement error in income data,
- Incorporation of the effects of indirect taxes, along with direct taxes and social benefits, in redistribution analysis.

All three projects are designed to improve the degree of comparability of measurement and analysis across countries. Each project will develop methodologies within a cross-national perspective and demonstrate their applicability to a wide range of research questions. The resulting data and method enhancements will be made generally accessible and re-useable by implementing them within EUROMOD.

The EUROMOD consortium also publishes a series of Working Papers describing applications of the model www.iser.essex.ac.uk/msu/emod/publications/emodwp.php provides web access to detailed statistics on income re-distribution in the EU-15 www.iser.essex.ac.uk/msu/emod/emodstats/ documents its work at the country level in Country Reports. www.iser.essex.ac.uk/msu/emod/countries/

Availability

EUROMOD is intended for use in academic and related research and is in principle available for use by any researcher. In practice, prospective users must gain permission to use the underlying micro-data and usually require some training and orientation in the practical use of the model, as its flexibility allows for choices in many more dimensions than is typical in a national model.

Technical Particulars

The model itself is written in C++. However, it is written in such a way that users, and in many cases developers also, do not need to access the code. The user manipulates building blocks of code through parameter files that are stored, accessed, documented and organised in Excel. The data are stored in Access. See Immervoll and O'Donoghue (2001) for more information. The model runs on a standard PC and has no particular system

Table 1: Data Sources

Country	Base dataset for EUROMOD	Date of collection
Austria	Austrian version of European Community Household Panel	1999
Belgium	Panel Survey on Belgian Households	1999
Denmark	European Community Household Panel	1995
Finland	Income distribution survey	2001
France	Budget de Famille (HBS)	1994/1995
Germany	German Socio-Economic Panel	2001
Greece	European Community Household Panel	1995
Ireland	Living in Ireland Survey	1994
Italy	Survey of Households Income and Wealth	1996
Luxembourg	PSELL-2	2001
Netherlands	Sociaal-economisch panelonderzoek	2000
Portugal	European Community Household Panel	2001
Spain	European Community Household Panel	2000
Sweden	Income distribution survey	2001
UK	Family Expenditure Survey (HBS)	2000/2001

requirements. The data sources currently used by the model are shown in Table 1.

Acknowledgement

The author thanks Horacio Levy for helpful comments.

References

Callan, T., O'Donoghue, C. and O'Neil, C. (1996). *Simulating Welfare and Income Tax Changes: The ESRI Tax-Benefit Model*, ESRI, Dublin.

Immervoll, H. and O'Donoghue, C. (2001). *Towards a Multi-Purpose Framework for Tax-Benefit Microsimulation. A Discussion by Reference to EUROMOD, a European Tax-Benefit Model.* EUROMOD Working Paper EM2/01.

Immervoll, H., O'Donoghue, C. and Sutherland, H. (1999). *An Introduction to EUROMOD*. EUROMOD Working Paper EM0/99.

Levy, H., Mercader-Prats, M. and Planas, M. (2001). An Introduction to ESPASIM: A Microsimulation Model to Assess Tax-Benefit Reforms in Spain. *Brazilian Electronic Journal of Economics*, 4(1), 1–23. http://www.beje.decon.ufpe.br/

Redmond, G., Sutherland, H. and Wilson, M. (1998). *The Arithmetic of Tax and Social Security Reform: A User's Guide to Microsimulation Methods and Analysis.* Cambridge University Press, Cambridge.

Sutherland, H. (2000). EUROMOD: A Tax-Benefit Model for the European Union. *Transfer*, 6(2), 312–316.

Viitamäki, H. (1998). *TUJA-mallin kehittäminen. (Developing the TUJA-Model.)* VATT-paper 32.

Model 11

PSSRU Long-Term Care Finance Model and CARESIM: Two Linked UK Models of Long-Term Care for Older People

Raphael Wittenberg[a], Ruth Hancock[b], Adelina Comas-Herrera[a], Derek King[a], Juliette Malley[a], Linda Pickard[a], Ariadna Juarez-Garcia[c] and Robin Darton[d]

[a]*London School of Economics, UK*
[b]*University of Essex, UK*
[c]*University of Birmingham, UK*
[d]*University of Kent, UK*

Introduction

This chapter describes two linked simulation models which project long-term care financing in the UK. The Personal Social Services Research Unit (PSSRU) long-term care finance model makes projections of future long-term care demand and expenditures. CARESIM analyses the current and projected future distributional effects of alternative ways of financing long-term care. They are linked for two purposes. The first is to improve the apportionment of total expenditure between the private and public sectors in the PSSRU model. The second is to weight CARESIM results to take account of the fact that older people who need care are not a random sub-sample of the older population.

The PSSRU Long-Term Care Finance Model

The aim of the PSSRU long-term care finance model is to make projections of future demand for long-term care for older people and associated expenditure. The model was constructed as part of a project on long-term care finance, which is funded by the Department of Health (England's health ministry). The project is concerned with two related policy issues on the

International Symposia in Economic Theory and Econometrics, Vol. 16

ISSN: 1571-0386 DOI: 10.1016/S1571-0386(06)16030-5

funding of long-term care for older people. The first is whether expenditure, and specifically public expenditure, on long-term care will remain sustainable over the coming decades. The second is what should be the balance between public and private expenditure on long-term care.

The PSSRU at the London School of Economics started development of the model in 1996. The core model makes projections for England to 2041. A variant makes projections for the United Kingdom to 2051.

The model and its variants have been used to make projections for the Department of Health, the Royal Commission on Long-Term Care, the Institute for Public Policy Research, the European Commission, the National Assembly for Wales, the Nuffield Foundation and the Joseph Rowntree Foundation. A variant has recently been completed to produce projections for the Wanless Social Care Review.

Coverage

The PSSRU model aims to make projections of four key variables: the future numbers of disabled older people, the likely level of demand for long-term care services and disability benefits for older people, the costs associated with meeting this demand and the social care workforce required.

The model covers informal care by family and friends, formal long-term health and social services (both publicly and privately funded) and cash disability benefits. The health services include long-stay hospital care, day hospital care, community nursing, nursing in care homes and therapy services. The social services include residential care, home care, day care, meals and assessment and care management. The disability benefits comprise cash payments that may be used to purchase care and/or for other disability-related expenditure.

Model Structure

The PSSRU model is a cell-based, or macrosimulation, model. It is a large Excel spreadsheet with Visual Basic features. It comprises sheets for data entry, base year estimates, projection years, summaries of results and menus for scenarios.

The model base year and projection sheets consist of five main parts:

- The first part estimates the numbers of older people with different levels of disability by age group, gender, household type and housing tenure. The number of older people by age and gender are divided by disability category, in terms of ability to conduct domestic and personal care tasks. They are then divided by marital status and within marital status by household composition and receipt of informal care. They are then divided by housing tenure.

- The second part of the model projects the volumes of services demanded by combining the output of the first part of the model (the projected numbers of older people by disability, household type/informal care and other characteristics) with functions that assign receipt of services to each sub-group of the older population. The probability of receiving health and social care services is estimated for each sub-group through analysis of the PSSRU survey and General Household Survey data listed below.
- The third part projects the total expenditure on the formal services demanded by applying unit costs of formal care to the volume of services projected in the second part of the model.
- The fourth part of the model breaks down projected aggregate expenditure by source of funding: health services (NHS), social services, service users and disability benefits. Output from the CARESIM model is used for this purpose.
- A fifth part of the model makes projections of the numbers of social care (but not NHS) staff required to provide the projected volume of social services, for different groups of social care staff.

The PSSRU model has been used for various studies on paying for long-term care in combination with the CARESIM microsimulation model.

Data

The model is regularly updated as new data become available. The latest version uses the following main data sources:

- Government Actuary's Department 2004-based population projections by age and gender and 2003-based marital status and cohabitation projections;
- Department of Health data on numbers of recipients of publicly funded social services at March 2003 and on gross and net expenditure on social services in 2002/2003;
- 2001 Census data on the numbers of older people in long-stay hospital care;
- General Household Survey 2001/2002 data on disability rates and receipt of informal care and of home-based services by older people in private households;
- PSSRU 1996 Survey data on the characteristics of older people in care homes;
- PSSRU and Laing & Buisson data on the unit costs of services, deflated to 2002 prices;
- Department for Work and Pensions 2003 data on numbers of older recipients of disability benefits;

- Department of Health data and estimates of the social care workforce caring for older people.

Scenarios

The model does not make forecasts about the future. It makes projections on the basis of specific assumptions about future trends in drivers of demand for long-term care. A set of assumptions is used as a base case. The base case projections take account of expected changes in factors exogenous to long-term care policy, such as demographic trends. The base case projections hold constant factors endogenous to long-term care policy, such as patterns of care and the funding system. The base case is used as a point of comparison when the assumptions of the model are subsequently varied in alternative scenarios.

The main assumptions of the base case are as follows:

- The number of older people by age, gender and marital status changes in line with the latest Government Actuary's Department official projections;
- Prevalence rates of disability by age and gender remain unchanged;
- Home-ownership rates change in line with CARESIM projections;
- The proportions of older people receiving informal care, formal community care services, residential care services and disability benefits remain constant for each sub-group by age, disability and other needs-related characteristics;
- Health and social care unit costs rise by 2 per cent per year in real terms (but non-staff revenue costs remain constant in real terms). Real Gross Domestic Product rises in line with HM Treasury assumptions;
- The supply of formal care will adjust to match demand and demand will be no more constrained by supply in the future than in the base year.

These base case assumptions can be varied in alternative scenarios.

CARESIM

CARESIM aims to provide information relevant to assessing the distributional effects of alternative care charging regimes. It is a dynamic microsimulation model which uses data on a sample of older people's income and assets to simulate what each older sample member would be required to pay towards his or her care costs should he or she need care. The results can then be analysed by income level and other socio-economic characteristics to see how alternative charging regimes affect the incidence of care costs. The initial sample of people aged 65 and above is aged but it is not refreshed with new entrants. This means that projections for 20 years ahead can be made only for people then aged 85 and above. However, since care needs are concentrated in this age group, this limitation is not as significant as might seem at first sight. In future work we hope to develop a method for refreshing the sample and so extending the model's time horizon.

CARESIM's development started in 1998 with a grant from the Nuffield Foundation. However, it grew out of a pre-existing static tax-benefit model for older people which also had the facility to analyse the interaction of equity release schemes (reverse mortgages) for older people (Hancock, 1998). The development from a static tax-benefit model to a dynamic care charging model involved making the model dynamic by ageing the sample and constructing routines to simulate the UK's complex care charging rules and potential reforms to them.

CARESIM has no core funding but is maintained and developed through grants for applications of the model.

Data

CARESIM uses microdata on older participants in the Family Resources Survey (FRS). The FRS is a nationally representative sample of British households carried out for the Department for Work and Pensions (see e.g., Department for Work and Pensions, 2005). It contains detailed information on the incomes, wealth, housing and other relevant characteristics of sample members, sufficient to make good estimates of their liability for care charges. The FRS excludes people living in care homes and therefore represents the population from which future entrants to care homes will come, but may provide a less accurate picture of the incomes and assets of people already resident in care homes.

Ageing the Sample

Sample members are aged in the following steps:

1. Predict stochastically according to age and gender, whether each member of all FRS households containing a member of the simulation sample[1] will be alive in the future year of interest up to a maximum of 20 years from the base year, and increase the age of those who are predicted to be alive.

[1] The simulation sample consists of all unpartnered people of age 65 and above and one partner in all couples where both are over state pension age (65 for men and 60 for women). The default in the case of couples is for care charges to be modelled for the older partner.

2. Predict whether each simulation sample member will have become a widow or widower in the year of interest. This is done deterministically once survival of each partner has been predicted.
3. Simulate how the income and wealth of each simulation sample member and partner will have changed by the year of interest using simple assumptions about changes relative to assumed increases in prices and earnings.
4. Model any inheritance of income and capital of the surviving partner if there is one including inherited pensions.

Divorce, remarriage or other changes in household composition are not currently modelled. The onset of disability is not modelled but is taken into account by a re-weighting process (see below).

Technical Details

CARESIM is written in SAS, reading weights provided by the PSSRU model from Excel files and writing results used by the PSSRU model into Excel files.

Linkages between the PSSRU and NCCSU Models

CARESIM provides projections of four variables for incorporation in the PSSRU model

- The proportion of care home residents and home care clients eligible for local authority support under the current or an alternative charging regime.
- For care home residents, the proportion of gross costs of care met by disability benefits in the case of those not eligible for local authority support.
- The proportion of gross costs met by users, in the case of those eligible for local authority support.
- The proportion of gross costs of home care met by disability benefits, for those eligible for local authority supported home care.

CARESIM calculates what each person in a representative sample of older people would be required to contribute to the costs of residential or home care. However, the PSSRU model shows that, controlling for age, care home residents and recipients of care at home are not a random subset of the older population. Home care users are disproportionately likely to live alone and care home residents are disproportionately likely to have lived alone and to have rented rather than owned their homes. Housing tenure and whether previously living alone are both characteristics which affect liability for care home charges. CARESIM results are therefore reweighted according to projection year, housing tenure and marital status within gender and 5-year age group. The weights are based on the PSSRU model projections of the (previous) housing tenure and household type of service users, by age and gender. They are used as grossing-up factors which reflect the PSSRU model projections of the composition of the population in these age groups in each of seven care categories including not receiving any chargeable care. Members of the simulation sample are assigned seven grossing-up factors to allow them to be grossed-up to the population in each of these categories. For future years, grossing-up factors are assigned only to those FRS respondents for whom the simulation remains valid.

People aged 16–64 are included in analyses of tax-raising options for the base year. Grossing-up factors which vary by gender but relate to the single-age group 16–64 are used for FRS respondents in this age group.

Further Information

A detailed account of the long-term care projections model and of the data and assumptions used can be found in Wittenberg et al. (1998), a report that describes the first version of the model. The model has been regularly updated and expanded. A description of the most recent version of the core model can be found in Wittenberg et al. (2006).

More details on CARESIM can be found in Hancock et al. (2006) and Hancock (2000).

References

Department for Work and Pensions. (2005). Family Resources Survey Statistical Report 2003–2004. Available at http://www.dwp.gov.uk/asd/frs/2003_04/index.asp

Hancock, R. (1998). Can Housing Wealth Alleviate Poverty in Old Age? *Fiscal Studies*, 19, 249–272.

Hancock, R. (2000). *Charging for Care in Later Life: Analysing the Effects of Reforming the Means Test.* Working Paper no. NF86, University of Leicester, Nuffield Community Care Studies Unit.

Hancock, R., Pickard, L., Wittenberg, R., Comas-Herrera, A., Juarez-Garcia, A., King, D. and Malley, J. (2006). *Paying for Long-Term Care for Older People in the UK: Modelling the Costs and Distributional Effects of a Range of Options.* PSSRU Discussion paper 2336.

Wittenberg, R., Comas-Herrera, A., King, D., Malley, J., Pickard, L. and Darton, R. (2006). *Future Demand for Long-Term Care, 2002 to 2041: Projections of Demand for Long-Term Care for Older People in England.* PSSRU Discussion Paper 2330, March 2006 (available free online at www.pssru.ac.uk/pdf/dp2330.pdf).

Wittenberg, R., Pickard, L., Comas-Herrera, A., Davies, B., and Darton, R. (1998). *Demand for Long-Term Care: Projections of Long-Term Care Finance for Elderly People.* PSSRU, University of Kent.

Model 12

Social Policy Simulation Database and Model (SPSD/M)

Chantal Hicks and Brian Murphy

Statistics Canada, Canada

Introduction

Statistics Canada's Social Policy Simulation Database and Model (SPSD/M) has been in use by policy analysts in Canada since 1985. Prior to the SPSD/M, microsimulation modeling in Canada was restricted to government analysts using large mainframe models in federal departments and their emphasis was on specific tax/transfer programs. The SPSD/M was developed by Statistics Canada, with participation of other federal government departments through a steering committee, in order to provide state-of-the-art microsimulation capability to the wider policy-making community. The model examines the combined impact on households of a large number of interrelated tax and transfer programs at two levels of government. The development of SPSD/M within Statistics Canada benefited from access to a range of key sources of confidential microdata, though the resulting database and model are fully in the public domain.

The SPSD/M was first developed in 1985 on a mainframe computer in SAS and then converted into a PC platform in C+ in 1986; the first major PC-based model in the world. It was released to the public in 1987. Since that time it has been widely used by federal and provincial policy analysts, private sector think tanks, lobby groups, consultants, academics, and students. It has been used to study every major change in the Canadian tax/transfer system since 1984 including several tax reforms, unemployment insurance reforms, and special issue areas such as intergenerational equity. It has formed the platform for detailed fiscal incidence studies and has been integrated in studies employing macro-economic forecasting models.

International Symposia in Economic Theory and Econometrics, Vol. 16

ISSN: 1571-0386 DOI: 10.1016/S1571-0386(06)16031-7

Overview

The SPSD/M is a static microsimulation model. It is comprised of a database, a series of tax/transfer algorithms and models, analytical software, and user documentation. The development of the model to date has focussed on accuracy, speed, flexibility, and control. It requires skilled analysts to operate effectively.

Database

The SPSD is a non-confidential, statistically representative database of individuals in their family contexts, with enough information on each individual to compute taxes paid to and cash transfers received from both federal and provincial levels of governments.

The SPSD is constructed by statistically matching four different survey and administrative microdatasets. The host dataset is currently the Survey of Labour and Income Dynamics (SLID), an annual Canadian income survey of about 70,000 individuals in 30,000 households. Several variables on the original survey have known problems with underreporting, so the database construction process adjusts certain records to ensure agreement with other known administrative benchmarks. Administrative data on employment insurance claim histories are statistically matched to the SLID. Data on tax deductions as well as on the distribution of high income Canadians are statistically matched from administrative files of tax returns. Household expenditure survey data is statistically matched to provide the basis for calculating sales and commodity taxes.

The database supports processing and analysis for five different units of analysis in an integrated fashion (individuals, tax families, census families, economic families, and households). The SPSD contains over 300 variables with basic information on demography, family structure, income, tax deductions, expenditures, and unemployment history.

Static Database Aging

The SPSD has significant production lags due to the availability of administrative data and the complexity of the database creation process. However policy analysts are largely concerned with the future. The SPSD/M therefore includes user-controllable static database aging techniques to project (not forecast) the data to represent past/future years in line with broad demographic and economic trends and forecasts. As with most static database aging, the distribution of income tends to hold the same shape as the base year of the data. The most recent SPSD is based on 2002 data and static adjustment algorithms are capable of representing all years from 1991 through 2010 (in terms of age/sex/province demography, labor force participation, and broad indicators of economic growth).

Tax/Transfer Models

The SPSM is a static accounting model that processes each individual and family on the SPSD, calculates taxes and transfers using algorithms that simulate legislated or proposed programs, and reports on the results. Each algorithm can, depending on the input parameter set, simulate the rules of the tax or transfer system in all years from 1991 through 2010 though data limitations can affect the accuracy of results for previous years (e.g. we do not attempt to impute the data underlying a given tax provision in 1991 to the 2002 version of the database).

The tax algorithms simulate all major federal and provincial personal income taxes and payroll taxes. Cash transfers simulated include all major federal and provincial transfer programs such as employment insurance benefits, old age security benefits, guaranteed income supplement benefits, family allowance benefits, child tax credit and federal child benefit, and the goods and services tax credit. All algorithms operate on an annualized basis.

COMTAX is the name of the commodity tax model associated with the SPSM. COMTAX is a macro-economic input/output-based model that is not released with the SPSD/M package, but the results from it are provided in the form of input parameters to the SPSM. COMTAX provides estimates of effective federal and provincial retail sales-tax-equivalent commodity tax rates by province, household expenditure category, and tax type. This model is required because many commodity taxes are levied at intermediate stages of production, not at the final retail stage. Rates calculated by the COMTAX model can be used to obtain estimates of the commodity taxes paid, both directly and indirectly, by any given household. Commodity taxes modeled include federal import duties, federal excise duties and taxes, federal goods and services tax, provincial profits on liquor commissions, provincial fuel taxes, provincial retail sales taxes, and cascading effects between taxes.

There are few behavioral response capabilities incorporated into the SPSM. Rather the approach is to allow the user a great deal of flexibility permitting the identification of individuals most at risk of behavioral response, and to simulate changes in their behavior using a wide number of software tools.

Analytical Facilities

The SPSD/M software includes many features to provide the analyst maximum control over the results. A flexible programming language allows users to create statements and expressions manipulating both input and output variables. This language includes regular operators. As such, a familiarity with programming is essential for its efficient use. There are two broad classes of analytical features, database- and policy analysis facilities.

Database analysis features include a selection facility that allows a user to select a subset of records for analysis. A custom variable facility which allows users to create, name, and label new variables as a function of any other database or modeled variables from multiple scenarios. A custom tabulation facility allows users to create *n*-dimensional tables. Database construction utilities allow the user to make modifications directly to the database (e.g. imputing new microdata). A distribution analysis facility provides basic distributional statistics such as mean, median, various quantiles, values for minimum and maximum records, and can produce a histogram. The SPSD/M is also capable of writing microdata files either as a native SAS dataset or as an ASCII file in a number of different formats, which can be analysed using other software.

Policy analysis facilities include a flexible marginal tax rate calculator with control over the unit of analysis, income source, incremental amount, and so forth. A "turning point" facility calculates, for a given household(s), the continuous tax function for that household to assist analysts in identifying, among other things, where stacked marginal tax rates exceed 100 (or are high enough to provide a significant labour disincentive). A series of 10 default tables present the main aggregates and population reporting numbers by province, income level, family type, and income relative to the low-income cut-off. A goal seeking facility will iteratively run the model such that conditions specified by the user are met (e.g. change the benefit level of a new program until certain target aggregate or revenue neutrality is achieved). It is possible to calculate both a base and variant scenario during the same model run, and then through the use of a reference variable facility compare any number of previously calculated scenarios with the base/variant scenarios of the current run.

Mode of Use

There are two ways of running the SPSM: using the visual SPSM interface and using the classic SPSM interface. The visual SPSM interface provides a graphical user interface in which users can interactively modify parameter values, save simulations, run the model, and examine output. The classic interface runs in a command window and is intended for batch processing.

Recognizing that no system can anticipate all types of changes to the tax/transfer system, the SPSM provides flexibility to users by allowing access to the SPSM tax/transfer source code base. Glass-box use involves using a C++ compiler to directly modify the source C++ routines that define the rules of the tax/transfer system. Users can alter the source code and re-compile a new version of the SPSM that can then be run.

Technical Details

The SPSD/M is written in C++. The full program requires PC with 220 Mb available disk space running under Windows 2000 or Windows XP.

The database is stored in a binary format with customized compression algorithms. Parameter files are stored as ASCII files and are designed to be easily readable.

The SPSD/M is installed as a stand-alone application on a single PC. Such an installation can also be accessed widely through a network.

The structure of a model run involves first reading the data for an entire household and statically aging it to the desired year. The tax/transfer algorithms associated with a base scenario are calculated next and model results stored in a vector of about 450 variables. Optionally a second set of algorithms defining the variant scenario are applied and stored in a second output vector. As such users have access to all variables for both scenarios to assist in tracking the effects of various policy changes.

Typical Run Time

On a standard fast 2006 PC, the default single scenario model run will take less than 5 s.

Educational Use

The SPSD/M has had a number of educational applications. It is available at no charge to Canadian universities, which participate in the Data Liberation Initiative. The SPSD/M has been used as a central focus in both undergraduate and graduate policy analysis courses in a number of Canadian universities.

Availability

Since 1987 the SPSD/M has been available to the public. The database and model are provided on a licensed basis as either a single use version or a site licence (which may be used on any number of computers at one organization). In cases where an organization lacks the necessary resources to run the model, a number of private sector consultants and Statistics Canada are able to provide custom analysis.

Macro–Micro Links

The model is calibrated to results from a number of macro-economic models and aggregate data sources. For example, an input–output model provides estimates of effective rates of commodity taxation as input to the model. There is no built-in capacity to provide economic feedback to these models, however experiments of this kind have been conducted on an ad hoc project basis.

Model 13

The OECD Tax-Benefit Model and Policy Database[☆]

Herwig Immervoll

Organisation for Economic Co-Operation and Development

The OECD has used and maintained models of tax and benefit policies operated by its member countries since the mid-1990s. The purpose of these models is to provide a comparative perspective of social and fiscal policies affecting working-age individuals and their families, to monitor policy changes and to examine the effects of interactions between different policy measures.[1] Tax and benefit policy developments and current policy indicators are regularly reported in the OECD series *Benefits and Wages*.

The OECD tax-benefit model uses a "model household" approach. The effects of taxes and social benefits on household incomes are evaluated for a range of different family and labour market circumstances. Using similar "model households" for each country, the aim is to provide an unobstructed view on the mechanics of legal tax and benefit policy rules. Calculation models are based on detailed policy information provided by governments of OECD member countries. This policy database is continually updated. Individual "country chapters" describing each policy area in detail are publicly available through the OECD web site. The models, while primarily intended for internal use, are also available to researchers outside the OECD.

The model is currently in use at the OECD, the European Commission and by a number of researchers and policy analysts in governments, universities and research institutes. Recent model applications have included analyses of work incentives, income poverty and adequacy of benefit

---

[☆] *This work reported here is the result of a joint project between the OECD and the European Commission. It has been produced with the financial assistance of the European Commission. The views expressed are entirely those of the author and do not represent the official opinion of the European Commission, or the OECD.*

[1] A separate model exists for calculating old-age pension entitlements. See OECD (2005).

International Symposia in Economic Theory and Econometrics, Vol. 16

ISSN: 1571-0386 DOI: 10.1016/S1571-0386(06)16032-9

entitlements, the net incomes of minimum-wage workers, as well as the cost of non-parental childcare. Details on these and related studies are available on the Internet at www.oecd.org/els/social/workincentives

Scope

The OECD model currently covers 29 OECD countries and the time-period is from 1995 to 2005.

Following the OECD *Jobs Study* in 1994, the model was initially developed in order to provide an improved basis for measuring financial work incentives. The primary focus was on comparing net (after-tax) values of unemployment benefits with net incomes of working individuals.

The models have since developed into a more generalised tool for tax-benefit analysis covering:

- income taxes,
- social security contributions,
- unemployment insurance benefits,
- unemployment assistance benefits,
- social assistance and minimum-income benefits,
- cash housing benefits,
- employment conditional or "in-work" benefits,
- family benefits,
- childcare fees, and
- childcare benefits.

Combining calculations for each of these elements, it is possible to derive net income measures for a range of different family situations (such as single persons and one- or two-earner couples with and without children) and at any level of gross earnings. The resulting net incomes can be broken down to separately show the influence of each policy element.

Calculations take into account the age, marital status and incomes of each household member, as well as hours of work, employment durations and, where applicable, the time spent out of work. The OECD generally relies on a set of standard assumptions for these characteristics although alternative scenarios can be specified.

The "model household" approach provides a useful complement to population-based approaches such as incidence studies based on micro-data or microsimulation models capable of simulating the effects of fiscal and social policy instruments on representative samples of actual households. By computing tax and benefit amounts using existing policy rules, calculations based on stylised households are helpful for understanding the features of these instruments. And by repeating these calculations for a number of different household situations, they can be used to assess under which circumstances each of these features becomes relevant.[2]

Model Architecture and Operation

The models are written in STATA®, a statistical analysis program, which was chosen primarily for its ease of use and data-editing features. At the most basic level, the models allow a user to calculate taxes, benefits and net incomes for a particular family type, either in a steady state — employed or unemployed — or a changing state — moving into or out of unemployment.

The models can be operated in two ways, either using a basic user interface, or in "batch mode", with multiple options. The menu-driven option allows users to select a country and policy year and make various choices concerning family type and the nature of individual work or unemployment situations. The batch mode reads all options from a control file, and allows for a faster and more automated generation of data for a large number of different family and work/unemployment circumstances. The batch mode is useful for complex analyses and reduces the scope of user errors when repeating model runs across a number of different countries.

Access

Country-by-country documents containing detailed descriptions of tax-benefit policies are available at www.oecd.org/els/social/workincentives. Those interested in using the models for their own work can also obtain copies of the relevant programs through this same web site where program files (STATA® source code) along with very brief instructions are available.[3] A PC with STATA® (version 7 or above) installed is required to run the tax-benefit models.

Access to the models, which is currently free of charge for non-commercial uses, is subject to agreement with the relevant terms of use. This includes indicating the source of the numbers along with any results derived from the OECD tax-benefit models. The terms of use also specify a requirement to provide the OECD with copies of any published and unpublished reports making use of the models.

[2] See Immervoll et al. (2004) for a discussion of the family types covered and the scope of the "model family" approach more generally.

[3] Models for the years 2001 and later are currently publicly available. Updates for a given policy year usually become available during autumn of the following year.

The programs are often complex and their proper operation requires a minimum degree of familiarity with both STATA® and the tax-benefit systems operating in the countries of interest. While the OECD welcomes feedback, we are, unfortunately, unable to offer user support. Users of the programs who wish to report errors or provide suggestions for future modelling innovations are invited to contact us at social.contact@oecd.org

Tax-Benefit Calculations On-Line

As an alternative to installing and operating the full version of the tax-benefit model, we are currently developing a web-based interface, which will allow users to perform simple tax-benefit calculations on-line. This feature will be accessible to non-expert users and is intended to be useful for journalists, researchers or members of the public who are looking for a simple way to compare tax burdens and benefit entitlements across OECD countries. The web-based tax-benefit calculator is planned to be released during the second half of 2006. Further details will be announced at www.oecd.org/els/social/workincentives

References

Immervoll, H., Marianna, P. and Mira D'Ercole, M. (2004). *Benefit Coverage Rates and Household Typologies: Scope and Limitations of Tax-Benefit Indicators.* OECD Social, Employment and Migration Working Paper No. 20, OECD, Paris (available through www.oecd.org/els/workingpapers).

OECD (2005). *Pensions at a Glance*. OECD, Paris.

Model 14

Pharmasim model ☆

Anil Gupta

Microsimulation Modelling and Data Analysis Division, Applied Research and Analysis Directorate, Health Canada, Canada

Introduction

The Microsimulation Modelling and Data Analysis Division (MSDAD) has built a microsimulation model to facilitate Pharmacare policy analysis. The Pharmacare Simulation Model (Pharmasim) provides means of analyzing current and future policy on drug coverage and drugs cost for Canadian.

Pharmasim can estimate the aggregate and distributional impacts of changes to existing provincial drug plans and simulate a hypothetical national plan. With Pharmasim, it is possible to create entirely new plans or modify existing plans and see the effects on various subpopulations and the total cost to the government. Pharmasim is built as an extension to the Canadian Health Tax Simulation Model (CHTSIM), an existing microsimulation model developed by MSDAD which simulates the health tax system on the Canadian population.

This chapter reflects the work done by the MSDAD team over the years to give a well-rounded look at the Pharmasim model. It illustrates the implementation, uses and data sources to demonstrate the utility of such a tool in the policy development process.

Overview

The CHTSIM and Pharmasim models are health-oriented microsimulation models which use highly customized parameters to give policy makers a flexible

☆ *The original model was built in the late 1980s by Vishnu Kapur and Anil Gupta. Over the years, many analysts have contributed to a variety of forms of the model. The present model is built with the help of the Microsimulation Modelling and Data Analysis team at Health Canada under the supervision of Anil Gupta. Loan Nguyen, Stéphane Paré and Kisalaya Basu along with a number of summer students have contributed to the present model.*

International Symposia in Economic Theory and Econometrics, Vol. 16

ISSN: 1571-0386 DOI: 10.1016/S1571-0386(06)16033-0

and powerful tool to accurately model the Canadian health tax system and Pharmacare plans. The Pharmasim model can analyze the effects of raising, lowering, adding or taking away from deductibles, co-payments, and maximum limits. These changes could be easily modeled through parameters, or the model could be modified to take on an entirely new benefit system. Another capability that is supported by Pharmasim is the ability to create a new hypothetical drug plan or to apply one province's plan onto another province and then compare the impacts of the new and old plans across provinces. In addition, Pharmasim/CHTSIM continues to allow changes to existing health and tax-related parameters to simulate health benefits under the tax system.

Data Sources

At the heart of CHTSIM and Pharmasim is a database representative of the Canadian population. This database is created using the Survey of Labour and Income Dynamics (SLID) as a backbone, with the 2000 data aged to 2006. Work is underway to update the underlying data with the SLID 2003 data to be grown to 2008. Other sources of data include tax information (T1) and data from the Survey of Household Spending (SHS) and National Population Health Survey (NPHS).

The Pharmasim System

Pharmasim uses FlexFiles to achieve unprecedented flexibility in terms of creating and modifying Pharmacare plans. These files allow easy creation and modification of provincial or national plans. Within, these allow policy makers to specify which group should receive a benefit then specify the actual formula used to calculate the benefit. Using these files, any plan based on the standard principles of Pharmacare is easy to create.

Pharmasim Flow

Pharmasim's operations can be divided into three stages as shown in Figure 1.

1. *Pre-pharmasim stage*

   - Input from database and parameter files is gathered
   - Variables later to be used by Pharmasim are calculated by CHTSIM (e.g. Guaranteed Income Supplement benefit)
   - Gross drug expenditures and premiums coverage are imputed
   - Income and taxes are calculated.

Figure 1: Three Stages of Pharmasim Operations

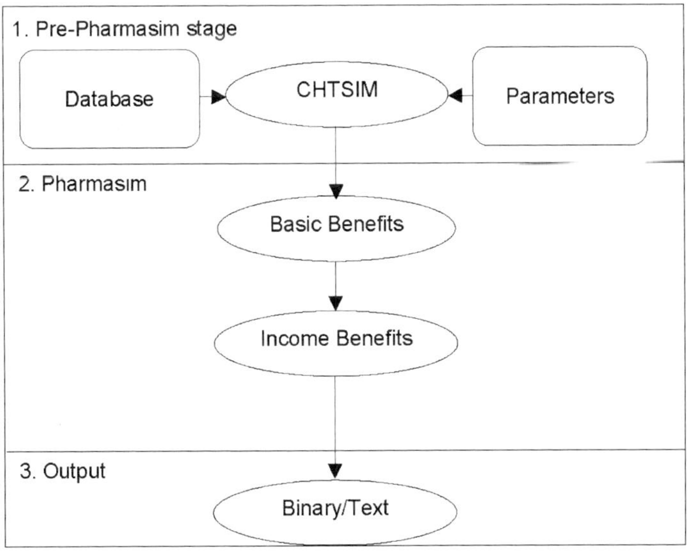

2. *Pharmasim*

- Provincial Pharmacare benefits assigned to individuals based on sub-populations (based on factors including province, senior status, social assistance)
- If an income-based component exists or has been selected this is applied separately to the family.

3. *Output*

- An aggregate summary of the simulation showing totals and impacts
- Total benefits through both income and basic plans are output to the binary and test files.

Pharmasim Output

After running through all the parameters and program files and over 80,000 individual records, the simulated output is saved under different formats. These include:

1. The binary output file, containing raw data for each individual
2. CHTSIM aggregate totals displayed on screen

Table 1: National Public Drug Benefit by Subpopulation

National Public Drug Benefit by Subpopulation

Subpopulation	Base Case				Option				Difference	
	Amount ($ '000)	Amt/Recip ($)	Amt/Per ($)	Recipients	Amount ($ '000)	Amt/Recip ($)	Amt/Per ($)	Recipients	Amount ($ '000)	Recipients
1 Newfoundland	70235	663.85	123.35	105800	79276	680.06	139.22	116572	9041	10772
2 P.E.I	13561	442.38	78.92	30653	16413	601.84	95.53	27272	2852	-3381
3 Nova Scotia	131971	770.50	130.31	171280	127716	764.45	126.11	167070	-4255	-4210
4 New Brunswick	91377	786.59	110.58	116169	90534	734.91	109.56	123191	-843	7022
5 Quebec	1553517	525.82	210.70	2954444	1264048	886.96	171.44	1425141	-289469	-1529303
6 Ontario	2148748	1005.57	182.86	2136848	1724592	1023.23	146.76	1685444	-424156	-451404
7 Manitoba	142833	963.49	130.63	148246	142833	963.49	130.63	148246	0	0
8 Saskatchewan	103389	493.90	105.18	209334	128637	958.68	130.86	134181	25248	-75153
9 Alberta	379329	525.44	133.11	721930	324008	818.98	113.70	395622	-55321	-326308
10 British Colombia	592240	694.01	154.29	853354	472732	939.03	123.16	503424	-119508	-349930
11 Tot Drug Exp < 250	207515	65.48	9.26	3169247	96200	76.35	4.29	1260011	-111315	-1909236
12 Tot Drug Exp 250 - 499	255475	260.68	104.94	980045	136514	233.22	56.07	585339	-118961	-394706
13 Tot Drug Exp 500 - 999	491719	493.58	225.36	996224	295493	411.55	135.43	718002	-196226	-278222
14 Tot Drug Exp 1000 - 2499	1635341	1107.13	675.21	1477094	1327062	1000.00	547.93	1327059	-308279	-150035
15 Tot Drug Exp 2500 - 4999	1568868	2435.67	1908.90	644121	1466639	2250.76	1784.52	651620	-102229	7499
16 Tot Drug Exp > 4999	1068283	5891.47	5149.87	181327	1048880	5696.35	5056.33	184132	-19403	2805
17 Drug Benefit < 250	309497	80.58	11.52	3840738	215704	120.75	8.03	1786313	-93793	-2054425

3. Pharmasim aggregate totals displayed separately
4. Test and aggregate data sent to files
5. Difference between base and option parameter files.

Table 1 displays a snapshot of the output on the computer screen. Shaded lines indicate differences between the base and option. From here, the user may export this as an HTML file, print the aggregate totals, get help, or start a new simulation, in which case the opening dialog is brought back up and the process recommences.

Figure 2 illustrates the implementation of the Pharmasim model. It shows how the Pharmasim model processes the information to generate the final output.

Usage and Usability

Pharmasim model is an ideal tool to simulate the impact of changes to various provincial prescription drug plans on the population while at the same time providing overall revenue and distributional impacts of such changes. The model shows this impact by age, sex, and province for alternative drug plans.

Recently, the model was used to estimate the costs of two catastrophic drug plans under the national pharmaceutical strategy for Canada.

Figure 2: Pharmasim Model Implementation

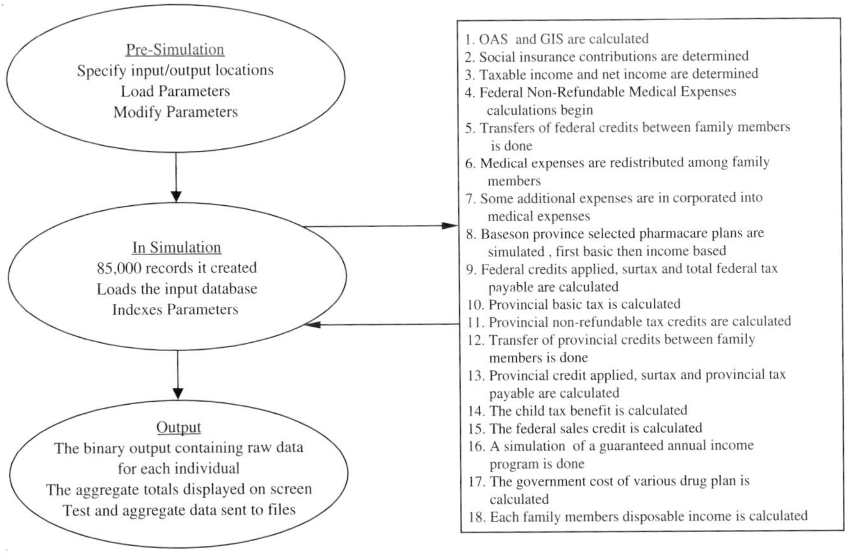

The model was also used to estimate the costs of a health promotion program to promote physical activity among younger children as part of the Budget 2006 for Canada that will allow families to claim a \$500 tax credit per child under the age of 16 for membership in organizations promoting physical activities.

Model 15

LOTTE — The Norwegian Tax-Benefit Model System

Jørgen Aasness, John K. Dagsvik and Thor O. Thoresen

Statistics Norway, Norway

Introduction

The Norwegian tax-benefit model LOTTE is a microsimulation model developed to predict distributional and revenue effects of changes in the taxation of individuals in Norway. The model is static in the sense that it is developed to simulate short-term effects, in contrast to the dynamic microsimulation model MOSART, which is capable of performing simulations into the distant future.

The LOTTE model system (currently) consists of three modules: a module for simulations of personal income taxes, LOTTE-Skatt, a module for indirect taxation, LOTTE-Konsum, and a module describing the labor supply effects of changes in the personal income tax, LOTTE-Arbeid. The latter module has just been developed. In the following, we will describe the three parts of the LOTTE model. More detailed descriptions and examples of applications can be found in Statistics Norway (2006).

LOTTE-Skatt

The first version of the LOTTE-Skatt model was developed early in the 1970s. Since then Norwegian policy-makers have extensively used it, and it is fair to say that the model has been a key tax policy tool over the last decades. The model is non-behavioral; we return to this issue shortly when presenting the LOTTE-Arbeid module.

The staff of the Ministry of Finance use the model throughout the year. For instance, they now (February 2006) have started preparing the budget proposal for 2007, to be put forward in early October 2006. After the budget

International Symposia in Economic Theory and Econometrics, Vol. 16

ISSN: 1571-0386 DOI: 10.1016/S1571-0386(06)16034-2

proposal is made public, the other political parties in Parliament use the model extensively when developing alternative budget proposals.

As the model is physically located at Statistics Norway, a standard process of running the model often starts with contact between the Ministry of Finance or members of Parliament and the dedicated model operator at Statistics Norway. After running the model, the results are reported back to the "customer" rather promptly, often within hours. Usually results are presented in contrast to a baseline simulation. For instance, when the policy-makers now start preparing the 2007 budget, they will usually compare various tax-law changes to a simulation based on the 2006 tax-law projected to 2007. The Ministry of Finance has had access to a version of the model in the ministry, but it has rarely been used. Early in 2006, we make arrangements to let the staff at the Ministry of Finance run the model at Statistics Norway through the Internet. For security reasons they have access to a version of the model that is placed on a separate computer in the bureau.

LOTTE is written in SAS and basically consists of four parts: individual income data, a program that projects data to the year of interest, a set of tax-laws, and a simulation routine that applies tax rules to individual records. Standard model results include aggregate revenue effects and various descriptions of distributional effects.

The main data source of the model is individual income tax returns. The income tax returns are now electronically available for all citizens. However, as many questions concerning income and taxes are best understood on the household level, we need to establish households. For that reason Statistics Norway has developed the income and property statistics for households, which is a sample survey, where information from various registers is combined with household composition data from interviews. Besides information from income tax returns, the income and property statistics for households also includes income data from the National insurance administration and other sources. The sample weights to readjust to national level results reflect that the sample is stratified and that weights have been calibrated to fit information from registers. Presently, the model is based on data from 2003, which implies that simulations are carried out for about 17,000 households. From 2007 and onwards, we will employ the National Register of ground addresses and buildings for household composition information, which means that all data are derived from registers. We can then (in principle) simulate tax burdens for the whole population.

The data are projected to the current year and to future years in accordance with macroeconomic predictions for income growth, income composition, etc. These estimates are derived in close collaboration with the Ministry of Finance, and by contributions of Statistics Norway's macro models.

Detailed tax rules for different years are compiled in the tax-law module of the model. The user can easily make tax rule changes, such as altering statutory tax rates and income deductions. For more advanced tax system changes, for instance changes in tax bases, one usually has to change the simulation routine. The simulation routine joins tax rules and data, in that various tax bases are defined and tax laws are applied to data in that part of the model.

We have recently seen a few examples of applications of the LOTTE-Skatt model in more academic orientated work. For instance, both in Thoresen (2004) and Lambert and Thoresen (2005) the model is employed in order to describe trends in tax progressivity.

LOTTE-Konsum

This model is based on theory of consumer behavior and standard of living, and theory of aggregation of consumption and standard of living over households and individuals in a population. There is no observed consumption data in the LOTTE database, so the microsimulation model is calibrated based on microeconometric relations and macro consumption data, giving a synthetic total expenditure, and allocated to a detailed set of commodity groups, of each household in the population. The main commodity grouping in current use consists of 30 commodities, but it may easily be changed depending on the purpose of the analysis and on the available econometric studies.

The expenditures for each household are derived from a system of Engel functions with demographic variables, satisfying adding-up and non-negativity constraints. This non-linear system, with many corner solutions, is calibrated through an iterative algorithm, such that the sum of expenditures over all households are exactly equal to macro household expenditures, for each commodity, given by an external source for the reference year (baseline simulation). For each household the budget shares are calculated in the reference situation and used to calculate a household-specific price index, using Laspeyres formula. This index is approximately equal to any "true cost of living index" for small price changes from the reference situation, for each household. This last approximation is usually satisfactorily, since we change the baseline simulation according to the problem at hand. Otherwise we may use a more advanced price index formula. The Engel functions are based on econometric studies of the Norwegian household budget surveys, see e.g. Aasness, Biørn and Skjerpen (2003).

The standard of living for each household, and every individual within the household, is defined as the household's total expenditure divided by the household's price index and the household's number of consumer units in the reference period. It can be shown that this can be interpreted as a money metric utility, see Aasness (1995). This measure is aggregated to different inequality and welfare measures and used for policy analysis, see e.g., Aasness (1997) and Aasness et al. (2002).

The revenue effects of changes in indirect taxes is not calculated by LOTTE–Konsum, but by a corresponding microbased macromodel called KONSUM, see e.g., Nygård and Aasness (2003) and the references within, with a corresponding commodity grouping which can be aggregated to different levels. The Ministry of Finance uses a selection of the $60 \times 60 = 3{,}600$ price elasticities from KONSUM in their procedures for calculating the revenue effects of indirect taxes in their national budget proposals to the Parliament. We can construct and calibrate the macromodel KONSUM and the microsimulation model LOTTE-Konsum in pairs, so they are both calibrated to exactly the same macro data and to the same reference period.

Schroyen and Aasness (2006) perform a marginal indirect tax reform analysis, combining output from the microsimulation model LOTTE-Konsum, in terms of expenditure tables for household deciles (according to standard of living), and output from the macromodel KONSUM, in terms of a complete system of demand elasticities, in the reference situation. According to standard optimal tax theory this is all the information needed to perform a marginal tax reform analysis. This is based on the same type of reasoning as is behind the well-known property of Laspeyres index being equal to the true cost of living index for infinitesimal price changes (cf. the envelope theorem). The optimal tax theory assumes that the household data adds exactly up to the macro data, which is fulfilled in our pair on simulation models, but which are usually not the case in other similar empirical tax analysis.

The microsimulation model LOTTE-Konsum can also be used in combination with a full-scale general equilibrium model, see Åvitsland and Aasness (2004).

LOTTE–Arbeid

Neither estimates of revenue changes that work through changes in consumption and indirect taxes, nor estimates of changes that work through labor supply effects, are usually included when discussing the composition of changes in the personal income tax in Norway. It means that the Parliament usually passes budgets without any detailed information on possible effects of the various tax scheme changes on behavior. Especially during the preparation of the last Norwegian tax reform, the reform of 2006, this practice came under pressure. The reason was that the reform involved substantial reductions in marginal tax rates, which most likely imply differences between cost measures with and without behavioral effects.

At Statistics Norway we have over the years developed substantial knowledge and experience on labor supply estimation for simulation purposes; see for instance Aaberge et al. (1995), Dagsvik and Strøm (2006), and Kornstad and Thoresen (2004). The latter study is the first attempt to employ an estimated labor supply model in combination with LOTTE-Skatt. However, the discussion of labor supply effects due to means testing was based on a labor supply model for married female wage earners only.

The module currently being established within the LOTTE system includes separately estimated labor supply models for married/cohabiting, single males and single females, based on the econometric approach laid out in Dagsvik (1994). We still restrict to wage earners, but we work on establishing a labor supply model for the self-employed too. In the near future this module will be made available to the Ministry of Finance and the Parliament as a tool in the budget planning process. However, we expect that this module will be less frequently used, compared to the LOTTE-Skatt module.

References

Aaberge, R., Dagsvik, J.K. and Strøm, S. (1995). Labor Supply Responses and Welfare Effects of Tax Reforms. *Scandinavian Journal of Economics*, 97, 635–659.

Aasness, J. (1995). *A Microsimulation Model of Consumer Behavior for Tax Analyses*. Paper presented at The Nordic Seminar on Microsimulation Models, Oslo, May 1995.

Aasness, J. (1997). Effects on Poverty, Inequality and Welfare of Child Benefit and Food Subsidies, in Keilman, N., Lyngstad, J., Bojer, H. and Thomsen, I. (eds), *Poverty and Economic Inequality in Industrialized Western Countries*, Scandinavian University Press, Oslo, pp. 123–140.

Aasness, J., Benedictow, A. and Hussein, M.F. (2002). *Distributional Efficiency of Direct and Indirect Taxes, Report 69 in the series Economic Research Programme on Taxation*. Norges forskningsråd, Oslo.

Åvitsland, T. and Aasness, J. (2004). Combining CGE and Microsimulation Models: Effects on Equality of VAT Reforms, Discussion Papers 392, Statistics Norway.

Dagsvik, J.K. (1994). Discrete and Continuous Choice, Max-Stable Processes, and Independence from Irrelevant Attributes. *Econometrica*, 62, 1179–1205.

Dagsvik, J.K. and Strøm, S. (2006). Sectoral Labor Supply, Choice Restrictions and Functional Form. *Journal of Applied Econometrics*, 21, 803–826.

Kornstad, T. and Thoresen, T.O. (2004). Means-Testing the Child Benefit. *Review of Income and Wealth*, 50, 29–49.

Lambert, P.J. and Thoresen, T.O. (2005). Base Independence in the Analysis of Tax Policy Effects: With an Application to Norway 1992–2004, Economics Discussion Paper No. 2005-13, University of Oregon, 2005 (http://econpapers.repec.org/paper/oreuoecwp/).

Nygård, O.E. and Aasness, J. (2003). Effects on Revenue and Consumption Patterns of Changes in Excise Taxes on Goods Exposed to Cross Border Shopping (in Norwegian), in NOU (2003:17), *Særavgifter og grensehandel* (Excise taxes and cross-border shopping), Oslo, Akademika, pp. 113–130.

Schroyen, F. and Aasness, J. (2006). Marginal Indirect Tax Reform Analysis with Merit Good Arguments and Environmental Concerns, Norway 1999, Discussion paper nr. 455, Statistics Norway. (http://www.ssb.no/publikasjoner/DP/pdf/dp455.pdf).

Statistics Norway (2006): The Norwegian tax-benefit model LOTTE, http://www.ssb.no/vis/english/research_and_analysis/models/lotte_en/hovedside.html

Thoresen, T.O. (2004). Reduced Tax Progressivity in Norway in the Nineties. The Effect from Tax Changes. *International Tax and Public Finance*, 11, 487–506.

Health Human Resource Models

Model 16

IPDSM (Integrated Physician Demand and Supply Model)

Kisalaya Basu and Anil Gupta

Microsimulation Modelling and Data Analysis Division, Applied Research and Analysis Directorate, Health Canada, Canada

Introduction

The Microsimulation Modelling and Data Analysis Division (MSDAD) of the Applied Research and Analysis Directorate at Health Canada started developing a physician supply model in 2000. Initially, the model used data for one year and projected the supply of physicians by headcounts for all of Canada.

In 2001, MSDAD started building a physician in-hospital demand forecast model for the province of Alberta in collaboration with Alberta Health and Wellness, Alberta's Ministry of Health, Canada. The model for Alberta was completed by 2003.

In 2003, MSDAD started building physician supply forecast models for each province of Canada. These models used historical trends for many of the variables using the full force of Southam Medical Database (SMDB), a list of all active physicians in Canada, from 1974 to 2002. During the same period, we started building a physician demand forecast model for Nova Scotia, which was different from the Alberta physician demand forecast model in that the new model forecasts demand for physicians, both in-hospitals and out of hospitals.

Once the physician demand model for Nova Scotia was built, it was linked with the physician supply forecast model for Nova Scotia.

Overview

IPDSM forecasts the demand and supply of physicians by three broad categories of specialization: General Practitioner, Medical Specialty, and Surgical Specialty for the province of Nova Scotia in Canada. The model

International Symposia in Economic Theory and Econometrics, Vol. 16

ISSN: 1571-0386 DOI: 10.1016/S1571-0386(06)16035-4

parameters are determined through extensive in-house analysis of a host of data sources and from existing literature and work of various professional associations. The model, even though static in nature, captures behavioural implications through an extensive list of parameters. The model can project demand of physicians by age, sex, and most responsible diagnosis (MRD) of the patient for the three broad categories of specializations. The model also projects the supply of physicians by the three broad categories of specializations. The model forecasts are based on historical trend analysis and policy parameters (Basu and Rajbhandary, 2004).

Data Sources

Demand

In general, Canada does not have good data on health human resources (HHR). The notable exception, fortunately, is for physicians. We use Nova Scotia's physician billings data to calculate the full-time-equivalent (FTE) of physicians by three broad categories of specialty in the base year. In particular, we use the following information: physician's ID (scrambled), physician's specialty, amount paid to a physician for each service, patient ID (scrambled), patient's age, patient's sex, primary diagnosis of the patient, and finally, a variable indicating whether the service was performed inside or outside of a hospital.

The model accommodates four options for the Nova Scotia population projection — Statistics Canada's 'high central', 'high west', 'medium' and 'low' growth population projections are used to forecast the future FTE requirements of physicians.

Supply

For the most part, we used the *Southam Medical Database* (SMDB), and information available through the *Canadian Medical Association.* The SMDB contains annual information for the period 1974–2002 on most physicians in Canada including: a unique physician ID, sex, year of birth, province of residence, postal code, activity status, the location of their medical school, year of graduation from medical school, and medical specialty. Since physicians are uniquely identified in the SMDB, we were able to use the SMDB to follow Canadian physicians through time. In particular, we can see their 'career transitions', such as (i) entry into practice (first entry in the database), (ii) change of specialties, (iii) illnesses, (iv) temporary absence from active practice, (v) emigration, (vi) inter-provincial migration, (vii) retirement, and (viii) death.

One limitation is that SMDB has no information on physicians before they start practice. To fill this need, we resorted to the *Canadian Post-M.D. Education Registry* (CAPER) and the *Canadian Medical Association* to provide information about medical students. Immigration information is obtained from *Citizenship and Immigration Canada* (CIC).

Finally, the model also requires data on the work intensity of physician's practice, as it is necessary to measure delivered services. The intensity of practice, measured in terms of FTE, is derived from the *National Physician Database* (NPDB).

The time-series characteristics of SMDB allow us to incorporate historical trends for many non-policy variables such as specialty switching and mortality rates. Along with the policy parameters such as the emigration rate, immigration rate, and new entrants to medical schools, the model provides a powerful tool to test sensitivity of new proposed policy options.

Methodology

The methodology (Basu and Gupta, 2005) for estimating the demand for physicians' services involve three steps:

(i) Establish the FTE for each physician. To this end we calculate the income of each physician using Physician Billings Data and then identify the 40th and 60th percentile income levels for each of the 40 specialties. The income levels are then used to calculate the FTE using a formula developed at Health Canada.
(ii) Calculate the FTE for each service by distributing the FTE of each physician at the service level (i.e., by patient age, sex, most responsible diagnosis, and hospital status group).
(iii) Use Statistics Canada's population projections to project future demand for three broad medical disciplines: general practitioners, medical specialist, and surgical specialists.

The supply side of the model employs a stock/flow approach and exploits time series and other data for variables, such as emigration, international medical graduates (IMGs), medical school entrants, retirements, mortality, and so on, which in turn allow us to access a host of policy parameters.

How the Model Works

On the demand side, the model is rendered more flexible by allowing the user to change the base FTE requirements of Physician Specialty for three categories: Age Group, Sex, and MRD. The model also accommodates any change in the incidence rates of diseases and thereby the potential changes to the demand side of the market under study. On the supply side, first the model calculates the stock by age, sex, and specialty and then translates it into FTE for projection. It is important to note that most of the policy levers (new entrant to the medical school, immigration, retirement) reside on the supply side of the model.

The demand is utilization based and physicians' full-time-equivalents (FTE) are projected up to the year 2020. Physician supply is determined by a stock/flow approach. The new entrants to the medical schools and immigration are the inflows, while emigration, retirements and deaths are the outflows. Interprovincial migration could be either an inflow or an outflow. The net flow for the current year is added to the stock of the previous year to determine the stock of the current year. Stock and flow of each year is calculated by province, age, sex, and specialty of the physicians. Headcounts of each category are transformed into FTE, so that the demand and supply are measured in the same unit.

The model also allows for comparative analysis of two competing options in a policy environment. This feature is very useful during a policy development process.

The following is the list of outputs from the model under the status quo and potential policy changes:

- Distribution of supply by physician age and specialty (both existing and projected);
- Distribution of flows by physician age and specialty (both existing and projected);
- Distribution of demand by patients' age, sex, primary diagnosis, hospital status, and specialty of the physician providing the service (both existing and projected);
- Integrated projection of supply and demand from 2002–2020 by physician specialty;
- Projected physician supply from 2002–2020;
- Projected flows from 2002–2020; and
- Projected demand from 2002–2020.

Technical Details

IPDSM is a Microsoft.NET application created in Visual Basic designed to work with Microsoft Excel.

All the stock and flow variables for the first year are stored in an Access database for each combination of province, specialty, gender, and age. The model makes a working copy of the database so the user can modify the flow variables using a custom interface. After the simulation calculates the new stock values the working database is saved as an Excel spreadsheet in the background. However, the user is allowed access to the data through a customized Pivot table that allows him/her to display any combination of the above categories. The user is also able to graph any combination of the data categories as well.

The model allows the user to project the future supply of family physicians, medical specialists, and surgical specialists. The supply projections are demographically rich. The output is displayed[1] by physicians' age and specialty.

The primary focus of the model is the integration of supply and demand. Unlike the case of physician supply, policy makers do not have direct control over the variables and factors that affect demand. The policy levers, therefore, lie mainly on the supply side.[2] However, the demand model is highly parameterized and can accommodate certain changes in the incidence of diseases by different age–sex groups.

The demand can be projected by patients' age (12 groups), sex (2), hospital status (2, in or out of hospital), physician specialty (3) and the most responsible diagnosis (17).

The model produces tables and graphs, which can be used in another application, or exported to Microsoft Excel.

Usage and Usability

The model offers an interactive interface, which allows policy makers to identify the gap between demand and supply of physicians in Nova Scotia. Also, the model allows policy makers to identify different policy options to close that gap.

Since IPDSM forecasts both demand and supply of physicians by three broad categories of specialization, the model can identify the gap in demand and supply immediately and then different policy levers can be used to close that gap. The gap is shown in FTE and the policy levers from the supply side determine how many headcounts of physicians entering the market through graduating from medical school, immigration, delaying retirement, etc., are required to fill that gap.

[1] Since female physicians constitute an insignificant portion of Nova Scotia's physician labour force, physicians are not classified by sex.

[2] The demand model is driven by specialty, age, and MRD. None of these are policy levers. However, the incidence rates of diseases are parameterized so that the model can immediately accommodate the information about a change in the incidence rate of certain diseases.

The supply side of the model was recently used in evaluating the impact of increasing the number of new entrants to medical schools in Canada on the future supply of physicians and in turn on the wait times.

IPDSM is a prototype model for physician demand and supply projection. The model can be easily modified to accommodate the information from other provinces. Some results from the model are cited in *The World Health Report 2006*, published by the World Health Organization.

References

Basu, K. and Gupta, A. (2005). Un Modèle Prévisionnel de l'offre et de la Demande de Médecins en Nouvelle-Écosse. *Cahiers De Sociologie et Démographie Médicales*, 45(2–3), 255–286.

Basu, K. and Rajbhandary, S. (2004). Building a Supply Model for Physicians. *Health Policy Research Bulletin*, (8), 36–38.

Model 17

Registered Nurses Supply and Demand Models (NSM & NDM)

Steve Tise and Marilyn B. Biviano

National Center for Health Workforce Analysis, Bureau of Health Professions, Health Resources and Services Administration, USA

Overview

The mission of the National Center for Health Workforce Analysis (NCHWA) in the Bureau of Health Professions (BHPr), Health Resources and Services Administration (HRSA), is *to collect, analyze, and disseminate health workforce information and facilitate national, state, and local workforce planning efforts*. To meet this mission as it pertains to the nurse workforce, NCHWA collects data on the nurse workforce through its quadrennial Sample Survey of Registered Nurses (SSRN) and maintains two models to project the supply of and demand for registered nurses (RNs): the Nursing Supply Model (NSM) and the Nursing Demand Model (NDM).

Nursing Demand Model

The model used to project the demand for registered nurses is the Nursing Demand Model (NDM). The NDM combines empirical analysis with input from health care experts regarding how the healthcare system operates and the role of nurses in the delivery of care.

The NDM forecasts future demand for health care services in six settings: inpatient, outpatient, and emergency departments in general and short-term hospitals; non-general and long-term hospitals; nursing facilities; and home health.

The workload measures used to model demand for health care services are inpatient days (for inpatient settings in short-term hospitals and for long-term hospitals); visits (for short-term hospital outpatient and emergency

International Symposia in Economic Theory and Econometrics, Vol. 16

ISSN: 1571-0386 DOI: 10.1016/S1571-0386(06)16036-6

department settings, and for home health); and nursing facility residents. Data limitations prevented the modeling of State-level estimates of the demand for ambulatory care in physician offices, occupational settings, at schools, and in public health clinics.

Nursing Demand Projections Process

To forecast future health care demands of the population and where patients are likely to receive services, the NDM first divides the population into 32 subgroups based on age, sex, and urban or rural location. For each subgroup, the current national per capita use of health care services was estimated for each of the six delivery settings. The NDM then applies these national rates to each State's population to obtain initial estimates of demand for health care services at the State level. Then, the NDM multiplies this initial extrapolation of health care utilization with a scalar that inflates or deflates the initial extrapolation to incorporate the projected impact on utilization of trends in the health care operating environment, economic conditions, and the overall health of the population.

To forecast the level of nursing services that patients will require and the mix of nurses to provide those services, the NDM forecasts future nurse staffing intensity. Staffing intensity is defined in terms of full-time equivalent (FTE) nurses per unit of health care services provided for the six delivery settings where future health care use is estimated (e.g., FTE RNs per 1,000 inpatient days at short-term hospitals). Staffing intensity is defined in terms of FTE nurses per population in the delivery settings where future health care use is not estimated (e.g., FTE RNs in public health per 10,000 population). Forecasts of future nurse staffing intensity are based on extrapolations of current staffing intensity and take into account projected trends in the health care operating environment, in acuity, and in economic conditions that affect staffing intensity.

Twenty-four equations in the NDM quantify the relationship between health care utilization and its determinants, and between nurse staffing intensity and its determinants. Twenty of these equations were estimated using multiple regression analysis with State-level data from 1996 to 2000, although most regression equations were estimated using a subset of these years based on data availability. Six equations describe the relationship between health care utilization and its determinants for the six health care settings modeled.

Eighteen equations describe the relationship between nurse requirements and its determinants for each nurse type in each setting modeled. In four settings, poor data or poor regression results led to the decision to model future requirements using an alternative approach. RN and licensed practical nurse (LPN) requirements in the "all other" category are modeled as a fixed ratio of FTE nurses per population. RN requirements in the "school health" category are modeled as a fixed ratio of FTE RNs per population age 5–17. RN requirements in nurse education are modeled as fixed percentages of total RN requirements in the other 11 settings.

Nursing Supply Model

The model used to project the supply of registered nurses captures the age-specific dynamics of the flow of nurses in and out of licensure and the work force, their progression from one educational level to another, and their State-to-State migration. Data are developed for each State on: (1) the population of nurses — all those with licenses to practice on a given date; (2) the supply — all those employed or available for employment (if sufficient positions are not available at the time being considered); and (3) the full-time equivalent supply that expresses employment independently of full- or part-time status. The United States summary is an aggregation of the State data.

Nursing Supply Projections Process

Projections of first-time licensees from United States schools are derived from projections of graduates. For these current projections of graduates from each of the three main types of basic nursing programs — diploma, associate degree (AD), and baccalaureate — statistical regression models were used to determine those factors most likely to predict the numbers of graduates. Historical data on graduations, from the National League for Nursing, annual surveys of schools of nursing, provided the trend information on the number of graduates from each type of program. Independent variables representing the availability and attractiveness of nursing as a career were considered for each of the models. These included measures of job availability, salaries, and healthcare expenditures. Also considered were data on the female population within the age groups found among nursing students and on the proportion of female high-school graduates enrolling in higher educational institutions.

In order to capture the changes brought about by registered nurses taking additional education after their initial entry into nursing, statistical regression models were developed to project annual graduations from post-RN baccalaureate and master's degree programs. National League for Nursing annual survey data provided the historical data on graduations used in the models. Projections of graduations from post-RN baccalaureate programs were based on graduations from basic AD and diploma programs and data from the National Sample Survey of Registered Nurses on the length of time between when nurses graduated from the generic program and the baccalaureate program. Similar variables on prior education graduations and intervening time were used in projecting post-RN master's degree graduates.

New licensees represent additions to the nurse population. Of critical importance to determining the overall nurse population in any one year is a measure of those who no longer have licenses as registered nurses. Most of the population consists of those who have entered nursing over a period of years and have continued their licensure. Losses to the RN population occur through death, failure to renew licenses, or in some instances, disciplinary action that would revoke all licenses. The model accounts for deaths by using measures derived from the life tables of white females developed by the National Center for Health Statistics. However, there is no direct measure of nurses who failed to renew their licenses. Therefore, "net losses" are derived. They measure the net change in the RN population, which is caused by those who drop all licenses minus those RNs who become relicensed after having dropped all their licenses.

To identify the supply of registered nurses, "activity rates" are developed using data from the National Sample Surveys of Registered Nurses on the proportion of the nurse population within a specific age group that is employed in nursing.

The derivation of the full-time equivalent RN supply was dependent upon data in the March 2000 National Sample Survey of Registered Nurses that identified the nurses working full-time and those working part-time and the number of scheduled hours for each nurse. A ratio was developed of the number of nurses within each age group cohort who were working on a full-time basis plus the full-time equivalent of those working on a part-time basis to the total number of working nurses. The full-time equivalent for part-time nurses was determined by the ratio of average scheduled hours of part-timers to average scheduled hours of full-timers.

Application and Limitations of the NSM and NDM

The state-based nursing supply and demand models (NSM and NDM) are used to project supply, demand, and shortages for the United States. Because the state-based supply is based on nurse training program production data by state and recent historical migration between states, the model is well suited for testing the impact of a change in nurse education capacity at the state level. Also, because extensive information is available from the National (U.S.) RN Sample Survey on employed versus licensed registered nurses by State, estimates of the potential supply of re-employed registered nurses can be made to inform policy makers.

Distribution within a state cannot be projected using the NSM and NDM. Further, shortages across the major employing sectors (e.g., hospitals and nursing homes) cannot be projected. Technologies that may affect nursing demand are assumed static. Finally, the NSM and NDM are independent models and neither model has a price variable. Historical nursing wage elasticities may be used as a proxy for a price variable.

Model 18

MediSim (Static Microsimulation Model of the Australian Pharmaceutical Benefits Scheme)

Annie Abello and Laurie Brown

NATSEM, University of Canberra, Australia

Introduction

NATSEM models the Australian Pharmaceutical Benefits Scheme (PBS) using the static microsimulation model, MediSim. The first version of MediSim was completed in 1998. Since then, the model has been developed in successive stages, up to the most current, MediSim version 04-05. MediSim simulates, at the level of the individual and the family, the current and future use and costs of PBS medicines under existing and different policy settings. It also estimates the distributional effects of policy changes. By altering the drugs included in the model, their assigned prices and script volumes, MediSim is capable of simulating the impact of inclusion of new drugs on to the list; restriction on the drugs listed on the scheme or on the pricing of drugs; increased restrictions on drugs by indication; increased use of generics at more competitive prices; or an increased emphasis on the quality use of medicines as reflected in changes in doctor prescribing behaviour; as well as changes to co-payment and safety net arrangements. The model could be used to provide answers to relatively simple issues such as the impact of expected changes in PBS subsidised drug prices and scripts over the next 5–10 years on government PBS outlays, or patient out-of pocket expenditures and related revenues to industry. It could be used to measure the likely impact of, for example, the introduction of new PBS-listed drugs, the effects of demographic and socio-economic changes upon outlays, or the distributional and revenue impact of certain changes in the rules of the PBS (e.g., introduction of differential copayment levels).

International Symposia in Economic Theory and Econometrics, Vol. 16

ISSN: 1571-0386 DOI: 10.1016/S1571-0386(06)16037-8

Overview

The model has two components: the Medicines Module that generates macro projections (of the total number of scripts and the average cost per script for 19 drug classes), and the Patient Module, whose main input dataset is at the person level. NATSEM developed the first version of MediSim for the Pharmaceutical Benefits Branch of the Commonwealth Department of Health and Family Services in 1998. Since then, MediSim has been developed and updated in successive stages by NATSEM in partnership with Medicines Australia, an association of pharmaceutical companies. In 2001, the model was revised to include an updated drug classification and a forecasting component called the Medicines Module with a five-year projection capability. Other changes include improved alignment to actual PBS scripts, and the ability to handle drugs dropping out of the PBS.

In 2003–2004, further work was undertaken to update the model and improve its capability, principally, to develop a facility within the model to evaluate not only the costs, but also the benefits, from the use of medicines. A necessary step to modelling both the costs and benefits of medicines is the inclusion of diseases and health conditions in the model's basefile. This entailed the development of a new input dataset that involved statistically matching two sample surveys. The model population and modules in MediSim were revised to enable an improved modelling of the PBS safety net, such that now the impact of the PBS can be estimated for a full year rather that on a fortnightly basis. The work also involved imputing the yearly pattern of short-term health conditions and yearly drug use based on the two-week 'window' captured in the National Health Survey (NHS). Other technical improvements included the introduction of a distributional approach to drug pricing (use of a distribution of prices for each of the 19 drug classes at a greater level of disaggregation); broadening the focus of the model, from PBS users only to the entire Australian population excluding veterans (the latter have their own version of the PBS called the RPBS or Repatriation Pharmaceutical Benefits Scheme); and simplifying the Medicines Module to be based on annual, rather than monthly data.

Data Sources

The basefile for MediSim was constructed using the following data sources:

1. 2001 NHS Basic CURF;
2. STINMOD 01A (which is based on the 1998–1999 Household Expenditure Survey Basic CURF);
3. 1995 NHS Basic CURF, to retrieve information on the distribution of short-term health conditions and drug usage; and

4. Medicare Australia (formerly Health Insurance Commission or HIC) administrative data sets, for imputation and benchmarking purposes:

   - PBS scripts/person by concession card status, gender, age, and drug class (2003)[1]
   - Scripts and government costs, by PBS item code (1992–1993 to 2004–2005)
   - PBS co-payments and safety net thresholds, used to estimate patient costs.

The 2001 NHS constituted the main input dataset, while the other datasets were used for imputation purposes. The process of combining the datasets is outlined in Figure 1. The four data sources were combined at the unit-record level — that is, the combined dataset is comprised of individuals, each described by a set of pooled relevant characteristics. Links between individuals and families were maintained in the dataset because the PBS rules regarding safety nets concerned total expenditures by families on PBS benefit drugs.

Projection Component

The Medicine Module produces a set of macro projections on the rate of growth in scripts, and average cost per script, for each of the model's 19 drug classes. The script usage for each individual in the base file is scaled up (or down), year-by-year, based on annual growth forecasts for each of the 19 drug classes. Average cost projections are applied to script projections, to get an estimate of the total cost of PBS medicines. Projections of PBS co-payments for the forecast period were made by updating the most current PBS co-payments in line with expected changes in the consumer price index, while to be consistent with current government policy, safety nets were increased by the dollar equivalent of two scripts per year. The co-payment rates and safety nets were used to estimate patient cost, while government cost is the residual between total cost and patient cost.

[1] 2003 is the first calendar year for which the HIC has data on the distribution of scripts per person by gender, age group, and drug classification for both concession cardholders and non-cardholders. Previous to this, data were only collected on concession cardholders that had not yet reached the safety net.

Figure 1: Combining the NHS, STINMOD, and PBS Datasets

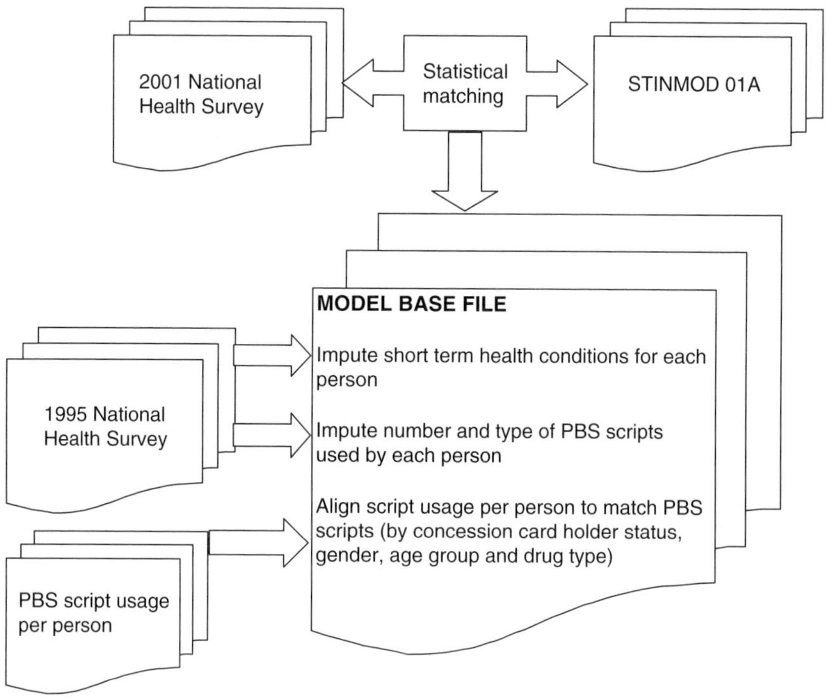

Data Ageing

The model's base population is as of 2001. It constitutes that part of the Australian population living in private dwellings, and excludes about 3 per cent of the population that lives in institutions — for example, hospitals and nursing homes, and veterans. The data records were reweighted to be representative of the entire Australian population (excluding veterans). They were reweighted for each year over the five-year forecast period, in line with Australian Bureau of Statistics projections of the Australian population (series b, intermediate growth assumption), less projections on number of veterans, by gender and five-year age group. Income was updated using the long-term growth in average weekly earnings.

Imputation

MediSim was built using the 2001 NHS as the main input dataset. The 2001 NHS contains the latest person-level information in Australia on long-term health conditions, drug usage for national health priority conditions, and health-risk factors. However, it has a number of limitations as the base data for a microsimulation model. These include the incomplete coverage of families (as the survey structure is person-based); lack of data on short-term health conditions; and lack of data on prescribed drug usage for short term and non-priority long-term conditions. A number of steps were taken to overcome these limitations. First, we statistically matched the NHS with another dataset — STINMOD 01A — to create synthetic families and get a complete record for every individual within each family, as family level information is needed to model PBS safety nets. The statistical matching allowed the retention of the health information available on NHS 2001, while borrowing the family structure from another survey. Short-term health conditions were imputed based on more detailed information in the previous (1995) NHS, and taking into account age group, gender, government concession cardholder status, and self-assessed health status. The 1995 prevalence rates were updated to 2001 levels. To assign short-term health conditions across the model dataset with a sufficient level of precision, it was necessary to *clone* records (i.e., create multiple records of the same person in the dataset). Annual drug usage for short-term and non-priority long-term health conditions was also imputed.

Estimating fortnightly drug usage involved a two-step procedure of first, estimating the probability of taking prescribed drugs given that one has a specific health condition; then, given that one takes prescribed drugs, the next step was to model the number and type of drugs one would take. For short-term conditions, the described procedure was done six times using prevalence rates for two-monthly periods, such that the imputed short-term conditions were what would have prevailed for a whole year. For long-term conditions, this was done only once. To convert the fortnightly long-term drug usage into an annual figure, each person with a long-term condition requiring the use of drugs was assigned 12 scripts for the year for each type of drug used, on the assumption that a person with a chronic condition requiring the use of prescription drugs will use the drug(s) regularly throughout the year, and that scripts are generally issued for a one month's supply. The initial estimates of drug usage were then modified such that the overall distribution of scripts was consistent with administrative data on the usage of PBS benefit drugs.

The availability of a variable on annual (rather than fortnightly) drug usage in the model basefile was the major change that made possible the improved modelling of the PBS safety net in MediSim. Having a realistic measure of annual drug usage at the person level enabled us to more closely approximate the annual drug usage of families in the model dataset, and after applying the PBS rules, to identify which families would reach the safety net and when during the year that would occur. Other features of the base file that facilitated modelling the safety net were that the model basefile covered the total Australian population, and that no records had overly large weight. The latter was achieved by taking records with large initial weight and *cloning* them, that is, creating multiple observations with proportionally smaller final weight. Having the whole Australian population in the basefile, we were able to identify the scripts reaching safety net and ensure that these matched administrative numbers.

Technical Details

Language: The Medicines Module is in Excel; the Patient Module is SAS-based.

System requirements/type of computer: Dual-processor 833 Mhz CPU with 2 Gb RAM.

Typical run time: A one-year simulation would take about 2 h to run, while the production of standard output tables would be a matter of minutes.

Interactivity: Simulations run using MediSim are run in a batch mode, although custom analyses involving SAS may be done interactively.

Conclusions

MediSim's chief utility has been in quantifying the use and cost of PBS medicines under different policy settings, and the distributional effect of such policy changes. It could be used to measure the impact of changes in other model parameters such as medicine prices or supply, or demographic changes (such as population ageing). The most recent use of the model was to model and quantify the distributional impact of various changes to the rules of the PBS, including differential co-payments, a means-based system of co-payments, among others. The only hands-on users of the model are the members of the MediSim team. To date, results from the model have been used primarily by Medicines Australia.

References

Abello, A., Brown, L., Walker, A. and Thurecht, L. (2003). *An Economic Forecasting Microsimulation Model of the Australian Pharmaceutical Benefits Scheme*, Technical Paper no. 30, NATSEM, University of Canberra, Canberra.

Brown, L., Abello, A., Phillips, B. and Harding, A. (2004). Moving Towards an Improved Micro-Simulation Model of the Australian Pharmaceutical Benefits Scheme. *Australian Economic Review*, 37(1), 41–61.

Harding, A., Abello, A., Brown, L. and Phillips, B. (2004). The Distributional Impact of Government Outlays on the Australian Pharmaceutical Benefits Scheme in 2001–02. *Economic Record*, 80 (Special Issue), S83–S96.

Technical Working Group ABS-NATSEM Collaboration on Statistical Matching. (2004). *Statistical Matching of the HES and NHS: An Exploration of Issues in the Use of Unconstrained and Constrained Approaches in Creating a Basefile for a Microsimulation Model of the Pharmaceutical Benefits Scheme*, ABS Methodology Advisory Committee Paper, Canberra, June 2004.

Walker, A. (2000). Distributional Impact of Higher Patient Contributions to Australia's Pharmaceutical Benefits Scheme. *Australian Health Review*, 23(2), 32–46.

Walker, A., Percival, P. and Fischer, S. (1998). *A Microsimulation Model of Australia's Pharmaceutical Benefits Scheme*. Technical Paper no. 15, National Centre for Social and Economic Modelling, University of Canberra, Canberra.

Walker, A., Percival, P., Fischer, S. and Harding, A. (2000). The Impact of Demographic and Other Cchanges on Expenditure on Pharmaceutical Benefits in 2020 in Australia, in Mitton, L., Sutherland, H. and Weeks, M. (eds), *Microsimulation Modelling for Policy Analysis: Challenges and Innovations*, Cambridge University Press, UK, pp. 149–171.

Spatial Microsimulation

Model 19

SVERIGE

Einar Holm, Urban Lindgren, Erling Häggström Lundevaller and Magnus Strömgren

Umeå University, Sweden

Introduction

SVERIGE is the name given to a family of related models. The original model (System for Visualizing Economic and Regional Influences Governing the Environment) is a spatial, dynamic microsimulation model representing all individuals and families in Sweden with high spatial resolution (Holm et al., 2002). SVERIGE-2 is a simplified version, especially targeting labour supply experiments while the SVERIGE-3, currently under construction, extends the former models with endogenous labour demand and labour market clearing modules.

The main purpose of the SVERIGE models is to facilitate experiments revealing detailed impact on mortality, fertility, migration, mobility, place of living, regional population composition, personal and regional income, work and welfare and transfer consumption. In an experiment, such impacts are simulated as the consequence of changed structural conditions, labour demand, individual behaviour and new governmental policy alternatives. The dynamic, partial impact is calculated as the difference in outcome between a reference scenario and an experiment scenario deviating in assumptions from the reference only with respect to one chosen factor (like benefit level in transfer programmes).

Another ambition is to develop and test modelling techniques (for storage, representation, estimation and administration) enabling efficient execution of large samples of interacting actors while maintaining high resolution in time, space, attributes and behaviours.

The scope of the models is national but it allows analysis and results for any spatial divisions; counties, municipalities and (for some versions) $100\,m^2$. Also, when the target application primarily relates, for example, to a municipality, the full nationwide model is executed. This is the simplest way to maintain consistent impact of domestic mobility on the selected

International Symposia in Economic Theory and Econometrics, Vol. 16

ISSN: 1571-0386 DOI: 10.1016/S1571-0386(06)16038-X

municipality. It is possible, but in most cases not advisable, to run the models for a hundred years.

Overview

The spatial microsimulation model SVERIGE was not only partly inspired by the Cornell Micro-simulation Model (CORSIM) but also by time geography and agent-based modelling. It adds geography in the form of detailed migration and location to the set of modules also appearing in CORSIM (Caldwell and Keister, 1996). During the development at Spatial Modelling Centre in Kiruna (1998–2002), the structure was gradually changed into an entirely Swedish setup. The spatial resolution of place of living is hectare grids. Geographical mobility is modelled in a two-step procedure. Firstly, an interaction model allocates each moving family on destination labour market regions. Secondly, within the regions, the movers are matched against a multidimensional mobility table.

Hence, SVERIGE is a spatial microsimulation model. It is mainly time driven, beginning with an empirical start population for a selected year, then running its modules annually until a selected time horizon, at most a hundred years ahead. Within the years, however, certain modules are rather operating in an event-driven mode. Family formation and mobility are often inevitably intertwined and trigger each other directly. Almost all model behaviour derives from individual probability equations estimated on Swedish longitudinal individual register data. Individual action is determined by comparing the calculated context — and individual-specific probability with a random number — it is a stochastic model constrained as much as possible by deterministic behaviour equations.

The simplified SVERIGE-2 version of the model does not contain families or family-formation events, just individuals (children are moved to the same region as their mothers), nor does it locate migrants and people to squares, just to 80 labour market regions. It, however, contains updated versions of all equations and expands on individual income sources by including modules with estimated equations for seven transfer payment programmes (for retirement pension, early retirement, sick leave, unemployment, training, studies and parental leave).

Current developments include the reintroduction of families, family formation and location of population and movers to $100\,m^2$. As compared to SVERIGE and SVERIGE-2, this version, named SVERIGE-3, contains modules for labour demand and individual labour market clearing. Based on exogenously given assumptions about general and sector growth of income, production and productivity, a partly endogenously driven development of each individual place of work (localised subsidiaries of individual juridical firms) in Sweden is modelled. This module produces annual demand for labour by profession and 100 m^2. The labour market module then matches each vacancy and job seeker in the country (constrained by distances and other attributes of firms and job seekers) by help of an event-driven algorithm.

A first version of SVERIGE-3 utilizes plain object constructs just as SVERIGE-2 does. Therefore, this model uses a stratified sampling mechanism. For a selected focus region, all inhabitants might be selected for the running sample while a considerably smaller fraction can be used for the rest of the country. As a consequence, in- and out migrants from the focus region has to be re-sampled accordingly during simulation. Later, the Turbo machinery of SVERIGE-1 (see Technical Details) will be used again, partly removing this sampling necessity. The reintroduction of Turbo is planned to be implemented as a model generator enabling users to specify sample, model, equations and experiment at runtime rather than being forced to reprogramme the simulation engine for every new model version.

Data Issues

All models in the SVERIGE family utilise the ASTRID longitudinal individual database for selection of start sample, for estimating behaviour and for validating the models by running counterfactual simulations for historically observed periods. ASTRID contains some hundred demographic and socio-economic attributes for each inhabitant in Sweden including the locations of place of living and workplace with 100 m resolution. Some individual demographic information is available for each year (1968–2003) while most socio-economic attributes are obtainable annually at least for 1985–2003. Data for each firm and workplace are in place annually since 1990. Some information regarding location, size, type and value of individually owned land properties are also usable since 1995. All data in ASTRID derives from administrative registers at Statistics Sweden (SCB) and are used under special conditions not to reveal any individual information outside the laboratory.

For most applications, there is no need for other data sources or imputation, merging etc., except when attitude information from surveys is needed or if, for instance, alignment to other projections like the national population projection by Statistics Sweden for some odd reason would be required.

Access to rich longitudinal, biographical information about all inhabitants provides some advantages. Firstly, there is no need for sampling for other reasons than enabling rapid simulation runs during development. Secondly, most individual behaviour is heavily contingent on the particular individual's intrinsic history. Including a large set of lagged drivers in the equations increases prediction precision considerably compared to only utilizing attributes from the last year. Thirdly, while a large sample might work for some attributes it considerably distorts relational attributes, that is, individual properties pointing at other individuals or objects like mother, father, sister, partner, family, workplace, school, place of living etc. Such relations become inevitably broken in a random sample. In addition, representing all individuals in the simulation facilitates a more accurate modelling of competition and cooperation than otherwise is possible. The partner market, labour market, housing market and education market are so inherently scale dependent that anything less than full scale often considerably truncates the choice sets and forces the model to produce biased and inconsistent results due to the combination of "normal" behaviour.

Technical Details

The original SVERIGE model and its simulation engine Turbo is programmed in C++, while SVERIGE-2 and SVERIGE-3 uses C# within the NET platform. SVERIGE is executed via commands in a DOS window. The Turbo engine does not utilize threads internally. It is tight and small (180k), packs data compactly and is very fast on a one-processor machine. The present version enables the model to run 9 million individuals (annual updating) on a 2 Gh machine with 1 GB memory within 1 min. The basic mechanism for scanning big population samples during the simulation is to compact the data and keep them in the primary memory. Earlier versions run on UNIX and conversion is still easy by recompiling source code.

SVERIGE-2 and SVERIGE-3 are developed as plain Windows applications and used interactively via user interfaces. For all models there is a choice of storing population data as text or binary files. All models run on standard Windows PC with at least 1 GB of memory. A version of SVERIGE-3 is developed for running on a 64 bit machine with 16 GB ram enabling representation of the entire population of 9 million people in core memory without compression of objects. With the entire Swedish population as the starting "sample", the original SVERIGE model with the Turbo engine runs for around 60 s per simulated year due to its customized data storage and representation. SVERIGE-2 requires about 10 times as much memory per person. Object and runtime duration per person per year is also about 10 times larger.

Usage and Usability

The model was developed in a research environment without immediate requirements on specific applications, and thus apart from policy analysis, the models also aim at exploring and testing more theoretical statements and questions like: effects of spatial and individual heterogeneity (i.e., small/large samples) on aggregated output, effects of scale dependence in social and economic choice processes, ecological fallacy or socio-deterministic fallacy, the class-ghetto question, and, generally, the question whether the origin of revealed spatial behaviour, conditions and performance is related to population composition or selective migration and place attraction and amenities.

The main constraint on using the models is not technical but administrative. As developed, all models so far require start populations containing subsets of individual records from the database ASTRID. The conditions for using this data preclude any use for model experiments outside our laboratory. So far, this has not severely constrained use since potential users are affiliated to the laboratory. For a wider use, however, other schemes have to be developed. One possibility is to scramble the user database, so no single person would be possible to recognize. That would inevitably deteriorate results. Another possibility is to develop a client-server setup with the server containing individual data and the model located behind a firewall in the laboratory. It is not easy, however, to invent unbreakable precautions against clever persons fishing out individual data while concurrently maintaining a reasonably usable and user-friendly interface to the simulation model for the client.

An Application

The developed microsimulation models can be utilized for a large set of policy evaluation studies. In this example application, the SVERIGE-2 model version was used for analysing the relationship between labour supply and seven major social security programmes. One hypothesis put forward in the study was that payment levels in the different programmes affect the propensity to participate in the programme and thereby indirectly the propensity to work and, in turn, the amount of labour supplied into the economy. Are people on sick leave only because they are sick and therefore cannot work? Are they receiving unemployment benefits only because they are unemployed and cannot get a work? Or is there some space for individual choice? If so, to what extent is it used and influenced by payment level? What are the consequences of a change in level on labour supply (and on the performance of the economy)?

On a micro level, income from work is compared with incomes from seven transfer payments: retirement pension (age ≤ 65), early retirement pension, sickness benefit, unemployment benefit, income from labour market measures, parental allowance and student grants. The individuals' participation in, and incomes from, each of these income sources are reproduced by equations estimated on the longitudinal micro database ASTRID for the period 1990–1999. A probit equation provides the probability of participating in the income source, and a linear regression (OLS) generates the amount of income from the same source. The equations are intertwined by the Heckman two-step estimator that adjusts for possible selection bias.

We use an experiment variable that annually indicates the individual's perceived alternative income from each of the transfer payments. This is the amount of money the individual would receive if he/she fully was supported from this particular programme. This is estimated by a regression based on similar individuals who were observed to change into this income source.

The needs of the individual and his/her use of social programmes may also be affected by a number of other reasons than simply levels of benefits. This is indicated in the equations by control factors such as sex, age, education level, industry and country of origin. Moreover, characteristics of the region where the individual lives are controlled for, such as occupation-specific unemployment, population density, economic growth and levels of benefit utilization in the previous year. The results of the analyses show that the selection into the different social programmes is stronger than the discriminating effects of the mentioned control factors. Therefore, we have chosen to integrate the benefit history of the individual in the analysis; in every equation the income from a specific benefit is determined also by the level of work income and levels of benefits from of each of the programmes in the previous year. It was shown that the single-most influential factor explaining incomes from benefits is the income from the same source last year.

The model is supposed to reflect a choice situation not only affected by regional and individual characteristics in the previous year. Choices are to a large extent exclusive because the individual cannot participate in several programmes at the same time. As a consequence, a variable reflecting an individual budget restriction is needed. The implementation of the budget restriction variable is made by using the summed incomes from all programmes as an additional variable in the work income equation. Unlike most other variables, this one is based on estimations and refers to current year (not previous year).

The experimental effect of changing a certain benefit level (everything else equal) appears when making comparisons to a reference scenario of unchanged levels. Experiment and reference scenarios are generated by the model — they are run separately and deliver two different population developments.

The results reveal that the perceived level of benefit has a strong positive effect on participation as well as benefits, except for sickness benefit (with particularly bad data). Economic incentives clearly play an important role for explaining the number of participants in, costs for and distribution between the studied programmes.

The general result is that small changes in benefit levels do have substantial effects on participation and labour supply, and that such effects become much more obvious and visible by help of a simulation compared to just inspecting parameters in the estimated equations. The full effect of a change does not emerge until after several years because of the cumulative dynamic side effect of different partial causal chains.

To answer the question if, and to what extent an increased labour supply actually results in larger work participation is however beyond the scope of the current model.

References

Holm, E., Holme, K., Mäkilä, K., Mattsson-Kaupi, M. and Mörtvik, G. (2002). *The SVERIGE spatial microsimulation model – Content, validation, and example applications*. Gerum Kulturgeografi 2002:4, Umeå Universitet.

Caldwell, S. and Keister, L.A. (1996). Wealth in America: Family Stock Ownership and Accumulation 1960–95, in Clarke, G.P. (ed), *Microsimulation for Urban and Regional Policy Analysis. European Research in Regional Science 6*, Pion, London, pp. 88–116.

Model 20

NSW Hospitals Model

Linc Thurecht

NATSEM, Australia

Overview

The New South Wales (NSW) Hospitals Model comprises a census of all in-patient separations from both public and private hospitals over the four-year period 1996–1997 to 1999–2000.[1] While these records contain many diagnoses and administrative details related to the treatment received by patients, information pertaining to the socioeconomic status (SES) of patients is scant. The major contribution of this model is to impute SES onto patient records by matching the empirical distribution of a proxy for SES (equivalent family income) at the level of sex, age and very small area. This contrasts to the standard approach in the literature of attaching a socio-economic indicator to a spatial area, thus implying a uniform SES for all people within the areal unit. The Hospitals Model also has modules that project future use of hospitals in addition to the take-up and use of private health insurance in the presence of various government incentives. The Hospitals Model has been used to

- perform distributional analyses of patients treated in NSW hospitals;
- project future hospital use and the related cost;
- determine the split of use between public and private hospitals; and
- model the take-up and use of private health insurance by hospital patients.

[1] A separation is the formal process whereby a hospital records the completion of an episode of care for an admitted patient.

International Symposia in Economic Theory and Econometrics, Vol. 16

ISSN: 1571-0386 DOI: 10.1016/S1571-0386(06)16039-1

Data Sources

There are three main sources of data for the Hospitals Model. The first is the NSW Health Inpatient Statistics Collection, which contains all in-patient separation records. There were around 1.9 million unit records in each year representing all separations from around 1.2 million patients. The second is the NSW Hospital Cost Data Collection, which enables a cost to be attached to each separation. The third is the 1996 Census of Population and Housing from the Australian Bureau of Statistics (ABS) from which the empirical distribution of equivalent family income (EFI) by age, sex and small area level was extracted.[2] A full list of the data items is provided in Thurecht et al. (2003).

An important issue is that a person may have multiple visits to NSW hospitals over the course of a year. Although a common patient identifier is not used for separations from different hospitals in NSW, the linking of patient records was undertaken by the NSW Department of Health and was achieved through probabilistic matching of details contained within each separation record (such as the date of birth, country of birth, sex and marital status of the patient — refer to Thurecht et al. (2003) for further details). All records were de-identified to ensure confidentiality.

A data item that assumed critical importance for our process of imputing SES (described below) was the *Census Collection District* (CD) in which the patient lived. CDs are the lowest level of spatial aggregation available in Australia with each containing on average around 200 households. This areal unit was chosen as it was expected that the SES of people would be more homogenous within a CD than at higher levels of spatial aggregation (such as a suburb).

Imputing Socioeconomic Status onto Administrative Records

In Australia, the imputation of SES to individuals captured within administrative data is traditionally carried out through the use of ABS geographic area-based socioeconomic indexes for areas (SEIFA). An important consequence with the use of these indexes is that a single SEIFA value is assigned to all individuals living within the geographic area (often at the level

[2] EFI measures the economic resources available to a family related to its size and composition. For example, a single person earning $60,000 a year has relatively greater economic means than a couple with three children earning the same income. To calculate EFI, we used the modified OECD scale which divides the gross family income by an equivalence factor equal to the sum of 1.0 for the first adult, 0.5 for the second adult and 0.3 for each dependent child.

of statistical local areas, SLA),[3] thus potentially reducing the apparent strength of any links between SES and health service usage. In reality, SES can vary greatly between individuals living within a geographic area, especially across age groups. Such an approach clearly removes any underlying heterogeneity that may be present within the spatial unit.

In contrast, the main innovation of the NSW Hospitals Model was the imputation of SES onto patient records in a way that allowed variation to occur among patients within the CD by age and gender. The first step in imputing the SES of hospital patients was to obtain the actual distribution of EFI for NSW residents on Census night. EFI was chosen as our proxy for SES as health need has been shown to be related to income (e.g., refer to the National Health Strategy, 1992), with an equivalence scale being a widely used method of improving the comparability of relative economic well-being.

For each CD within NSW, a separate EFI distribution was obtained by sex and age. To preserve confidentiality, age was defined in 10-year age groups from 0–9 up to 70 years old and over, and EFI was reported in quintiles. With around 11,500 CDs in NSW at the time of the 1996 Census, this suggests that over 180,000 unique combinations, each with their own distribution of people across EFI quintiles could be obtained. However, in practise not all of these combinations were populated.

SES was imputed onto each patient record, by assuming that those who used hospitals within a particular CD were representative of the sex–age group–EFI quintile distribution of all people living within that CD. For example, suppose that the NSW hospitals dataset for a given year contained eight 0–9-year-old males from a particular CD and that the 1996 Census showed that there were twenty 0–9-year-old males living in that CD, with half in EFI quintile 2 and half in EFI quintile 5. Our imputation method stochastically assigns four of the 0–9-year-old male patients to quintile 2 and the other four patients to quintile 5.

Distributional Analysis of NSW Hospital Patients

Owing to the richness of administrative and diagnostic information contained within the patient separation records, having imputed individually each patient's SES, it has been possible to examine distributional differences in the use of hospitals in a number of ways.

[3] Statistical local areas (SLA) are the next highest level of spatial aggregation after CDs that are defined by the ABS. Within NSW at the time of the 1996 Census, the average SLA population was around 32,000. The SLA with the largest population included around 180,000 people.

For example, the Hospitals Model has been used to examine whether the 'inverse care law' applies to patients treated in NSW hospitals.[4] In this study, after controlling for age, Thurecht et al. (2005) found that per-patient treatment costs were similar for low- and high-SES patients, suggesting that the 'inverse care law' did not apply within NSW hospitals over the period examined. As an example of the type of more focussed analysis that the model can be used to perform, patients that were treated for coronary heart disease (CHD) were also specifically examined. Among those treated for this condition, there was little distributional difference found among patients in public hospitals, but some differences were evident among patients treated for CHD in private hospitals.

Projections and Ageing Module

A module was also constructed to provide the capacity to project future hospital use, including the split between public and private hospitals. This module was based on ABS population projections and trend growth in hospital separations by service category. The population projections take account of both population growth and the ageing of the population while the trend in hospital use by service category enabled the evolving mix of treatments provided by hospitals to be captured. Thurecht et al. (2005) provides a detailed description of the projection methodology.

In Thurecht et al. (2005) it was found that while ageing of the population is commonly thought to be the main driver of increased health costs, this had a relatively minor effect — with the increasing cost of providing hospital services being the dominant contributor. It was also found that the majority of the projected increase in hospitals expenditure would be due to increased use of private hospitals.

Private Health Insurance Module

To supplement the main Hospitals Model and Projection and Ageing Module, a Private Health Insurance (PHI) Module was also developed. This module used various predictive variables and major policy changes to predict the probability that a person of given sex, age and income quintile would be covered by PHI.

The PHI Module was applied to assessing the distributional consequences of recent changes to government policy as it relates to the take-up and use of PHI. In Walker et al. (2005), distributional differences in the response to

[4] Hart (1971) first proposed the 'inverse care law' in which those of higher SES receive more extensive and costly medical treatment than those of lower SES.

policies designed to encourage increased take-up of PHI was examined. This also included a 10-year projection of how different socioeconomic groups would respond to the withdrawal of various government incentives that have been put in place to encourage the take-up of PHI.

Spatial Analysis of Hospital Use and Cost

Spatial differences in the use of hospitals by NSW residents and the associated cost of treatments was also examined using the Hospitals Model. In Thurecht et al. (2004), differences in the use of hospitals and the cost of treatment between patients of low and high SES was examined at the SLA level, with considerable differences in hospital use and the cost of treatment found between low and high socioeconomic patients at lower levels of spatial aggregation. In general, lower socioeconomic patients were found to use hospitals less as remoteness increased. However, more remote areas of the state also had higher than expected rates of hospital usage, given the sex and age composition within the area.

Technical Particulars

The NSW Hospitals Model was developed using SAS version 8 running in a Windows environment. The model was constructed using a desktop computer with a 2.5 GHz processor and one gigabytes of RAM. A user interface was created to enable the distributional characteristics of hospital patients across various variables to be easily examined.

Conclusions

The NSW Hospitals Model makes a unique contribution to our understanding of the characteristics of NSW hospital patients. By imputing a patient-based measure of SES onto administrative records, it has been possible to assess distributional differences in the use of public and private hospitals at the patient level. This contrasts with approaches using an area-based measure of SES in which any heterogeneity in the SES of the underlying population within the areal unit is discarded.

The model has been used to examine distributional differences in the use of hospitals and the related cost of treatment. This has been across a number of dimensions including between public and private hospitals, for specific medical conditions and by considering regional differences across the state. Ten-year projections of future hospital use and the associated cost have also been developed, including the separate impact on the public and private hospitals sector. The distributional effect of recent government policy changes intended to encourage the take-up of PHI has also been examined including how people of varying SES might respond to the removal of key government policies in this respect.

References

Hart, J.T. (1971). The Inverse Care Law. *Lancet*, 297(7696), 405–412.

National Health Strategy (1992). *Enough to Make You Sick: How Income and Environment Affect Health*. National Health Strategy, Research Paper No. 1, Melbourne.

Thurecht, L., Bennett, D., Gibbs, A., Walker, A., Pearse, J. and Harding, A. (2003). *A Microsimulation Model of Hospital Patients: New South Wales. Technical*. Paper No. 29, National Centre for Social and Economic Modelling, University of Canberra.

Thurecht, L., Harding, A. and Walker, A. (2004). *Equity and Hospitals: Do Usage and Treatment Costs Vary with Socioeconomic Status and Locality?* Paper presented at the 28th Australia New Zealand Regional Science Association International Conference, Wollongong.

Thurecht, L., Walker, A., Harding, A. and Pearse, J. (2005). The 'Inverse Care Law', Population Ageing and the Hospital System: A Distributional Analysis. *Economic Papers*, 24(1), 1–17.

Walker, A., Percival, R., Thurecht, L. and Pearse, J. (2005). Distributional Impact of Recent Changes in Private Health Insurance Policies. *Australian Health Review*, 29(2), 167–177.

Model 21

Customer Service Projection Model (CuSP): A Regional Microsimulation Model of Centrelink Customers

Ben Phillips

NATSEM, University of Canberra, Australia

Introduction

Centrelink is the agency in Australia that has responsibility for the delivery of a range of Australian government services including income support payments and associated services. As such, it has a large infrastructure devoted to contact with customers through a variety of channels — ranging from walk in offices to e-mail. A constant challenge for Centrelink is the need to 'tune' this infrastructure in response to government policy direction, changing customer patterns, changes in customer behaviour, and new modes of access.

With the aim of more efficient service delivery Centrelink embarked in 2000 on a regional Microsimulation Modelling project. Centrelink is undertaking the project with the National Centre for Social and Economic Modelling (NATSEM) at the University of Canberra. The core model for the project — the Customer Service Projection model (CuSP) — has been developed by NATSEM.

Overview and Data

The Task for the CuSP Model

The aim of the CuSP Model is to provide a tool that can generate small-area projections of:

- Centrelink customer numbers and characteristics; and
- Associated channel use.

International Symposia in Economic Theory and Econometrics, Vol. 16

ISSN: 1571-0386 DOI: 10.1016/S1571-0386(06)16040-8

Figure 1: CuSp Model – Overall Structure

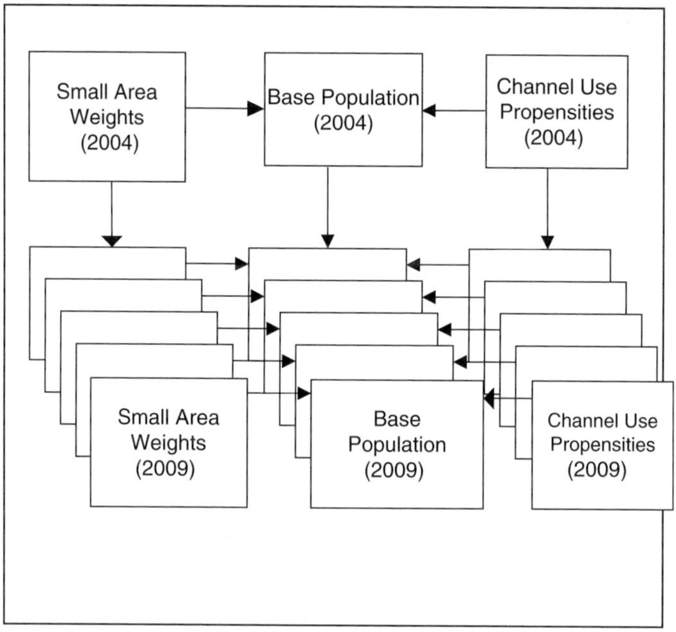

The time horizon for the projections is generally five years into the future, and the projections need to be made under scenarios that can capture alternative views about the future environment. The Model needs to be able to accommodate changes in the demographic and economic environment, changes in government policy, changes in service delivery directions, and changes in customer behaviour.

Structure of the CuSP Model

Essentially, the model is a static regional microsimulation model that involves the generation and linking of three datasets based on common characteristics between cohort groups (Figure 1):

1. A base population file (which includes a pool of detailed records for individuals[1]).

[1] These records are based on Australian Bureau of Statistics (ABS) survey data of real, but unidentifiable, Australians.

2. Small area weights (which specify the prevalence of each individual in the pool in each small area).
3. Channel use propensities ('channels'' are the available methods of contact between Centrelink and its customers, and the propensities specify expected channel use given a person's characteristics).

Application of the weights to the base population file gives the estimate of the numbers and characteristics of Centrelink customers in each small area. Application of the channel use propensities to the customer estimates then gives the estimate of channel use. These three datasets are produced for the base year (currently 2004) and then each is updated for the projection years.

The Model draws together the following data from Centrelink, the Australian Bureau of Statistics (ABS) and other sources:

- amalgamated Centrelink customer data;
- amalgamated Centrelink channel use data;
- small-area data from the Census of Population and Housing;
- detailed data on population characteristics from the ABS household expenditure survey (HES); and
- various data for the construction of projection scenarios,
- and also incorporates elements of two established NATSEM models:

o STINMOD — a 'microsimulation' model which allows for the detailed identification of entitlements to income support; and

o MarketInfo — a 'regional microsimulation' technique that is used to generate a detailed picture of the characteristics of the population in small areas.

Projection and Ageing Module

Given the three component parts of the CuSP Model for June 2002 — base population, small-area weights, and channel use propensities — projections are then made by adjusting each of these datasets to reflect particular aspects of the future environment. For example:

- Changes in the size of the population and its demographic and labour market structure, at the Statistical Local Area (SLA) level, can be incorporated by changing the small-area weights. This changes the assumed number of people of a given type in the area.
- Changes in the income support system, or the impacts of earnings and CPI growth on means-testing, can be simulated in the base population by using the 'outyears' facility of STINMOD.
- Changes in channel use propensities — which may stem from changes in

the options made available by Centrelink, changes in Centrelink requirements, or possible behavioural changes on the part of customers — are handled by altering the channel use propensities dataset.

A particular projection scenario can thus range from a simple scenario involving change in just one aspect of the future environment through to a more complex scenario that combines changes in many aspects of the future environment. Scenarios can also be specified at different levels of geographic detail. For example, different labour market prospects can be specified for particular parts of the country.

Once a projection scenario has been designed, the required amendments are made to the CuSP Model elements (base population, weights, and propensities), and running the Model then generates:

- the projected number and characteristics of customers;
- the amount of associated channel use;
- for each of the 1340 SLAs; and
- for the base year and each of the projection years.

Data Ageing

The survey file that underlies the CuSP model is the ABS' 1998 HES. The CuSP model has projection years between 2004 to 2009 and 2014. To use the HES for these projection years the HES is aged using static microsimulation techniques. The base population for each projection year is reweighted to reflect current and future populations as predicted in the ABS' Statistical Local Area population projections. The population projections are detailed enough to allow the HES data to be reweighted by SLA and age by sex categories.

The HES data is updated to each projection year using NATSEM's STINMOD microsimulation model. STINMOD updates the social security programs, wages and other prices in line with appropriate inflators.

Technical Particulars

The CuSP model is constructed using PC SAS version 9 and relies on SAS' ability to handle large data sets. As the construction requires the processing of the HES for every SLA the model is computationally intense. The user however only needs to run simulations on the final datasets and computer run-time becomes somewhat trivial.

The model has not yet been made interactive by the use of an interface, simulations require the analyst to run their own SAS code to create results. The model is fully documented with a list of variables, their related categories, and datasets.

The model was last updated in 2005 by NATSEM and is currently being used by Centrelink. The model is owned by Centrelink and is strictly for their use only. Centrelink have most recently been using the model as a basis for scenario building. In particular they have been interested in predicting the likely impact on customer usage patterns and numbers in response to different unemployment scenarios for Australia.

Conclusions

The CuSP model is primarily used by Centrelink as a decision support tool. The model enables them to predict into the future the usage of Centrelink's many services down to the small area level. Centrelink is also able to simulate the impact on these services of changes to government social security policy and different demographic and economic conditions.

Model 22

SpatialMSM — NATSEM's Small Area Household Model for Australia

Shih-Foong Chin and Ann Harding

National Centre for Social and Economic Modelling (NATSEM), University of Canberra, Australia

Introduction

NATSEM's spatialMSM is a modelling system that produces synthetic small-area estimates for persons and households, which can be used for such purposes as estimating the current characteristics of households (such as poverty rates, housing stress, income tax paid or cash transfers received) and predicting the spatial impact of changes in taxes and transfers.

Overview

The spatialMSM system is a spatial microsimulation model that first re-weights a national sample survey to small area population targets to create a synthetic database of persons and households for each local area. This synthetic database is then used to generate estimates of household characteristics within small areas and to model the spatial impact of policy change in income tax and cash transfer programs. It was developed by the National Centre for Social and Economic Modelling (NATSEM) at the University of Canberra, starting in 2003, and represents part of NATSEM's continuing attempts to develop small-area microsimulation models. The spatialMSM system has been used to generate small-area estimates of such variables as wages and salaries, disposable income, income tax paid, social security and family benefits received, personal wealth, poverty rates, housing stress. Because data for individuals and households still underlies the model, the flexibility apparent in all microsimulation models still exists. For example, the characteristics of those in poverty can be analysed in detail and the impact of policy change on particular population sub-groups in each small

International Symposia in Economic Theory and Econometrics, Vol. 16

ISSN: 1571-0386 DOI: 10.1016/S1571-0386(06)16041-X

area can be modelled. In all these efforts, the small areas used were the standard statistical geography of the Statistical Local Area (SLA), maintained by the Australian Bureau of Statistics (ABS).

Data Sources

The two key sources of input data for the spatialMSM (Versions 01A and 01B) are

- The *1998–1999 Household Expenditure Survey* (HES) *Confidentialised Unit Record File* produced by the ABS in 2002, which is a national sample survey covering just under 9,000 households and providing information about incomes, housing tenure, socio-demographic characteristics, expenditure, etc.
- The *2001 Census Expanded Community Profile* datasets, produced by the ABS in 2003, which provided the census benchmark counts of particular population characteristics within each SLA.

Considerable efforts were expended in updating the monetary information in the 1998–1999 Household Expenditure Survey to 2001 and in making the various household descriptors contained within the HES match the Census variable categories (see Chin et al., 2006).

Technical Details

Methodology: The processes employed by the spatialMSM system involve two major steps. Step one creates household weights for small areas using a core technique called 'reweighting'. Step two applies the SLA household weights thus created to the selected output variables generated by NATSEM's static model STINMOD, to create the small-area (SLA) estimates of the desired outputs (such as housing affordability and household income poverty).

Step one: In step one, the national HES survey is reweighted to small area targets derived from the 2001 national population and housing census. As the name suggests, reweighting 'reweights' (or converts) a set of household weights from a larger spatial unit (the nation) into a smaller spatial unit (the SLA). The spatialMSM system uses the reweighting algorithm called *GREGWT*. This is a generalised regression routine written as a macro in the SAS programming language. GREGWT was developed by the ABS (Australian Bureau of Statistics, 2000). It conducts iterative calculations, SLA-by-SLA, to derive an 'optimal' set of household weights for each SLA.

This is achieved by using a regression approach to minimise the difference between the estimated count and the known census count for each of the benchmark classes, until the difference between them (known as a 'residual') is within a defined tolerance. The iterative process stops when the residuals are zero or approaching zero. When this happens, *convergence* is said to have been achieved. In this study, convergence entails the matching of the synthetic estimates to *all* the benchmark targets (which are the census counts of those selected variables that are common to the national survey and the census, and were used for 'constraining' the reweighting process). The end result of step one — when convergence is reached — is the production of 'optimal' sets of 2001 household weights for SLAs, with one set of weights for each household for each SLA.

Step two: The small area household weights for each SLA are merged onto the HES household level output from NATSEM's STINMOD static microsimulation model (which replicates the rules of the income tax and cash transfer systems in 2001 and allows possible changes to those rules). The output provides household level results for every SLA, which can be summed to produce totals (e.g. total income tax paid by all households living in a particular SLA) or used to calculate averages (e.g. average reduction in income tax due to a specified change in the income tax schedule for households living in a particular SLA).

So far two versions of the spatialMSM system have been produced, both for 2001. Version /01A has been specially created to produce estimates of housing affordability and housing-related issues, with the HES data being reweighted to detailed Census housing targets. Version /01B has been created to provide regional estimates of poverty and the spatial impact of tax and transfer change. We have now commenced work on the production of spatialMSM/04A, which will reweight the newly released 2003–2004 ABS Household Income and Expenditure Survey to an updated version of the 2001 Census.

We have validated the reliability of the small-area estimates generated by spatialMSM against available independent sources of information, either in the form of commissioned data obtained from the ABS, or administrative data supplied by the various government agencies such as the Australian Taxation Office, the welfare payment agency — Centrelink, and the Department of Families, Community Services and Indigenous Affairs (Chin et al., 2005). The small area estimates of housing affordability closely matched those produced for us by the ABS in each of the four states and territory (Chin and Harding, 2006b). For the small-area estimates of household income poverty, the closeness of fit was also good — about two to three percentage-point differences — in each of the four jurisdictions (Chin and Harding, 2006c).

The spatialMSM methodology is very complex. The above discussion is but a very brief overview. Interested readers are advised to consult the two technical papers (Chin and Harding, 2006a; Chin et al., 2006), available on NATSEM's website at www.natsem.canberra.edu.au

Usage

The development of the spatialMSM spatial microsimulation modelling system has been supported by the Australian Research Council (LP349152), the ABS, and five departments from four states and territories (the New South Wales Premier's Department, the Queensland Department of Premier and Cabinet, the Queensland Treasury, the Victorian Department of Sustainability and Environment and the Chief Minister's Department of the Australian Capital Territory). Apart from providing funding support, these state and territory government departments have also been users of the detailed, spatial microdata generated by NATSEM using spatialMSM, to support their needs-based analyses and regional policy decision processes. Access to the output data can be arranged for researchers within these states and territories, with the approval of the original agencies involved.

In the future, we hope to make a wide range of data about the characteristics of households at a small-area level freely available through the web to Australian and other researchers.

References

Australian Bureau of Statistics. (2000). *GREGWT and Table Macro — Users Guide,* Commonwealth of Australia, Canberra.

Chin, S.F. and Harding, A. (2006a). *Regional Dimensions: Creating Synthetic Small-Area Microdata and Spatial Microsimulation Models.* Technical Paper no. 33, NATSEM, University of Canberra.

Chin, S.F. and Harding, A. (2006b). *Housing Stress in 2001: Estimates for Statistical Local Areas.* Conference Paper CP0601, NATSEM, University of Canberra.

Chin, S.F. and Harding, A. (2006c). *A Spatial Portrait of Disadvantage: Income Poverty by Statistical Local Areas.* Conference Paper (forthcoming), NATSEM, University of Canberra.

Chin, S.F., Harding, A. and Bill, A. (2006). *Regional Dimensions: Preparation of the 1998–1999 Household Expenditure Survey for Reweighting to Small-Area Benchmarks.* Technical Paper no. 34, NATSEM, University of Canberra.

Chin, S.F., Harding, A., Lloyd, R., McNamara, J., Phillips, B. and Vu, Q.N. (2005). Spatial Microsimulation Using Synthetic Small-Area Estimates of Income, Tax and Social Security Benefits. *Australasian Journal of Regional Studies*, 11(3), 303–336. (See also NATSEM Online Conference Paper CP 0516 for the version of this paper with detailed maps.)

Subject Index